MW00658569

Emergency Health

PRACTICAL APPLICATION OF PUBLIC HEALTH PRINCIPLES

For access to digital chapters,
visit the APHA Press bookstore (www.apha.org).

Emergency Health

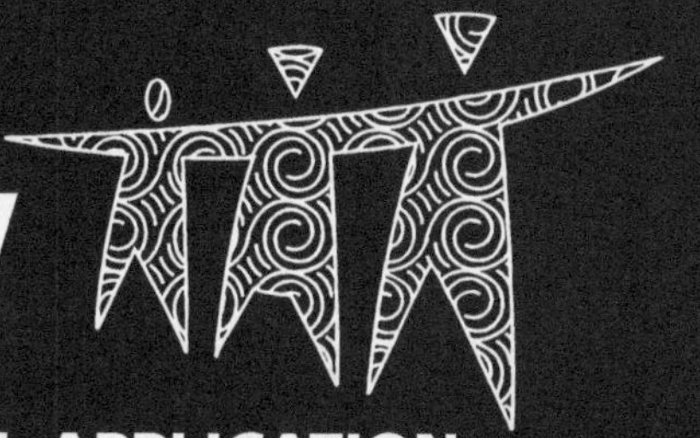

PRACTICAL APPLICATION OF PUBLIC HEALTH PRINCIPLES

Mark Keim, MD, MBA

APHA PRESS
AN IMPRINT OF AMERICAN PUBLIC HEALTH ASSOCIATION

American Public Health Association
800 I Street, NW
Washington, DC 20001-3710
www.apha.org

Georges C. Benjamin, MD, MACP, Executive Director

Printed and bound in the United States of America
Book Production Editor: Maya Ribault
Typesetting: KnowledgeWorks Global, Ltd.
Cover Design: Alan Giarcanella
Printing and Binding: Sheridan Books

Library of Congress Cataloging-in-Publication Data

Names: Keim, Mark, 1959- author. | American Public Health Association, issuing body.
Title: Emergency health : practical application of public health principles / by Mark Keim.
Description: Washington, DC : American Public Health Association, [2023] | Includes bibliographical references and index. | Summary: "For the past 50 years, the US approach to managing environmental health emergencies has been mostly reactionary and curative, rather than precautionary and preventive. This book proposes "emergency health" as a new paradigm-a more equitable and effective application of public health practice as applied to disasters"-- Provided by publisher.
Identifiers: LCCN 2022051395 (print) | LCCN 2022051396 (ebook) | ISBN 9780875533346 (paperback) | ISBN 9780875533353 (Adobe PDF)
Subjects: MESH: Disasters | Public Health Practice | Emergencies | Environmental Health | Disaster Medicine | United States
Classification: LCC HV553 (print) | LCC HV553 (ebook) | NLM WA 295 | DDC 363.34--dc23/eng/20230113
LC record available at https://lccn.loc.gov/2022051395
LC ebook record available at https://lccn.loc.gov/2022051396

This book is dedicated to my lifelong friend Jerry Bush.

Contents

Foreword ix

Preface xi

Introduction xiii

I. SOUNDING THE ALARM

1. The Current State of Disaster Science 3

2. An Introduction to Emergency Health 13

II. DEFINITIONS OF DISASTER-RELATED DISEASE

3. The Definition of Disease 25

4. The Definition of Disaster 37

5. Hazardous Exposures 45

6. Natural Disasters 57

7. Technological Disasters 79

III. THE ETIOLOGY OF DISASTER-RELATED DISEASE

8. Causes of Disaster-Related Disease 101

9. Upstream: Causal Pathways of Disaster-Related Disease 125

10. Downstream: The Natural History of Disaster-Related Disease 131

IV. THE EPIDEMIOLOGY OF DISASTER-RELATED DISEASE

11. Public Health Consequences of Disasters 141

12. Global Patterns of Disaster-Related Disease 151

V. PRINCIPLES OF EMERGENCY HEALTH

13. Wellness 163

14. Health Equity 169

15. Determinants of Emergency Health 175

16. Disaster Risk Management 181

17. Risk Assessment 191

18. Risk Communication 201

VI. THE PRACTICE OF EMERGENCY HEALTH

19. Tenets of Emergency Health 207

20. Disease Prevention 215

21. Health Promotion 223

22. Health Protection 233

23. Provision of Care 241

24. Target Capabilities of Emergency Health 253

25. The Role of Public Health Professionals 261

26. Performance Management 267

VII. OPPORTUNITIES FOR EMERGENCY HEALTH

27. Opportunities for Research, Education, Intervention, and Integration 277

VIII. APPENDICES

Appendix A: The Etiology of Disaster-Related Disease 285

Appendix B: Glossary of Key Terms 311

Afterword 333

About the Author 335

Index 337

Foreword

Emergency Health is a great book that I enjoyed reading immensely. I have great regards for Dr. Keim as an expert public health teacher and for his long, rich, and invaluable experience in the field of disaster management. No one else can present such complex concepts in such simple and understandable language.

Consider this book a primer for public health and disaster studies, written for students and professionals alike with the intent of applying foundational public health concepts in disaster-related health care. This book is also an excellent resource for instructors and faculty, offering ideas for discussion questions, anchors, activities, and assignments. The book has a didactic style, yet it is engaging for the audience. The book's strength lies in its flow of information, slow buildup of complex ideas, simplicity of language, and use of numerous tables, figures, and boxes to emphasize important messages and explain different frameworks by using original and clear illustrations.

This book helps both public health and emergency management professionals in reimagining disasters through the lens of public health. This book is transformational in the way it articulates and illustrates the principles and foundations of public health studies in the context of disasters and humanitarian emergencies. The topics are broad and highlight the complexity of the system we live in—the socioecological factors, proximal and distal determinants of health, policies, politics, and environment factors—that play a role in how hazards take form, could turn into incidents, and incidents could evolve into disasters. The reader is exposed to the basic concepts of disaster risk reduction from the standpoint of population health, social and environmental justice, and equity, all factors that play a role in differentiation of exposure versus vulnerability of a population against various hazards.

One unique aspect that readers will find very useful is the conceptualization of emergency health and "how health and well-being are produced in the context of emergencies." This is unlike emergency management, where provision of care is closely tied with disaster response. This book challenges the audience to think outside the box of disaster cycle to expand their understanding into the larger ecosystem determining the health outcomes of affected populations.

Another strength of *Emergency Health* is the introduction to cross-cutting interdisciplinary concepts such as risk management, health promotion, evidence-based decision-making, and disease prevention and control frameworks and to operationalization of these concepts for an audience whose primary focus is a population at risk of or at the receiving end of a potential natural or human-made hazard.

Any professional in emergency management who cares for population health and any public health practitioner whose focus is disasters and large-scale emergencies will find this book beneficial, relevant, and impactful in shaping their thought framework, setting goals, and refining strategies to care for the populations they serve.

Amber Mehmood, MBBS, MPH, FCPS
Associate Professor
University of South Florida, College of Public Health
Tampa, Florida

Preface

THIS I BELIEVE

I believe in public health.

Because of people like John Snow, I believe that disease does not occur randomly. Because of Edward Jenner, I believe that disease can be prevented, that we may act now to influence the incidence of future disease. And because of Edwin Chadwick, I believe that people should be protected from dangerous social and environmental conditions *before* these hazardous exposures cause disease.

I believe that social and environmental determinants of health influence modifiable risk factors for disease. I believe that public health's role is to engage multiple sectors and community partners to generate a collective impact and improve these determinants of health and risk factors for disease. I believe in the 10 essential public health services and in public health's purpose that includes prevention, protection, promotion, response, and equity of access and quality. I also believe that the highest degree of public health impact results from dealing with health determinants and risk factors compared with less effective clinical interventions, counseling, and education. Why do I believe these things? I do so because they are *proven.*

And yet, to this day, public health has still not applied even these most basic principles and practices to address morbidity and mortality caused by disaster-related hazards. The current reactionary approach is expensive, with unproven effectiveness. There are no validated models for predicting disaster-related health risks. Most disaster-related epidemiological investigations assess victim demographics without correlation with other critical risk factors, such as geographical location and dose of hazardous exposure. Considered in John Snow's terms, every year (for many decades now), we count the number of cholera cases without bothering to find the contaminated well, let alone remove the pump handle. More recently (after Hurricane Maria hit Puerto Rico and with the lack of COVID testing during the pandemic), some have noted that public health no longer even counts all the cases!

Over the past 50 years, the focus of the US approach to managing environmental health emergencies (as compared with managing infectious disease emergencies) has been mostly reactionary and curative, rather than precautionary and preventive. For this reason, we have very few measures of effectiveness for either public health preparedness or response after literally hundreds of millions of dollars in public and private investment.

For this same reason, we should *return* to the basics of public health to address this health problem. And it is also for this reason that I wrote this book. Here I propose emergency health as a new paradigm that is better aligned with public health principles and as a more equitable and effective application of public health practice as applied to disasters.

A special thank you goes to Gal Frey and Mickey Woolard for their love, healing, and belief.

Mark Keim, MD, MBA

Introduction

MATERIAL COVERED

The first half of this book includes an introduction to the basic principles behind emergency health. The second half includes a detailed description of emergency health interventions. The book is also accompanied by a series of simple mnemonics, easy-to-read tables and easy-to-understand graphics, and a glossary—all intended to facilitate practical usability of the book. *Emergency Health* is composed of 27 chapters, which are organized into seven parts, and two appendices. The two appendices include disease etiology tables for 20 disasters and a glossary of over 300 definitions for key terms and phrases used in the book.

HOW TO USE THIS BOOK

Emergency Health may be used both as a collegiate-level textbook and as an information source for professionals in the field. Prior knowledge of public health, medicine, and emergency management may be helpful but is not necessary.

The contents are presented within a logical progression that first introduces the basic principles of emergency health before describing its practical application. As such, one of the strengths of the book is that it describes many of the current practices of emergency management within the language of public health. For this reason, both public health and emergency management professionals will likely learn new information when viewing the process from this perspective.

The first part of the book, entitled Sounding the Alarm, sets out our problem statement and, as the part title implies, is intended to sound the alarm regarding the dangerously haphazard state of modern disaster science. The second part, Definitions of Disaster-Related Disease, then provides definitions of disaster-related disease within the context of hazardous exposures. The next two parts—The Etiology of Disaster-Related Disease and The Epidemiology of Disaster-Related Disease—explore the global causes and patterns of disaster-related disease. Principles of Emergency Health, which comes next, describes the public health principles that form the basis for emergency health. The practical application of emergency health is the subject of the next part, entitled The Practice of Emergency Health, while following this section comes Opportunities for Emergency Health, which describes opportunities for the future of the field. The final part of this book comprises the etiology tables and the comprehensive glossary.

Because of its placement as an appendix, however, it may be possible to overlook one of the most valuable resources within this book—the glossary. Every reader is encouraged to read the glossary in its entirety. For it not only defines the terminology for emergency health clearly and succinctly but also, consequently, stands alone as an effective review of the content and context of this entire book.

I. SOUNDING THE ALARM

1

The Current State of Disaster Science

LEARNING OBJECTIVES

Upon completion of this chapter, the reader will be able to

1. Define the following terms and phrases:
   - Determinants of health (DoH)
   - Emergency
   - Emergency management
   - Effectiveness
   - Efficiency
   - Functions
   - Morbidity
   - Mortality
   - Natural hazard
   - Population
   - Preparedness
   - Prevention
   - Program
   - Public health
   - Recovery
   - Resilience
   - Response
   - Sendai Framework for Disaster Risk Reduction, 2015–2030
   - Stakeholders
   - Technological hazard
   - Vulnerability
2. Recognize that human development has resulted in maladaptive and inequitable activities.
3. Recognize that disasters are increasing in frequency and magnitude worldwide.
4. Recognize that public health is chronically underfunded.
5. Recognize factors that have hindered the development of modern disaster research.

HEALTH AS A HUMAN RIGHT

As Dr. C.-E. A. Winslow rose to take the podium, he stood up for so much more. He stood up for public health. Dr. Winslow stood up for disease **prevention**, prolonging life, and promoting health. He stood up for a model of health that is not limited to a strictly clinical focus on the individual but also includes the importance of relationships and the environment. He stood up for health equity and every citizen's "birthright of health and longevity." And he stood up for public health's role in addressing the ecosocial **determinants of health (DoH)** through the "development of the social machinery to ensure everyone a standard of living that was adequate for the maintenance of health."[1]

You may ask yourself, "Why didn't I see Dr. Winslow on my smartphone? How did I miss a message that describes public health prevention, health promotion, and health protection as a birthright? And what about the *social machinery* that ensures everyone an *adequate* standard of living? How did this one slip by me?" These are good questions, considering Dr. Winslow's speech occurred over 100 years ago.

Much has changed in public health since Dr. Winslow's visionary oratory in 1920. Public health's "art and science" has grown into a global, multitrillion-dollar industry. Since then, the United States has built a system of allocations, infrastructure, and implementation for public health **emergency** preparedness and response programs. The US Department of Health and Human Services (HHS) annual budget has exceeded $1.7 trillion. The role of **emergency management** has since been elevated to the agency level at the Department of Homeland Security and HHS.

And yet, many things have remained the same in the United States since 1920. Consider these points:

- Unlike many other causes of death, there has been no significant change in disaster-related mortality rates during the entire past century.
- Most tax dollars allocated for public health emergencies are intended to respond to public health crises, not prevent them.
- Most public health emergency **functions** still involve a relatively narrow role of oversight (i.e., assessment, policy, and assurance) compared with interventions.
- Very few public health programs related to emergencies are intentionally designed to attain disease prevention or to measure intervention **effectiveness**.
- Most disaster-related public health risk assessments do not include exposure science.
- At-risk **populations** are characterized as inherently "vulnerable" and encouraged to take personal responsibility for being "resilient," as compared with having their "birthright of health and longevity."
- Unlike other public health programs (e.g., tobacco), government agencies are not expected to measure their effectiveness regarding the number of disaster deaths prevented.

- The state has no legal duty to protect its citizens from health hazards.
- There is no legal right to health, health care, or health insurance.

Dr. Winslow defined **public health** as "the science and art of preventing disease, prolonging life, and promoting health through the organized efforts and informed choices of society, organizations, public and private communities, and individuals."[1] In 1948, almost 30 years after Winslow's speech, 48 nations, including the United States, signed the Universal Declaration of Human Rights, the UN document declaring that "everyone has the right to a standard of living adequate for the health and well-being of oneself and one's family, including . . . medical care."[2]

In 2005 the United States and other UN member-states signed World Health Assembly Resolution 58.33, which stated that everyone should have access to health care services and not suffer financial hardship when obtaining them.[3] Today the United States is the only economically developed nation with no universal health care in practice. By contrast, over 70% of the world's countries have a right to health care specified in their national constitutions.[4]

In 2022 the United Nations also recognized "the right to a clean, healthy and sustainable environment as a human right" and called on "members states, international organizations, business enterprises, and other relevant **stakeholders** to adopt policies, to enhance international cooperation."[5]

> Environmental health is a human right.

DEVELOPMENT DRIVES DISASTERS

During the past century, humanity has achieved remarkable gains involving life expectancy, poverty, and child mortality. However, human development has also included maladaptive activities such as overuse of natural resources, pollution, biodiversity loss, and negative impacts of energy sources.[6,7]

Global warming has caused an increasing number of extreme weather events (EWEs).[8] Scientific consensus is now reportedly "virtually certain" that heat waves will increase in frequency. Predicted precipitation frequency and intensity increases are also considered highly likely. And the number of compound EWEs is also expected to increase.[7,9]

Added to the increasing problem of maladaptive activities (e.g., the overuse of natural resources, pollution, biodiversity loss, the negative impacts of energy sources), the successes of human development have not been shared efficiently nor distributed effectively among all stakeholders and contributors. Despite all its promise, the so-called Great Acceleration of the mid-20th century has yet to deliver an optimal and equitable health level for all, even among the richest of nations.[10] Significant disparities persist across many health conditions and outcomes, including life expectancy, infant mortality, and exposure to environmental pollutants. The gap in life expectancy between people with the highest and lowest incomes is narrow in some communities but broad in others.[11]

DISASTERS ARE INCREASING

This past century of rapid human development has seen a remarkable increase in the number of disasters occurring worldwide, as shown in Figure 1-1, which illustrates the increasing annual incidence of disasters caused by **natural hazards** as well as by **technological hazards** (i.e., those that are human-caused). The sharp upturns that begin in the mid-20th century are most notable among these data trends.

This increase in disaster frequency aligns with the simultaneous rise in an extensive range of human activity, first recorded in the mid-20th century, known as the "Great Acceleration."[10] This phrase refers to the rapid increase of humanity's impact on the earth's geology and ecosystems characteristic of this period. To that same point, recent studies have also suggested that the global incidence of weather disasters appears to be positively associated with world real gross domestic product (GDP) during 1961–2020.[7] Figure 1-2 depicts this association between world real GDP and the global incidence of weather-related disasters from 1961 to 2020.[12]

During 1961–2020, four out of five hydrological and meteorological (i.e., hydrometeorological) disasters positively correlated with GDP. Population-adjusted values for

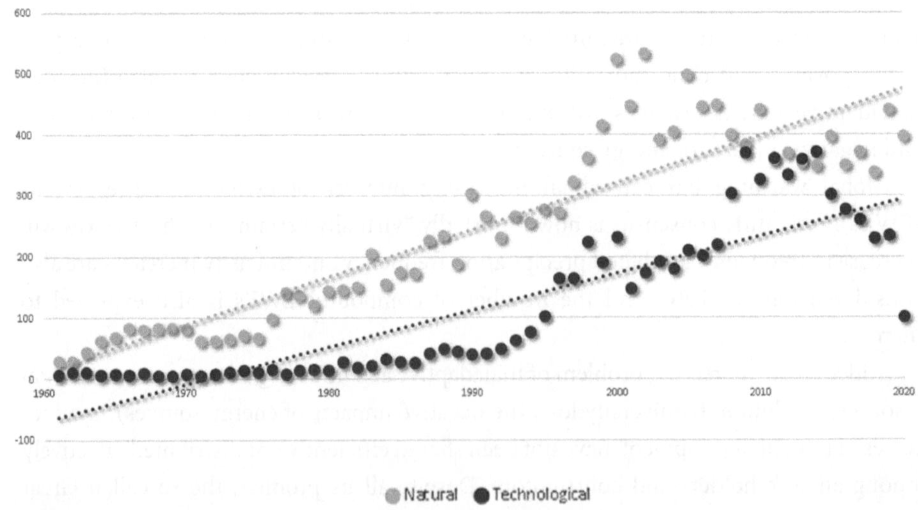

Figure 1-1. Annual Global Incidence of Disasters Caused by Natural and Technological Hazards, 1961–2020

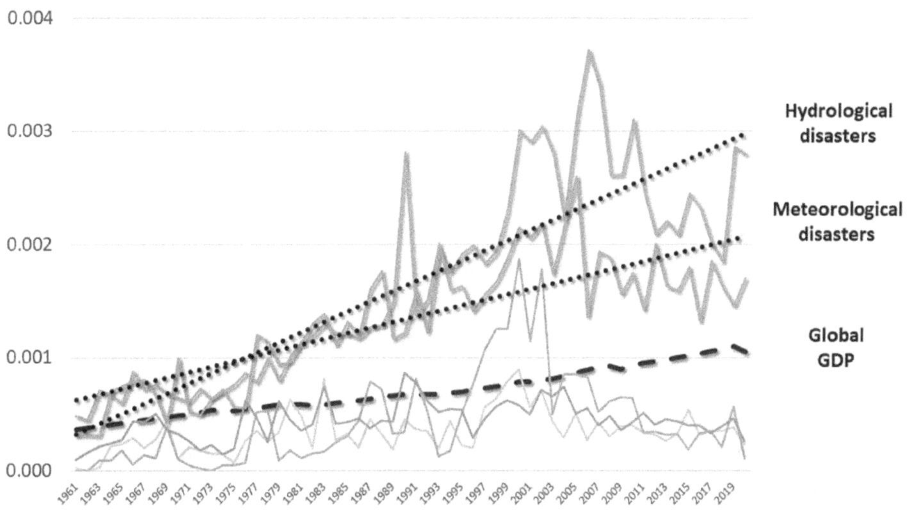

Source: Keim et al.[12] Adapted under the terms of the CC BY license (https://creativecommons.org/licenses/by/4.0).

Figure 1-2. World Real GDP and the Global Incidence of Weather-Related Disasters, 1961–2020

annual global incidence rates of flood and storm disasters appeared to correlate highly with world GDP. The yearly global incidence rates of heat waves and cold weather disasters also appeared to correlate positively with world GDP ($P = 0.002$ and $P = 0.007$, respectively).[7]

These four **hydrometeorological** (i.e., weather-related) disasters are exclusively the result of atmospheric conditions. The incidence of a fifth hydrometeorological disaster studied (wet landslides) not only depends on atmospheric conditions but also is influenced by inherent characteristics of the earth's surface, such as topography and geology. This fifth disaster type, however, showed no significant correlation with GDP ($P = 0.862$). Nor were significant associations found between the seven other individual types of biological, climatological, and geophysical disasters and GDP.[7]

PUBLIC HEALTH IS UNDERFUNDED

In 2002 the Institute of Medicine called for strengthening US governmental public health capabilities and requiring accountability from and among all public health system sectors.[13] Relative to health care spending, the United States has made minimal investments in nonmedical DoH such as social services, education, transportation, environmental protection, and housing programs.[14] This strategic lack of investment in addressing nonmedical DoH has detrimental effects on the general population's health.[15]

DISASTER SCIENCE IS UNDERDEVELOPED

Significant reductions in health risk have historically required a comprehensive approach to disease management that includes preventive and curative interventions. Disaster risk management serves as a primary means for the world's populations to address disaster losses, including health-related losses.[16]

Over four decades ago, world policymakers began formalizing relationships between health, climate, sustainable development, and emergency management and implementing this alignment within international strategies for risk management.[16] The outputs of these meetings were furthered by the subsequent development of international **standards** for risk management and have since contributed to a global doctrine for disaster risk management for all sectors, including health.[16] Today one of the world's "seven targets in seven years," as agreed upon in the **Sendai Framework for Disaster Risk Reduction**, is to reduce global mortality by 2030.[17]

And yet, to date, disaster-related health science remains in its infancy. Scientists report a severe lack of scientific rigor for public health interventions and research applied to disasters. One study of 709 consecutive peer-reviewed articles published during 2009–2014 reported that most outcome indicators were limited to process (e.g., number accomplished) rather than to effectiveness or **efficiency**.[18] Also, surprisingly, no randomized controlled trials, nonrandomized, comparative controlled trials, or systematic reviews were published in the journals in question during the five years examined.[19] This study and others have cautioned for decades that the evidence base for disaster-related health science is far from robust and is often disorganized, making the development of scientific evidence on which to base best practices difficult. This lack of scientific evidence and sufficient data for decision-making significantly hampers policymakers' ability to make well-informed, empirical decisions that result in measurable, cost-effective reductions in disaster-related mortality.

OUR UNDERSTANDING OF DISASTERS IS OUTDATED

The ability of the scientific community to effectively research disaster-related health effects is also integral to the health security of populations at risk. In 2011 the US National Biodefense Science Board called for scientific investigations as an essential component of emergency preparedness and response efforts.[15] In a subsequent report, the Department of Health and Human Services, Office of the Assistant Secretary for Preparedness and Response (HHS/ASPR), noted, "The U.S. and the U.S. Government have tremendous science research capabilities, but applying them for public health emergencies, especially using non-traditional public health science resources, has been challenging."[16]

According to the National Research Council, "Disaster research, which has focused historically on emergency response and **recovery**, is incomplete without the simultaneous study of the societal hazards and risks associated with disasters, which includes data on the **vulnerability** of people living in hazard-prone areas."[20,21]

However, despite over 25 years of global policy development, the National Academies of Sciences, Engineering, and Medicine recently noted that "while some disaster management and public health preparedness programming may be viewed as tangentially related, a multi-sectoral and inter-disciplinary national platform for coordination and policy guidance on involving disaster risk reduction in the United States does not exist."[21,22] Indeed, the majority of disaster-related policies, programming, and investments at the local, state, and national levels are customarily directed more toward responding to and recovering from disasters than toward investing in risk reduction and preparedness.[22]

Although in 2014 HHS/ASPR and the National Academies of Science conducted a joint workshop entitled "Enabling Rapid and Sustainable Public Health Research During Disasters,"[19] the workshop did not produce a list of recommendations. Nor have there been subsequent publications related to the workshop. Furthermore, although in 2014 HHS/ASPR established the Science Preparedness Research Interagency Team, that team has not been published to date.

After Hurricane Maria in 2017 an article published in the *New England Journal of Medicine* called for "a preventive approach to disasters, exemplified by international research on disaster risk reduction—which focuses on anticipating vulnerabilities, creating **resilience**, and mitigating consequences."[23] Earlier that same year the National Academies of Science noted that "few U.S. scientific investigations address the issue of disaster risk reduction."[19,24]

Again, many of these deficiencies may be traced to a chronic lack of academic and scientific investment. Recent studies of US disaster science identified five key findings. Federal funding of disaster research in the United States can be characterized as (1) deficient when compared with other federal investments in research and development, (2) highly variable according to year, (3) highly variable according to the scientific discipline of research, (4) highly variable according to target response capabilities, and (5) consistently awarded to relatively few recipients.[25]

In 2019, in an editorial published by the *American Journal of Public Health*, a group of national public health leaders reported that, despite billions of dollars spent preparing and responding to disasters, disaster-related mortality in the United States has remained unchanged for 50 years. They called for a comprehensive national strategy to reduce disaster-related mortality that is also consistent with the tenets of the Sendai framework for disaster risk reduction, 2015–2030.[24]

TOPICS FOR DISCUSSION

1. Draw a table comparing the advantages of human development on the left and disadvantages on the right. Draw lines between entries on the left and right sides that show significant associations between the two factors. Describe your reasoning.
2. Consider if the following curves may also be correlated with the Great Acceleration:
   - The global concentration of atmospheric CO_2
   - The global number of telephones
   - The global number of McDonald's restaurants
3. Disaster science has been considered an asset of national security and remains remarkably underfunded regardless of nation or political structure. List the factors that you feel affect public policy related to disaster science. Discuss your reasoning.

REFERENCES

1. Winslow C. The untilled field of public health. *Modern Med.* 1920;2:183–191.
2. *General Assembly Resolultion 217 A: Universal Declaration of Human Rights.* Paris, France: United Nations General Assembly; 1948.
3. World Health Organization (WHO). World health report 2013: research for universal health coverage. 2013. Available at: https://www.who.int/publications/i/item/9789240690837. Accessed November 19, 2022.
4. Comparative Constitutions Project. What's in constitutions? *Constitute.* 2022. Available at: https://constituteproject.org/topics?lang=en. Accessed November 19, 2022.
5. The human right to a clean, healthy and sustainable environment: resolution. Resolution adopted by the UN General Assembly, 76th session. 2021–2022. Available at: https://digitallibrary.un.org/record/3983329?ln=en. Accessed November 20, 2022.
6. Whitmee S, Haines A, Beyrer C, et al. Safeguarding human health in the Anthropocene epoch: report of the Rockefeller Foundation–Lancet Commission on Planetary Health. *Lancet* 2015;386(10007):1973–2028.
7. Keim ME, Smith TM, Burkle FM. The annual global incidence rate of extreme weather event disasters appears positively correlated with world GDP, 1961–2020. *Prehosp Disaster Med.* 2022;37(4):431–436. doi:10.1017/S1049023X22000966
8. Intergovernmental Panel on Climate Change (IPCC). *Climate Change 2007: Impacts, Adaptation, and Vulnerability.* Cambridge, UK: Cambridge University Press; 2007.
9. Intergovernmental Panel on Climate Change (IPCC). *The Physical Science Basis. Contribution of Working Group I to the Sixth Assessment Report of the Intergovernmental Panel on Climate Change (AR6).* Cambridge, UK: Cambridge University Press; 2021.
10. Steffen W, Broadgate W, Deutsch L, Gaffney O, Ludwig C. The trajectory of the Anthropocene: the Great Acceleration. *Anthropocene Rev.* 2015;2(1):81–98.
11. DeSalvo K, Wang Y, Harris A, Auerbach J, Koo D, O'Carroll P. Public health 3.0: a call to action for public health to meet the challenges of the 21st century. *Prev Chronic Dis.* 2017;14:170017.

12. Keim ME, Smith TE, Burkle FR. The annual global incidence rate of extreme weather event disasters appears positively correlated with world GDP, 1961–2020. *Prehosp Disaster Med.* 2022;(4):431–436.
13 US Institute of Medicine Committee on Assuring the Health of the Public in the 21st Century. *The Future of the Public's Health in the 21st Century.* Washington, DC: National Academies Press; 2002.
14. Bradley E, Elkins B, Herrin J, Elbel B. *Br Med J Qual Safety.* 2011;20(10):826–831.
15. National Biodefense Science Board. *Call to Action: Include Scientific Investigations as an Integral Component of Disaster Planning and Response.* Washington, DC: Dept of Health and Human Services; 2011:1–38.
16. Office of the Assistant Secretary for Preparedness and Response. ASPR Scientific Preparedness and Response for Public Health Emergencies Workshop. Washington, DC: Dept of Health and Human Services; 2012.
17. UN Office of Disaster Risk Reduction. *Sendai Framework for Disaster Risk Reduction, 2015–2030.* New York, NY: United Nations; 2015.
18. Birnbaum M, Adibhatla S, Dudek O, Ramsel-Miller J. Categorization and analysis of disaster health publications: an inventory. *Prehosp Disaster Med.* 2017;32(5):473–482.
19. Forum on Medical and Public Health Preparedness for Catastrophic Events; Board on Health Sciences Policy; Institute of Medicine. *Enabling Rapid and Sustainable Public Health Research During Disasters: Summary of a Joint Workshop by the Institute of Medicine and the US Department of Health and Human Services.* Washington, DC: National Academies Press; 2015.
20. National Research Council. *Facing Hazards and Disasters: Understanding Human Dimensions.* Washington, DC: National Academies Press; 2008.
21. Keim ME. Managing health in disasters. *Lancet.* 2003;362(9400):1947–2032.
22. National Academies of Sciences, Engineering, and Medicine. *Exploring Disaster Risk Reduction Through Community-Level Approaches to Promote Healthy Outcomes: Proceedings of a Workshop—in Brief.* Washington, DC: National Academies Press; 2016.
23. Shultz J, Galea S. Preparing for the next Harvey, Irma, or Maria—addressing research gaps. *N Engl J Med.* 2017;377:1804–1806.
24. Keim ME, Kirsch TD, Alleyne O, et al. The need for a national strategy to assess and reduce disaster-related mortality in the United States. *Am J Public Health.* 2019;109(4):539–540. doi: 10.2105/AJPH.2019.304975
25. Keim M, Kirsch TD, Lovallo A. A comparison of US federal government spending for research and development related to public health preparedness capabilities, 2008–2017. *Disaster Med Public Health Prep.* 2020;14(4):459–466. doi:10.1017/dmp.2019.66

2

An Introduction to Emergency Health

LEARNING OBJECTIVES

Upon completion of this chapter, the reader will be able to

1. Define the following terms and phrases:
   - Agent
   - Analysis
   - Approach
   - Community engagement
   - Control
   - Disaster medicine
   - Disease prevention
   - Emergency health
   - Environmental health
   - Environmental impact assessment
   - Evacuation
   - Evaluation
   - Health determinants
   - Health equity
   - Health promotion
   - Health protection
   - Humanitarian assistance
   - Mass care
   - Objective
   - Preventive control
   - Principles
   - Program logic model
   - Quality of life
   - Strategy
   - Wellness
2. Recognize the four pillars of emergency health:
   - Prevention
   - Promotion

- Protection
- Provision of care

3. Recognize a conceptual framework for emergency health.

ENVIRONMENTAL HEALTH

Emergency health, the topic of this book, is a new discipline of environmental health. It is in fact Dr. C.-E. A. Winslow's version of environmental health. So we must ask, What is environmental health? To answer, the World Health Organization has broadly defined environmental health as "those aspects of human health and disease that are determined by factors in the environment." Because environmental factors are known to influence all human health and disease, this definition posits environmental health as a foundational component of public health.

This book employs an environmental health perspective to study the relationships between human health and disasters. The National Environmental Health Association defines **environmental health** as "the science and practice of preventing human injury and illness and promoting well-being by (1) identifying and evaluating environmental sources and hazardous **agents** and (2) limiting exposures to hazardous physical, chemical, and biological agents in air, water, soil, food, and other environmental media or settings that may adversely affect human health."[1]

The Centers for Disease Control and Prevention describes the role of environmental health professionals as "protecting groups of people from everyday threats to their health and safety that result from elements in their environments."[2]

The National Environmental Health Association has described the role of environmental health professionals in creating and promoting the following public health interventions and outcomes:[1]

- **Hazard identification** and analytical risk assessment
- Protective interventions
- Public health guidelines and policies
- Health communications and education
- Public health leadership
- Systems **analysis**
- **Community engagement**
- **Environmental impact analysis**
- Interpretation of research
- Interpretation of data

EMERGENCY HEALTH

Emergency health is perhaps best defined as a discipline of environmental health; its goal is to prevent *disaster-related* injury and illness. Prevention is accomplished by (1) identifying and evaluating environmental sources and hazardous agents; and (2) limiting exposures to hazardous physical, chemical, and biological agents in air, water, soil, food, and other environmental media or settings that may adversely affect human health.

Emergency health prioritizes a complete and equitable state of health and wellness among individuals, families, communities, and society over time—before, during, and after disasters occur. Emergency health applies four key concepts of public health intervention related to disasters: prevention, health protection and promotion, and provision of care) related to disasters. (See Figure 2-1.)

This book's main themes mirror the four pillars of emergency health: prevention, promotion, protection, and provision of care. The book begins with a definition of emergency health that includes an overview of the causes, characteristics, and patterns of disaster-related disease. Then follows an investigation of the **principles** and practice of emergency health in terms of the role public health plays in disease prevention, health protection, health promotion, and the provision of clinical care and humanitarian assistance.

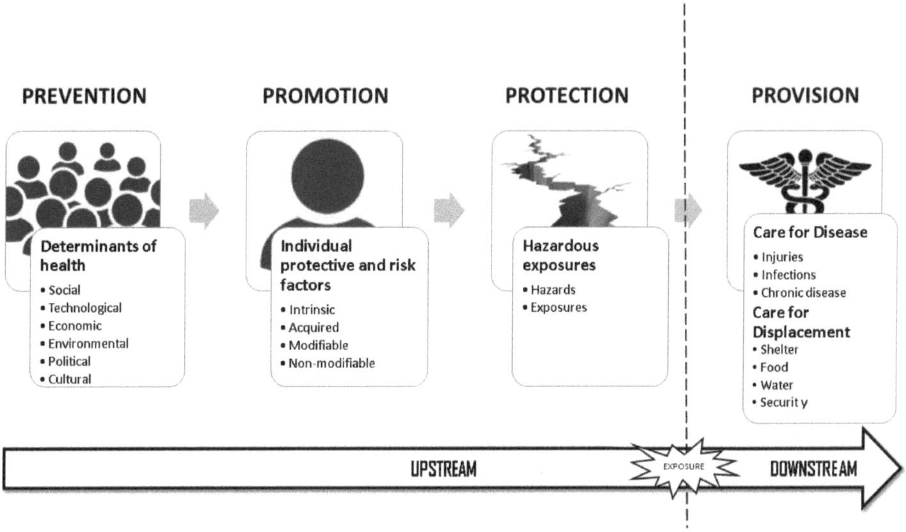

Figure 2-1. The Four Pillars of Emergency Health

DISEASE PREVENTION

Disease prevention is a component of disease management that involves elimination of disease-related risk factors. This **preventive control** of disease is based on the fundamental principle that disease does not occur randomly.

Disaster-related disease is caused by factors that may be identified and modified. Causation is considered the foundation of population health.[3] Pre-disaster **health determinants** cause post-disaster health impacts. Health, like other forms of human development, is affected by interactions between individuals, their relationships with others, and hazards in their environment.[4]

Disease occurs when individuals are exposed to health hazards.

Adverse health effects are prevented entirely when one of these three proximate causes no longer occurs. Let us consider the example of an epidemic disaster. Infections associated with an epidemic may be prevented by avoiding exposure to sick persons, thus preventing transmission. Examples of measures people can take to avoid exposure include engaging in social distancing and using personal protective equipment. Infections may also be prevented by modifying an individual's vulnerability to the disease. This modification is commonly accomplished by immunization. An immunized individual is considered much less vulnerable (i.e., susceptible) to the targeted infection than is someone who is not immunized. Finally, the hazard may be eliminated or avoided altogether. In the case of **infectious disease**, this is accomplished by eradicating the pathogen or markedly reducing its prevalence. Most laypersons recognize this process as a vital contribution to public health in this example. Now let us consider a different public health hazard, floods—the most common disaster worldwide. When individuals become exposed to flooded environments, they may experience a wide range of adverse health effects resulting from flood-related exposures. Injuries include drowning, electrocution, and heat illness. Infections include diarrheal illnesses and respiratory infections. Floods also exacerbate chronic diseases like emphysema, heart disease, and mental illness.

However, flood-related disease may be prevented by modifying exposure, vulnerability, and hazard risk factors. Exposure to flooding is dependent on an individual's location. Change the location, and we change the degree of exposure. Public **evacuation** actions designed to change the location of a population are called population protection measures (PPM). Like personal protective equipment, PPM is also intended to separate the individual from hazardous exposures. Vulnerability to flood-related exposures also varies among the population. Some individuals are more vulnerable because they cannot wade or swim through water, for example. Others are more susceptible to exacerbation of respiratory disease caused by inhalation of flood-related mold. Some may experience worsening mental illness, substance abuse, or violence resulting from stress related to the event. Some of these risk factors may be modifiable (e.g., swimming lessons, reasonable control of asthma, mental health interventions). Other factors, such as age, socioeconomic status, or disability, may require rendering additional PPM assistance (e.g., risk communication, social services, transportation, shelter, sanitation, nutrition).

This comparison offers a good lesson regarding our need to better appreciate the environmental causes of disaster-related morbidity and mortality and infectious etiologies. Our commonly held understanding of disease prevention for infectious diseases is nearly second nature compared with our lack of familiarity with applying these same principles to environmental hazards like floods. Instead, we often watch flood hazards cause exposures that result in disease among vulnerable populations. Typically, we then "respond" the next day by providing medical care to the sick and injured survivors with the hope of ending—not preventing—the suffering they have already experienced. by comparison, John Snow, the father of epidemiology, would surely plead with us to "Remove the pump handle already!"

Definition of Disease Prevention

The ultimate **goal** of disease prevention is to avoid the proximate cause of disease—that is, of avoiding exposing individuals to hazards. Disease prevention aims to address risk factors for disease incidence and prevalence. In the proximal setting, these risk factors include hazard incidence, exposure dose, and personal characteristics of the individual. In the distal setting, these include ecosocial factors—that is, the determinants of health (DoH)—that increase the likelihood of these proximate causes.

Table 2-1 describes the five prevention phases: primordial, primary, secondary, tertiary, and quaternary. **Primordial prevention** first seeks to avoid the ecosocial DoH. **Primary prevention** is then used to prevent hazardous exposures. Given that the

Table 2-1. The Five Stages and Corresponding Goals of Disease Prevention

Stage of Prevention	Goal	Example
Primordial	Prevent ecosocial determinants of health	Improving living standards in an impoverished river delta region
Primary	Prevent hazards Given hazards, prevent exposures	Preventing floods Evacuating communities
Secondary	Given exposure, prevent disease	Providing mass care
Tertiary	Given disease, prevent disability and death	Treating disease
Quaternary	Given illness with no disease, prevent medicalization of ecosocial health determinants	Preventing iatrogenic injury and overallocation

hazard still exists, primary prevention seeks to prevent exposures to the individual that may result in adverse health effects. Examples include taking PPM such as evacuation and **mass care**. In cases where it may be impossible to prevent exposures, **secondary prevention** is used to avoid disease (e.g., providing safe food, water, and shelter to homeless survivors). If exposures result in disease, **tertiary prevention** seeks to prevent further progression, disability, and death (e.g., providing emergency medical care). And finally, **quaternary prevention** prevents disease-free disaster survivors from developing iatrogenic disease resulting from treatment of illness (in absence of disease).

The goal of emergency health is to prevent the causes of disaster-related diseases. This goal is accomplished by preventing hazards (e.g., engaging in floodplain management); preventing exposures (e.g., taking PPM); preventing additional exposures to disease (e.g., providing safe food, water, and shelter). Ultimately, taking these measures can help prevent impairment, disability, and death.

HEALTH PROMOTION

Health promotion is "the process of enabling people to increase **control** over their health, and its determinants and thereby improve their health."[5] The goal of health promotion is to improve the health of everyone within a population by promoting modifiable risk and protective factors among individuals at risk. Health promotion is designed to engage and empower individuals, groups, and communities to reduce health risks. They may do so by improving their health, fitness, well-being, and capacity to function in society. Health promotion is an inclusive **approach** that seeks health equity for every individual regardless of demographic. Health promotion includes communications beyond risk communication and involves programs and systems for health marketing.

Health promotion encompasses three basic strategies: (1) advocate for factors that encourage health, (2) enable people to achieve health equity, and (3) mediate collaboration across all sectors.[6] These strategies are accomplished by promoting protective factors that help lower the risk of disease for the individual.

> Ensuring equity is a key component of health promotion.

Health promotion may also serve as a modifier of primary, secondary, and tertiary prevention. Let's consider floods as an example. Healthy people can better understand and inform land use and environmental policies involving nature and the built environment (i.e., primordial prevention). Healthy people can also better prevent their own exposures to flood hazards through their ability to communicate, ambulate, travel, and

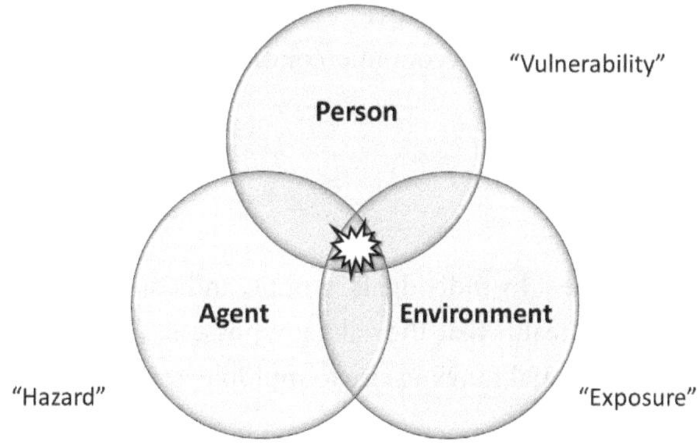

Figure 2-2. Three Proximate Causes of Disaster-Related Morbidity and Mortality

maintain social relationships such as those needed during self-evacuation and PPM during flooding (i.e., primary prevention). Healthy people are also less likely to suffer illness or injury even when exposed to flood hazards (i.e., secondary prevention). Finally, even when injured or ill, previously healthy people are more likely to recover (i.e., tertiary prevention). As such, health promotion also serves as a valuable model for preventing the multiple determinants directly attributable to the individual's health.

Extrinsic DoHs can influence risk and protective factors that are either inherent to or acquired by the individual. These risk and protective factors may also be modified through various behavioral, social, technological, economic, environmental, and cultural interventions. Medical interventions tend to prioritize technological solutions, whereas public health programs tend to prioritize social solutions. Health promotion is intended to create lifestyles and living environments that promote safe and healthy choices by default. Healthy options involve addressing technological and social factors and economic, environmental, political, and cultural differences.

Emergency health recognizes the range of ecosocial DoH affecting disaster-related health outcomes among individuals, groups, and communities.[7] Emergency health practitioners seek to promote human behaviors and living environments that are safe and healthy by default. Interventions involving health promotion must therefore consider a full range of DoH and must be applied across the individual's entire life cycle. Such interventions are designed to protect and promote health, **wellness**, **health equity**, and **quality of life** by addressing the proximate causes of disaster-related **morbidity** and **mortality** for all individuals (including the factors contributing to health disparity).

By its nature, health promotion requires interdisciplinary collaboration and community engagement to raise awareness, empower behavioral changes, and influence policy, systems, and the environment. Public health no longer defines its role as narrowly limited to that of the "assessor, policymaker, and assurer."[8] The role has evolved to become that of a community strategist, leveraging resources and partnering across multiple sectors to address social, environmental, and economic conditions that affect health and health equity.[9]

HEALTH PROTECTION

In addition to promoting healthy individuals, groups, and communities, it is also essential to protect the level of health that they already possess. Disasters create dangerous environments with the potential for exposure to multiple health hazards.

Definition of Health Protection

Health protection involves the effective collaboration of experts in identifying, preventing, and mitigating the impacts of infectious diseases and environmental, kinetic, chemical, and radiological hazards. It also involves risk assessment and communication strategies that inform individuals, groups, and communities how to protect themselves. Health protection also includes equitable resourcing and community engagement in assessing their needs, along with design, implementation, and **evaluation** of their solutions (compared with more paternalistic approaches that empower an external authority for "assessment, assurance, and policy").[8] Health protection encompasses the totality of personal, organizational, technical, social (including legal), economic, environmental, and political measures intended to protect the health of individuals, groups, and communities from harmful effects of the health hazards in their environment.

Emergency health seeks to convene expertise that will help groups and communities develop communication and implement sustainable strategies for self-protection. The entire community is engaged to ensure the equitable assessment of the community's needs, along with the design, implementation, and evaluation of potential solutions.

PROVISION OF CARE

In cases where disease and injuries cannot be prevented, providing care to disaster-affected individuals, groups, and communities is essential. This provision of care is usually directed downstream after exposures have occurred and toward addressing the two most critical human needs—namely, health care and mass care.

As illustrated in Figure 2-1, care addresses disease and displacement, the direct and indirect causes of disaster-related health effects. The provision of health care involves diagnosing and treating communicable and noncommunicable diseases and injuries associated with the event. Care for displacement consists of the provision of life-sustaining resources such as shelter, food, water, sanitation, hygiene, and security.

Emergency health provides disaster-related health care (i.e., **disaster medicine**) and health-sustaining resources (i.e., **humanitarian assistance**). These services and materials are provided within an overarching framework for the prevention of disease, the protection and promotion of health, and the provision of medical and public health care related to disasters.

A CONCEPTUAL FRAMEWORK FOR EMERGENCY HEALTH

Program logic models are schematic diagrams representing the logic underlying a program's design, indicating how various components interact with the goods or services they produce and how they generate the desired results.[10]

Throughout, this book builds a conceptual framework for emergency health, beginning with the DoH and extending into managing disaster-related exposures, diseases, and ensuring wellness and equity. This process concludes with overarching strategic goals related to the four pillars of emergency health. It also details target **objectives** to accomplish these **strategies** for disease prevention, health promotion, health protection, and provision of care associated explicitly with the disaster-related disease. (See Figure 2-3.)

TOPICS FOR DISCUSSION

Describe the social, technological, environmental, economic, political, and cultural factors that affect health outcomes in the following disasters:

- Hurricane
- Chemical spill
- Epidemic

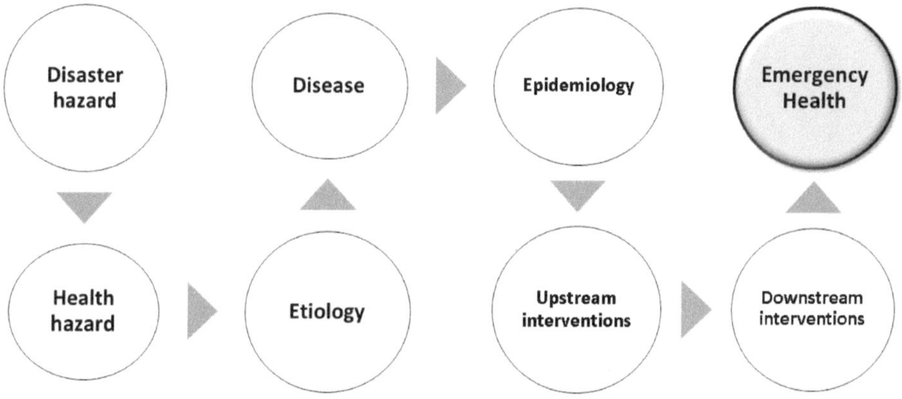

Figure 2-3. Building a Conceptual Framework for Emergency Health

REFERENCES

1. National Environmental Health Association. Definitions of environmental health. 2022. Available at: https://www.neha.org/about-neha/definitions-environmental-health. Accessed November 19, 2022.
2. Centers for Disease Control (CDC). What is environmental health? 2013. Available at: https://blogs.cdc.gov/yourhealthyourenvironment/2013/04/15/what-is-environmental-health. Accessed November 19, 2022.
3. Schultz J, Sullivan L, Galea S. *Public Health: An Introduction to the Science and Practice of Population Health*. New York, NY: Springer Publishing; 2021.
4. Bronfenbrenner U. Ecological systems theory. In: Vasta R, ed. *Six Theories of Child Development: Revised Formulations and Current Issues*. London, UK: Jessica Kingsley Publishers; 1992:187–249.
5. World Health Organization (WHO). *Health Promotion Glossary*. Geneva, Switzerland: World Health Organization; 1998.
6. World Health Organization (WHO). Ottawa Charter for health promotion. 1987. Available at: https://www.who.int/publications/i/item/ottawa-charter-for-health-promotion. Accessed November 19, 2022.
7. Stoffels J. *Strategic Issues Management: A Comprehensive Guide to Environmental Scanning*. Milwaukee, WI: Pergamon Press; 1994.
8. US Institute of Medicine Committee for the Study of the Future of Public Health. *The Future of Public Health*. Washington, DC: National Academies Press;1988.
9. DeSalvo K, Wang Y, Harris A, Auerbach J, Koo D, O'Carroll P. Public health 3.0: a call to action for public health to meet the challenges of the 21st century. *Prev Chronic Dis*. 2017;14:170017. doi: http://dx.doi.org/10.5888/pcd14.170017
10. Couillard J, Garon S, Riznie J. The logical framework approach—millennium. *Proj Manage J*. 2009;40(4):31–44.

II. DEFINITIONS OF DISASTER-RELATED DISEASE

3

The Definition of Disease

LEARNING OBJECTIVES

Upon completion of this chapter, the reader will be able to

1. Define the following terms and phases:
    - Bronfenbrener's ecosocial model of health
    - Causal factors
    - Clinical
    - Common cause variation
    - Communicable disease
    - Deterministic
    - Disease
    - Disease management
    - Ecosocial model of health
    - Environment
    - Epidemiological triad
    - Exposure
    - Hazard
    - Health
    - Health effects
    - Homeostasis
    - Illness
    - Incubation period
    - Infectious disease
    - Injury
    - Latency period
    - Natural history of disease
    - Noncommunicable disease (NCD)
    - Pathological
    - Process
    - Process-person-context-time (PPCT) model
    - Protective factors
    - Risk factor
    - Special cause variation

- Stochastic
- Subclinical
- Syndrome

2. Recognize that disease does not occur randomly.
3. Recognize three key components in the definition of disease.
4. Compare the definition of *disease* with that of *illness*.
5. Compare the definition of *disease* with that of *health effects*.
6. Recognize how special cause and common cause variation influence our definitions of health and disease.
7. Recognize the ecosocial model of health.
8. Recognize the process-person-context-time (PPCT) model of human development.
9. Compare the primary constructs regarding determinants of health (DoH).
10. Classify DoH according to the process-person-context-time (PPCT) model.
11. Recognize the three proximate causes of all disease.
12. Recognize how the epidemiological triangle (i.e., person, hazard, environment) refers to the proximate causes of disease.
13. Recognize major steps in a timeline for the natural history of disease.
14. Compare the terms *incubation period* and *latency period*.
15. Recognize three major disease categories and give examples of each.
16. Recognize that injury is a disease.

DEFINITION OF DISEASE

To establish a foundation for our discussion that embraces the terminology of public health, we begin by defining the terms used to describe the practice and principles for the discipline of emergency health. Let us start by defining disease.

Disease does not occur randomly.

Disease is a widely described process with etiologies and determinants that have been extensively studied. In short, disease is determined. **Disease** is defined as "a deviation from normal health that derives from an identifiable pathological process and which the patient experiences as an illness."[1]

This definition of disease includes several vital components. First is that disease is a measurable deviation from normal health. Second is that an identifiable process causes the condition. And third is that the patient subjectively experiences an illness. Thus, illness may exist without known disease, and disease may exist without illness. Disease processes may be clinical or **subclinical** and can present various signs and symptoms that may go unrecognized by the patient and the clinician. In comparison to the pathological

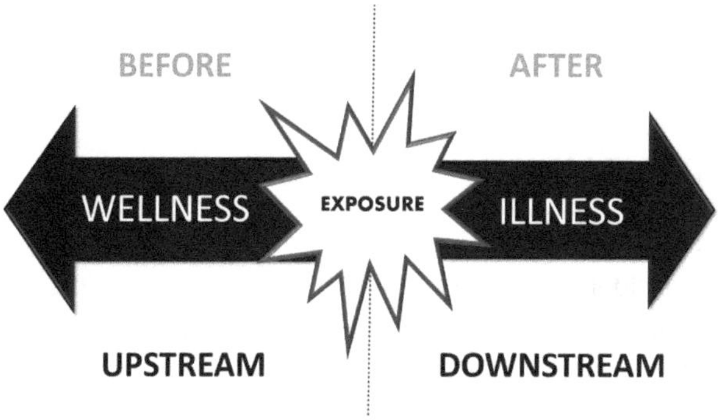

Figure 3-1. Wellness and Illness as a Continuum Affected by Hazardous Exposures

process of disease, **illness** is the "subjective sense of feeling unwell that often motivates a patient to consult a physician."[1] (See Figure 3-1.)

This definition of disease broadly refers to any condition that impairs the body's normal functioning. However, the distinction may not be practical, since patients can have a significant disease without experiencing illness (e.g., hypertension) or experience significant illness without an identifiable pathological process (e.g., infantile colic). Specific definitions of disease may also include inherent bias. For example, it is notable that these definitions of health and illness refer to the individual as a health care "patient." The definition of disease is based on an often tenuous premise that the patient *has* access to health care, which is not a foregone conclusion.

This book, however, recognizes the more inclusive definition of **health effects** among other related terms such as *disease, condition,* and *disorder*. Health effects are defined as "the causation, promotion, facilitation, and exacerbation of a structural and functional abnormality with the implication that the abnormality produced has the potential of lowering the quality of life, contributing to a disabling illness or leading to a premature death."[2]

The term *condition* is often used to describe a nonspecific state of health, describing someone as well or ill. A condition that involves illness might be further classified as a disease or a disorder. The definition of disease implies an identifiable cause and measurable change, as well as patient signs and symptoms that allow for clinical diagnosis. Again, disease denotes a condition characterized by functional impairment, structural change, and patient recognition of illness. However, subclinical and even some clinical diseases may not become evident to the patient or clinician. By contrast, a disorder denotes a condition characterized by functional impairment without structural change. Signs and symptoms need not be present for a condition to be termed a disorder.

By comparison, our discussion recognizes "adverse health effects" as a more inclusive definition that recognizes the role of determinants of health (DoH) in outcomes. It identifies multiple contributing factors and a variety of pathways. The term *health effects* also recognizes **deterministic** (i.e., dose-dependent) and **stochastic** (dose-independent) effects.

For these reasons, here the phrase *health effects* is used synonymously with the term *disease.*

DEFINITION OF HEALTH

Health-related studies typically seek to identify a pathological process as the specific cause of disease or to identify a measurable association between the special cause and variations from normal. Notably, many definitions of disease are based on a reference to health. These definitions often describe health as a standard baseline from which deviation (i.e., disease) may occur. As such, health is considered a homeostatic system that may be affected by both common cause (random) and special cause (nonrandom) "signals" or sources of variation.

Homeostasis is the tendency for a physiological process (e.g., health) to maintain a relatively stable equilibrium. Variations in homeostasis are typically measured as deviations from the central tendency (i.e., norm) of historical values.

It is possible to monitor human health surveillance data, whether from individuals or from populations, for signs of special cause variation that may be associated with disease. However, there are inherent difficulties when variations do not meet arbitrary thresholds, do not involve a recognizable pathological process, or do not occur frequently enough to establish an accurate normal baseline for comparison.

Our perceptions of health and wellness involve a complex balance of psychology, biology, and ecology. This definition of health is rooted in the development of the individual. And yet, we use the term *health* as an aggregate definition to describe a distribution of conditions we consider normal. Our public health surveillance systems are intentionally designed to detect these variances from "normal." But what is "normal" health?

According to the World Health Organization (WHO), "Health is a state of complete physical, mental and social well-being and *not merely the absence of disease or infirmity*."[3] Most important is that this language has broadened the medical definition of health beyond the simple absence of disease. This definition is based on an **ecosocial model of health** that reflects how people interact with each other and their environment.[4,5] Ecology is a branch of biology that deals with the relations of organisms to one another and their physical surroundings. The ecosocial model understands health to be affected by the ecology existing between the "individual, their close relationships, the community, and society."[6]

Bronfenbrenner originally conceived the **ecosocial model** as a framework for human development that includes the core physiology of the individual, a core influenced by five increasingly more extensive environments: micro, meso, exo, macro, and chrono.[7] (See Figure 3-2.) Bronfenbrenner's theory described how interactions between individuals and their environment form the basis for human development. This **process-person-context-time (PPCT) model** recognizes that proximal processes—that is, those directly involving the person—are the primary mechanism for human development.[7]

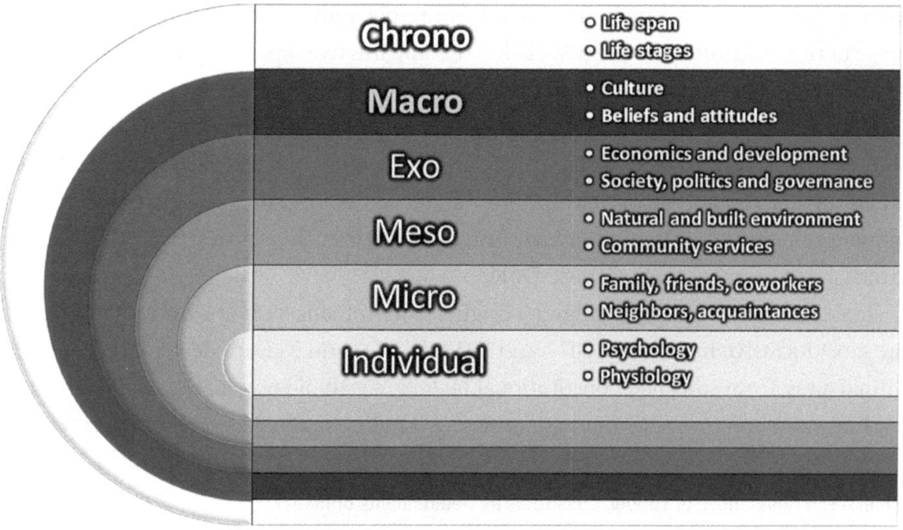

Source: Based on Bronfenbrenner.[7]

Figure 3-2. Bronfenbrenner's Ecological Systems Theory of Human Development

Bronfenbrenner's model recognizes the individual's physiological and psychological development as a core makeup. This makeup is modified by the immediate physical and social environment and subsequent interactions with more distal ones. These subsystems are then influenced by a broader set of social, political, and economic conditions. Finally, as shown in Figure 3-2, social, political, and economic conditions are influenced by the culture, beliefs, and attitudes (i.e., macrosystems) shared by members of the society.

An ecosocial model of health is based on the "health-producing" processes, personal characteristics, environmental context, and life stage.[5,7] This perspective emphasizes the multiple determinants (e.g., environments and persons), multiple social levels (e.g., individuals, groups, societies), and complexity of human situations (e.g., culture, history, conflict, beliefs). Also important is that an ecosocial model for health incorporates life span and life stage concepts that determine health.

Determinants of Health

Like disease, health does not occur randomly.

Health does not occur randomly.

Health is determined. It must be proactively promoted and potentiated. According to Schultz et al., health must be "produced."[5] Our health is determined by many factors, some more easily measurable than others. Multiple authors have described DoH as a range of risk and protective factors. Table 3-1 compares five separate (yet somewhat overlapping) constructs offered as DoH.[8-12]

Determinants of health may be broadly categorized as involving factors that are either extrinsic and collective or intrinsic and individual. Intrinsic factors can be either innate or acquired. Factors may be modifiable or nonmodifiable.[4] Extrinsic factors influence the health of the individual. In return, intrinsic factors can also influence the external environment and extrinsic DoH.[11]

Table 3-1 illustrates how Dahlgren's original conceptualization of DoH remains one of the most inclusive models. By 2017 and 2018, WHO's and Kaiser's descriptions of DoH shifted away from so-called constitutional factors (e.g., biology, genetics, gender, behavior, life stage) and from income, economics, and policy-making factors. The Centers for

Table 3-1. A Comparison of Various Constructs as Determinants of Health

	Constructs of Health Determinants				
Category of Determinant	Dahlgren 1991[8]	WHO 2017[9]	Kaiser 2018[10] (SDoH)	Healthy People 2020[11]	Healthy People 2030[12] (SDoH)
Behavior	■			■	
Biology	■			■	
Genetics	■	■		■	
Health services	■	■	■	■	■
Policy making	■			■	
Social	■	■	■	■	
Economic	■		■		
Cultural	■	■	■		■
Physical environment	■	■	■		■
Education	■	■	■		■
Economics	■	■	■		■
Food	■		■		
Community	■		■		■
Social support	■	■	■		■
Income	■	■			
Gender	■	■			
Life stage	■				■
War and military expenditures	■				

Note: SDoH = social determinants of health.

Disease Control (CDC) Healthy People 2020 program appears to reflect the narrowest range among this group, with determinants mostly related to constitutional factors like behavior, biology, and genetics, along with health services and policy making. Most recently, CDC's Healthy People 2030 program described "social DoH," or SDoH, by including several of Dahlgren's original determinants (e.g., community, gender, life stage) in place of constitutional factors.

Table 3-2 summarizes these and other reported DoH, categorized according to Bronfenbrenner's PPCT model. This approach recognizes that these factors occur within an ecosocial context and change with life stage. In other words, this approach addresses "the causation, promotion, facilitation and exacerbation of factors that have the potential of lowering the quality of life, contributing to illness, or leading to premature death."[2]

This ecosocial model characterizes a broad range of DoH according to their impacts on individuals, families, communities, and societies (including those related to disasters).

Table 3-2. Classification of Health Determinants According to an Ecosocial Model

	Determinants of Health				
	Person	**Context**			
Process	**Individual**	**Micro**	**Meso**	**Exo**	**Macro**
Producing health	**Demographic** Age Ethnicity Gender Race Sex **Psychological** Behavior Intellect Motivation **Physiological** Food Functionality Genetics Health Health status Hygiene Water	Advocates Antagonists Care providers Community Coworkers Criminals Educators Family and friends Health care workers Institutionalized persons Leaders Media Neighbors Patients Public safety Retailers Service providers	Built environment Clinics Ecosystem Home Hospitals Infrastructure Institutions Markets Natural environment Neighborhood School Shelter Workplace	Accessibility Commerce Communication Economics Education Employment Energy Finance Goods Government Health care Hospitals Housing Income Information Legal system Logistics Organization Sanitation Security Safety Social capital Socioeconomic status Technology	Bias Conflict Culture Discrimination Equality Equity Governance Human rights Humanitarianism Insularity Justice Norms Peace Religion Risk Sacredness Violence
	Chrono: Spanning all life stages: newborn, infant, child, adolescent, adult, elderly				

These DoH may be further characterized as risk or protective; innate or acquired; modifiable or nonmodifiable. Interventions may then be designed accordingly.

ROOT CAUSES OF DISEASE

Figure 3-3 depicts the epidemiological triad, the interaction between the individual, the hazardous **agent**, and their environment as the proximate cause of disease. Disease occurs when a person is exposed to an **environment** containing agents that are hazardous to health.

Disease incidence is based on the characteristics of the hazard, the individual, and the environment. These can increase the likelihood of disease (i.e., **causal factors**), or they can decrease its likelihood (i.e., protective factors). Studying the causal pathways involving the hazard, the person, and the environment is possible and may reveal both causal and **protective factors**. Causal factors include any behavior, omission, or deficiency that would have prevented the disease if corrected, eliminated, or avoided. Simply put, the goal is to prevent the convergence of these three proximate causal factors.

Let us consider how the epidemiological triad is applied using an **infectious disease** such as pneumonia as an example. In this case, the specific disease process is bacterial pneumonia. The causative hazard is the bacteria *Streptococcal pneumoniae. S. pneumoniae* is transmitted through the environment as an airborne droplet. Individuals become infected when exposed to contaminated air through a respiratory route. Characteristics of the individual influence susceptibility to infection and the severity of outcomes. Disease may be prevented by avoiding the hazard altogether (e.g., isolation, quarantine), avoiding **exposure** to the hazard (e.g., respiratory protection), and modifying the susceptibility of the individual (e.g., vaccination). If these steps are unsuccessful, health care is provided to treat the disease.

Now let us consider an example of a disaster-related disease. In this case, consider floods. The primary cause of death during floods is drowning. The specific disease process of drowning is an immersion **injury**. The causative hazard is water in a person's

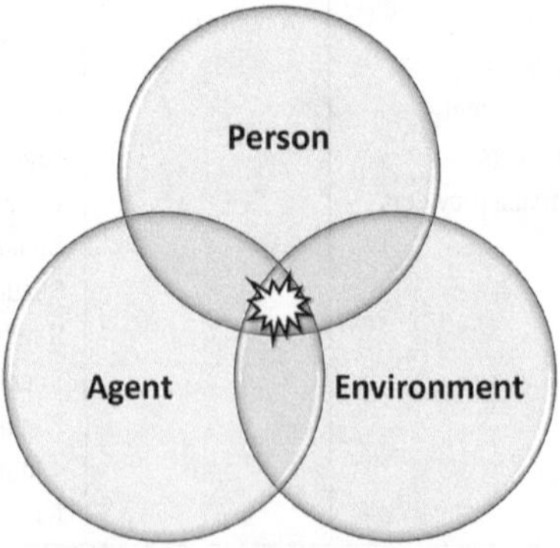

Figure 3-3. The Epidemiological Triad Model of Disease

airway that hinders respiration. Floodwater is transported through the environment according to topographical, hydrological, and meteorological factors. This process may also be affected by the built environment. Individuals become injured when they are exposed to floodwater immersion. Characteristics of the individual influence susceptibility to floodwater and the likelihood of drowning (e.g., age, functional ability, behavior). Drowning injuries may be prevented by avoiding the hazard altogether (e.g., floodplain management), avoiding exposure to the hazard (e.g., population evacuation), and modifying the susceptibility of the individual by way of education (e.g., personal awareness, swimming skills). If these steps are not entirely successful, health care is then provided for treatment of the injury.

THE NATURAL HISTORY OF DISEASE

Disease management recognizes distinct stages in the development of disease. If left untreated, a disease will evolve through a series of stages that characterize its natural history. But if an intervention is applied, the natural history is modified, producing a typical clinical course for the condition. Figure 3-4 represents this **natural history of disease**, the concept of disease as a process that unfolds in a series of steps over time.[13,14]

Effective disease management requires controlling the immediate problem and managing the person's underlying DoH. Figure 3-4 depicts the relationship between DoH, risk factors, and disease. After exposure to a hazard (or an accumulation of causal factors), there is a theoretical point at which the disease process may begin. Symptoms may appear after a delay that can vary from seconds (as with injury) to days (as with infections) to years (as with cancer). This stage of subclinical disease, extending from the time of exposure to the onset of disease symptoms, is called the **incubation period** for

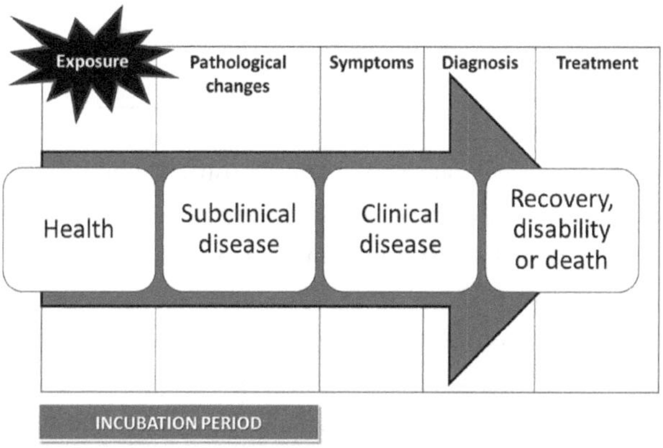

Source: Keim.[13] Adapted with permission of Cambridge University Press. © World Association for Disaster and Emergency Medicine 2018.

Figure 3-4. A Timeline for the Natural History of Disease

infectious diseases and the **latency period** for chronic diseases and injuries.[14] During this stage, disease is said to be asymptomatic. The onset of symptoms marks the transition from subclinical to clinical disease when most diagnoses are made. Patients may (or may not) interpret their symptoms as indicating an illness and seek clinical care. Therapy is usually initiated shortly after a clinical diagnosis, and short- and longer-term outcomes can be documented and reported.

Therefore, it is critical to understand a disease's natural history to intervene effectively at the earliest opportunity. The goal is to establish preventive control over every stage of a disease process that occurs over time. Early detection of hazardous exposures and their resultant health effects is associated with better health outcomes.[15]

MAJOR CATEGORIES OF DISEASE

Extensive systems have been developed to categorize diseases. Such systems classify any injury or disease according to a coded design.[16] Public health often classifies disease according to three general categories: **communicable disease**, **noncommunicable disease (NCD)**, and injury.

A communicable disease is an infectious disease that can be passed (i.e., transmitted) from person to person. Infectious disease is "caused by pathogenic microorganisms, such as bacteria, viruses, parasites, or fungi; the diseases can be spread, directly or indirectly, from one person to another."[17]

By contrast, NCDs are not passed from person to person. They are commonly associated with exposures related to lifestyle (e.g., diet, exercise, smoking, workplace) and are typical of long duration and generally slow progression. Significant NCDs include cardiovascular diseases (like heart attacks and stroke), cancer, respiratory diseases (such as chronic obstructive pulmonary disease and asthma), mental illness, and diabetes.

Injury is a disease.

Injury is a category of disease "caused by acute exposure to physical agents (i.e., kinetic energy, heat, electricity, chemicals, and ionizing radiation) interacting with the body in amounts or at rates that exceed the threshold of human tolerance."[18–20] Some experts consider that the interval between exposure and the appearance of injury can be relatively long. The shorter the time from exposure to a hazard to its physical effects, the more likely we are to call the resulting condition "injury" rather than "disease." This distinction is somewhat arbitrary but is conceptually helpful for classifying disaster-related diseases.

In part III, we will discuss disaster-related disease, according to these three main categories. Later, in part IV, we will discuss how disasters relate to these three categories and what public health and medical capabilities are necessary to address each.

TOPICS FOR DISCUSSION

1. Why is it important to recognize that disease and health do not occur randomly?
2. Using an ecosocial model, describe DoH for tobacco-related emphysema.
3. Using the epidemiological triad, describe the causes of tornado-related injuries.
4. Compare the latency period of traumatic injuries with the incubation period for infectious diseases.
5. People often do not consider injury as a disease. Offer your opinions regarding the reason.

REFERENCES

1. Donovan D, McDowell I, eds. *AFMC Primer on Population Health: A Virtual Textbook on Public Health Concepts for Clinicians.* Ottowa, ON: Association of Faculties of Medicine of Canada, University of Ottawa; 2018. Available at: https://phprimer.afmc.ca/en. Accessed November 19, 2022.
2. Sherwin R. What is an adverse health effect? *Environ Health Perspect.* 1983;52:177–182.
3. Grad FP. The preamble of the Constitution of the World Health Organization. *Bull World Health Organ,* 2002;80(12):981–984. World Health Organization. Available at: https://apps.who.int/iris/handle/10665/268691. Accessed December 17, 2022.
4. Birkhead G, Morrow C, Pirani S. *Essentials of Public Health.* 4th ed. Burlington, MA: Jones and Bartlett Learning; 2021.
5. Schultz J, Sullivan L, Galea S. *Public Health: An Introduction to the Science and Practice of Population Health.* New York, NY: Springer Publishing; 2021.
6. Centers for Disease Control and Prevention (CDC). *Principles of Community Engagement.* Atlanta, GA: Centers for Disease Control and Prevention, 2011:4–8.
7. Bronfenbrenner U. Ecological systems theory. In: Vasta R, ed. *Six Theories of Child Development: Revised Formulations and Current Issues.* London, UK: Jessica Kingsley Publishers; 1992:187–249.
8. Dahlgren G, Whitehead M. The Dahlgren-Whitehead model of health determinants: 30 years on and still chasing rainbows. *Public Health.* 2021;199:20–24.
9. World Health Organization (WHO). Determinants of health. Questions and Answers. 2017. Available at: https://www.who.int/news-room/questions-and-answers/item/determinants-of-health. Accessed November 19, 2022.
10. Friedman N, Banagas M. Toward addressing social determinants of health: a health care system strategy. *Permanente J.* 2018;22:18–095. Available at: https://www.ncbi.nlm.nih.gov/pmc/articles/PMC6207437. Accessed November 19, 2022.
11. US Department of Health and Human Services (HHS). Determinants of health. In: *Healthy People 2020.* Vol. 2022. Washington, DC: Dept of Health and Human Services; 2020.
12. US Department of Health and Human Services (HHS). Social determinants of health. 2020. Available at: https://health.gov/healthypeople/priority-areas/social-determinants-health. Accessed November 19, 2022.

13. Keim M. Managing disaster-related health risk: a process for prevention. *Prehosp Disaster Med.* 2018;33(3):326–334.
14. Centers for Disease Control and Prevention (CDC). Natural history and spectrum of disease. In: *Principles of Epidemiology.* 3rd ed. Atlanta, GA: Centers for Disease Control and Prevention; 2012.
15. Krug EG, Kresnow M, Peddicord JP, et al. Suicide after natural disasters. *N Engl J Med.* 1998;338(6):373–378.
16. World Health Organization (WHO). International classification of diseases. 11th revision. ICD-11. Classifications. 2022. Available at: https://www.who.int/standards/classifications/classification-of-diseases. Accessed November 19 2022.
17. World Health Organization (WHO). Regional Office of the Mediterranean Infectious disease. 2022. Available at: https://www.emro.who.int/health-topics/infectious-diseases/index.html. Accessed December 17, 2022.
18. Haddon W. A note concerning accident theory and research with special reference to motor vehicle accidents. *Ann N Y Acad Sci.* 1963;107:635–646.
19. Haddon W. The changing approach to the epidemiology, prevention, and amelioration of trauma: the transition to approaches etiologically rather than descriptively based. *Am J Public Health and Nation's Health.* 1968;58(8):1431–1438.
20. Gibson JJ. The contribution of experimental psychology to the formulation of the problem of safety: a brief for basic research. In: Gibson JJ, ed. *Behavioral Approaches to Accident Research.* New York, NY: Association for the Aid of Crippled Children; 1961:77–89.

4

The Definition of Disaster

LEARNING OBJECTIVES

Upon completion, the reader will be able to

1. Define the following terms and phrases:
   - Accuracy
   - Biological, climatological, hydrological, meteorological, and geophysical
   - Disaster
   - Disaster pathway
   - Governance
   - Incident
   - Incident command system (ICS)
   - Incident continuum
   - Toxic, thermal, and kinetic hazards
   - Uncertainty
   - Unified command
   - Validity
   - Variability
2. Describe five steps in a disaster pathway.
3. Describe five levels of an incident continuum.
4. Recognize that disasters are classified according to causative hazard.
5. Describe eight subgroups of disasters that compose natural and technological disasters.

DEFINITION OF DISASTERS

Etymology of Disasters

The term **disaster** has a complex, polysemic meaning that has changed throughout history. These events are often dramatic and life-altering. For that reason, lay perceptions of disaster phenomena often carry undertones of the beliefs and attitudes of the affected populations. And these perceptions change over time.

For example, we are reminded that the ancient Greek root of the English word *disaster* (i.e., "bad star") indicates an astrological cause of disasters. In some cultures, the word that describes disasters is associated with punishment for a tragic personal or societal flaw. By the mid-20th century, a more fatalistic approach replaced human blame for these events. This new approach considered such phenomena "acts of God" (caused by natural hazards) or "accidents" (caused by technological hazards). At the inception of the Anthropocene epoch, we have learned that human factors markedly influence not only so-called technological (i.e., human-made) disasters but also so-called natural disasters.[1]

Key Characteristics of Disasters

Disasters have been defined according to key quantitative characteristics related to resources available, degree of uncertainty, risk of additional losses, and the scale of the incident.

The definition of disaster means different things to different people. In one scenario, a crash occurs in a major metropolitan area. In another scenario, a crash occurs in a remote location in the mountains, miles from the nearest doctor. Let us consider an example involving a bus crash that has resulted in 20 severely injured patients. The major metropolitan hospitals will likely possess all the resources necessary to avoid excess mortality among these patients. However, this may not be the case in more remote rural areas. In this latter case, 20 severely injured patients would likely exceed the local capacity to care for them. Thus, we may appreciate how a disaster is determined by a mismatch of needs and resources, not by the sheer number of cases.

The Disaster Pathway

Hazards (e.g., drought) create incidents that result in consequences (e.g., health effects). In turn, these consequences characteristically create needs that exceed the affected population's resources (e.g., water). Thus hazards frequently result in a mismatch of needs and resources. Figure 4-1 represents disasters as a pathway resulting in this mismatch of needs and resources.[2]

The Role of Uncertainty

In addition to the mismatch of needs and resources, uncertainty is a key characteristic of all disasters. **Uncertainty** is defined as a state or condition that involves a deficiency of information and leads to inadequate or incomplete knowledge or understanding.[3] Statistical uncertainty is often estimated (in terms of **accuracy** and **validity**) around historical measures of central tendency. As discussed in Chapter 3, this uncertainty is compared with historical baselines using special cause and common cause variation.

Uncertainty is a state of limited knowledge where it is impossible to describe the existing state or a future outcome precisely. It is often difficult to identify potential disaster hazards and to accurately predict when, where, and how they will occur. Identifying or predicting the extent of disaster-related consequences and needs is even more challenging. Typically, the first assessment of disaster-related needs occurs immediately after the incident.

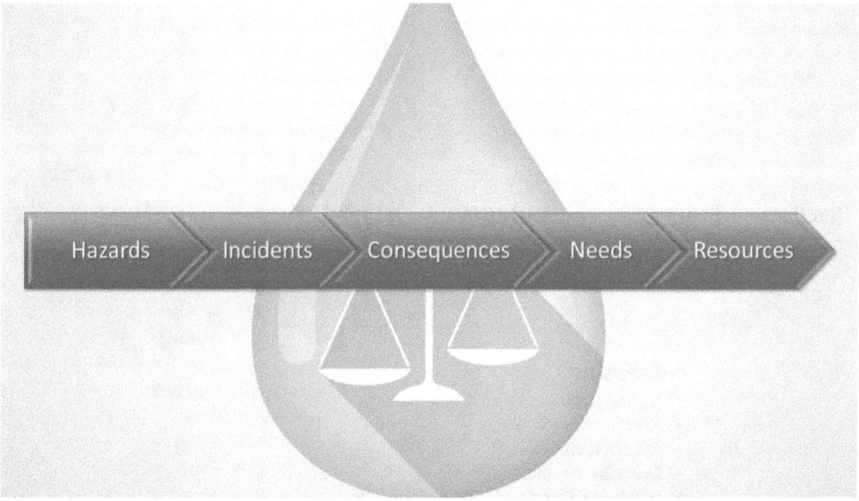

Source: Keim et al.[2] Reprinted with permission of Cambridge University Press. © Cambridge University Press 2021.

Figure 4-1. The Disaster Pathway

Many disaster managers instinctively consider uncertainty as a threat to successful emergency operations. Uncertainty increases operational **variability** and reduces the efficiency and effectiveness of emergency operations.

The Incident Continuum

The severity and scale of disaster incidents are known to occur along a characteristic continuum. Figure 4-2 illustrates how emergencies and disasters are part of a relative continuum of incidents that extend from routine events to **catastrophes.**[2] These incidents along the continuum are characterized by increasing degrees of scale, needs, uncertainty, operational variability, and risk. The boundaries between these various classifications are often obscured and overlap. It is also common for an incident to rapidly escalate to a higher degree of acuity, severity, and/or scale. These escalations do not necessarily occur in sequential order. It is not uncommon for routine operations to be abruptly interrupted and replaced by a full-scale disaster response (e.g., flash floods) or the less frequent extent of catastrophe (e.g., transpacific tsunami). Figure 4-2 also depicts how uncertainty increases with the scope of an incident.[2]

An **emergency** is a "sudden and usually unforeseen event that calls for immediate measures to minimize its adverse consequences." This definition involves several critical elements, including uncertainty, acuity, and the risk of additional losses. A disaster is "a serious disruption of the functioning of a community or a society causing widespread human, material, economic or environmental losses that exceed the ability of the affected community or society to cope using its resources."[4]

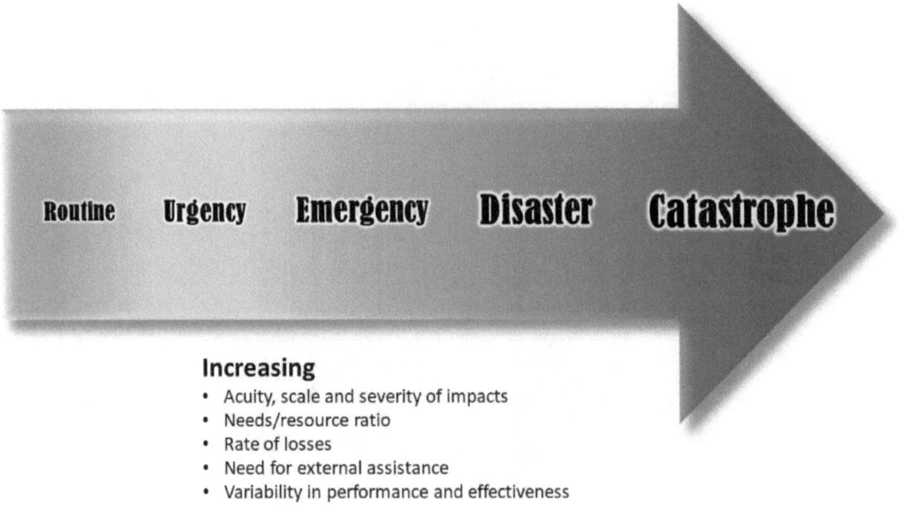

Source: Keim et al.[2] Reprinted with permission of Cambridge University Press. © Cambridge University Press 2021.

Figure 4-2. The Incident Continuum

Disasters create needs that exceed a society's ability to cope using its own resources. An event that does not exceed a society's ability to cope is then classified as an emergency.[5] Affected populations during disasters, compared with emergencies, are compelled to take a number of measures, among them these[5]:

- Quickly relate to many unfamiliar groups
- Adjust to shared command and decision-making
- Communicate, cooperate, and collaborate with a range of stakeholders
- Apply different standards and methods
- Operate within closer-than-usual interfaces with health and private sectors

Disaster responders utilize a unified incident command system to share power among leaders of the affected populations and outside assistance. For example, after a major disaster (e.g., tropical cyclone) an emergency response is often mounted by a variety of organizations and agencies. These groups typically work within a new organizational structure (i.e., an incident command system), where power for decision-making is shared among stakeholders.

Emergencies and disasters also tend to be conceptually differentiated from catastrophes. In a **catastrophe**, compared with emergencies and disasters, the following characteristics pertain[6]:

- Most or all of the critical infrastructure is heavily affected.
- A large portion of the affected population is killed or incapacitated.
- Affected public officials are unable to undertake their usual work roles.

- Nearly all routine societal functions are sharply and simultaneously interrupted.
- External assistance is either impossible or ineffective in alleviating the need.

For example, after a significant catastrophe (e.g., a nuclear detonation), emergency response options are characteristically limited because of ongoing environmental hazards, the relatively low number of survivors, and the relative absence of local **governance** and infrastructure. Humanitarian assistance may not be able to enter the area safely from the outside. And even if those assisting do so, they cannot implement a **unified command** system because of the lack of local decision makers and the prohibitively high risk-to-benefit ratio associated with most interventions. As was the case after the 1994 Indian Ocean tsunami, blanketing the location with an enormous number of resources does not significantly change the outcome. Sadly, those persons lost during a catastrophe remain so regardless of our best intentions.

DISASTER TYPOLOGY

Classification According to Causative Disaster Hazard

Environmental disasters may be further categorized according to the rapidity of onset. For example, hydrometeorological disasters such as flash floods and tornado disasters may occur abruptly, whereas droughts and heat waves may have a slower and more insidious onset. Technological disasters like chemical releases may occur slowly and insidiously or be explosively abrupt.

Technological disasters may also be categorized according to the presence or absence of willful human intent.[7] **Toxicological, thermal, kinetic** (and even some biological) disasters may occur as a result of intentional or unintentional human actions. Many technological hazards may occur as a result of human error and procedural means associated with the industry or as a result of a conflict (i.e., terrorism, sabotage, or warfare).[8,9] "In effect, the main difference between industrial disasters and those of chemical sabotage, warfare, and terrorism may be a distinction only of malicious intent."

Finally, environmental disasters may also be categorized as intensive and extensive risk events.[10] Disasters may be classified as intensive risks when extreme earthquakes—or tsunamis, volcanoes, floods, or major storms—strike densely populated areas. Disasters are categorized as an extensive risk when overall risk is associated with dispersed populations' exposure to repetitive or persistent hazard conditions of low or moderate intensity. These incidents (e.g., the drought-flood cycle) are often highly localized yet can lead to debilitating cumulative disaster impacts.

Given the myriad potential scenarios, it is helpful to classify disasters according to the causative agent or hazard. Disaster hazards are broadly grouped into three categories according to their origin. Environmental hazards or biological hazards cause natural disasters. By comparison, human-made hazards cause technological disasters.

Table 4-1. Definitions and Examples for Eight Disaster Subgroups Caused by Natural and Technological Hazards

Hazard Group	Hazard Subgroup	Definition
Technological	Toxic	Pertaining to poison
	Thermal	Pertaining to heat
	Kinetic	Pertaining to motion
Natural	Biological	Pertaining to living organisms
	Climatological	Pertaining to the climate: long-term atmospheric phenomena
	Geophysical	Pertaining to the earth's physical phenomena
	Hydrological	Pertaining to water: in the atmosphere and on the earth
	Meteorological	Pertaining to weather: short-term atmospheric phenomena

Source: Keim et al.[1] Adapted under the terms of the CC BY license (https://creativecommons.org/licenses/by/4.0).

By comparison, complex disasters are caused by a complex mix of biological, social, and environmental hazards related to conflict, displacement, and food insecurity. This group of disasters is also referred to as "complex emergencies" and is specifically addressed by the field of refugee health. This textbook (and the concept of emergency health itself) is intended to focus on disasters caused by natural and technological disasters, as defined in Table 4-1.[1] Table 4-1 also illustrates how the two categories of technological and natural disasters may be further categorized into eight subgroups. (Hydrological and meteorological are often combined to create seven subgroups.)[1]

Disaster subgroups are also further classified into individual disaster types. Table 4-2 represents a typology for common disasters, classified according to disaster subgroups.[11] According to this typology, four subgroups of natural disasters comprise 13 individual disaster types, and three subgroups of technological disasters include 9 different kinds of disasters.[10]

While the dividing lines between these classifications are helpful for purposes of comparison and discussion, it is essential to recognize that they are relatively arbitrary and have become less distinct over time. So-called natural disasters are often associated with human activity. Historical examples include the worsening of hurricane intensity as a result of climate change.[12] Technological disasters are also frequently exacerbated by natural weather and topography. One example is the spread of radioactive contamination by atmospheric winds after the Chernobyl power plant failure.[13] Another is food insecurity associated with drought-related crop failures and implicated as a contributing factor to complex emergencies in Syria.[14]

The World Bank has coined the phrase "natural hazards, but unnatural disasters" in recognition that disasters are symptoms of dysfunctional development resulting from human acts of omission and commission.[15] In effect, few natural disasters are caused

Table 4-2. A Typology for Disasters

<table>
<tr><th colspan="2">Natural</th><th colspan="4">Technological</th></tr>
<tr><th>Subgroup</th><th>Type</th><th>Subgroup</th><th colspan="3">Type</th></tr>
<tr><td rowspan="2">Climatological</td><td>Drought</td><td rowspan="6">Toxic</td><td colspan="2" rowspan="2">Poisoning</td><td rowspan="16">Industrial and Nuclear</td></tr>
<tr><td>Wildfire</td></tr>
<tr><td rowspan="4">Hydrometeorological</td><td>Cold weather</td><td rowspan="2">Spill/release</td><td>Chemical</td></tr>
<tr><td>Cyclone</td><td>Radiological</td></tr>
<tr><td>Heat wave</td><td colspan="2" rowspan="5">Fire</td></tr>
<tr><td>Storm</td></tr>
<tr><td rowspan="3">Biological</td><td>Outbreak</td><td rowspan="6">Thermal</td></tr>
<tr><td>Epidemic</td></tr>
<tr><td>Pandemic</td></tr>
<tr><td rowspan="7">Geophysical</td><td>Earthquake</td><td colspan="2" rowspan="3">Explosion</td></tr>
<tr><td>Landslide</td></tr>
<tr><td>Volcanic eruption</td></tr>
<tr><td rowspan="4">Tsunami</td><td rowspan="4">Kinetic</td><td colspan="2">Transportation</td></tr>
<tr><td colspan="2">Gathering</td></tr>
<tr><td colspan="2">Mining</td></tr>
<tr><td colspan="2">Structural collapse</td></tr>
</table>

Source: Keim et al.[11] Adapted with permission.

entirely by nature. In addition, the term *natural* is also polysemous and sometimes misconstrued to represent an inevitable event (as opposed to one derived from nature). However, it helps classify disasters that are amenable to comparison.

Note that the discussion here uses the terms *natural disaster* and *technological disaster* to categorize these events according to their associated hazard group.

TOPICS FOR DISCUSSION

Choose one type of disaster and describe the following:

1. The disaster group and subgroup
2. Five stages of the disaster pathway, to include hazard, incident, consequences, needs, and resources
3. Three critical characteristics of the disaster, related to
   - mismatch of needs and resources,
   - issues regarding uncertainty, and
   - the incident continuum.

REFERENCES

1. Keim ME, Smith TM, Burkle FM. The annual global incidence rate of extreme weather event disasters appears positively correlated with world GDP, 1961–2020. *Prehosp Disaster Med.* 2022;37(4):431–436.
2. Keim M. *Disaster Planning: A Practical Guide to Effective Health Outcomes.* Cambridge, UK: Cambridge University Press; 2021.
3. Standards Australia Committee OB-007. *AS/NZS 4360:2004 Risk Management.* Sydney, Australia, and Wellington, New Zealand: Standards Australia International; 2004.
4. United Nations International Strategy for Disaster Reduction (UNISDR). USDR terminology on disaster risk reduction. 2009. Available at: http://www.unisdr.org/files/7817_UNISDRTerminologyEnglish.pdf. Accessed November 27, 2022.
5. Tazmania: World Health Organization (WHO). *Health Sector Emergency Preparedness Guide.* Geneva, Switzerland: World Health Organization; 1998.
6. Quarantelli EL. Catastrophes are different from disasters: some implications for crisis planning and managing drawn from Katrina. June 11, 2006. Available at: https://items.ssrc.org/understanding-katrina/catastrophes-are-different-from-disasters-some-implications-for-crisis-planning-and-managing-drawn-from-katrina. Accessed January 27, 2023.
7. Keim M. Intentional chemical disasters. In: Hogan D, Burstein J, eds. *Disaster Medicine.* Philadelphia, PA: Lippincott Williams & Wilkins; 2002:340–348.
8. Lillibridge S. Industrial disasters. In: Noji EK, ed. *The Public Health Consequences of Disasters.* New York, NY: Oxford University Press; 1997:354–369.
9. Keim ME. Intentional chemical disasters. In: Hogan DE, Burstein JL, eds. *Disaster Medicine.* 2nd ed. Philadelphia, PA: Lippincott Williams & Wilkins; 2007:402–411.
10. Center for Research on the Epidemiology of Disasters (CRED). EM-DAT: the international disaster database. 2022. Available at: www.emdat.be. Accessed November 27. 2022.
11. Keim M. Environmental disasters. In: Frumkin H, ed. *Environmental Health: From Global to Local.* 3rd ed. San Francisco CA: Wiley & Sons; 2016.
12. Intergovernmental Panel on Climate Change (IPCC). *Climate Change 2007: Impacts, Adaptation, and Vulnerability.* Cambridge, UK: Cambridge University Press; 2007.
13. Paatero J, Hämeri K, Jaakkola T, Jantunen M, Koivukoski J, Saxén R. Airborne and deposited radioactivity from the Chernobyl accident: a review of investigations in Finland. *Boreal Environ Res.* 2008;15:19–33.
14. Selbya J, Dahib O, Fröhlich C, Hulmee M. Climate change and the Syrian civil war revisited. *Polit Geogr.* 2017;60:232–244.
15. World Bank. *Natural Hazards, Unnatural Disasters: The Economics of Prevention.* New York, NY: World Bank; 2012.

5

Hazardous Exposures

LEARNING OBJECTIVES

Upon completion, the reader will be able to

1. Define the following terms and phrases:
   - Biohazard
   - Casual pathway of disease
   - Consequences
   - Dose
   - Dose rate
   - Dose-response modeling
   - Etiology of disease
   - Exposure
   - Exposure science
   - Hazard characterization
   - Hazardous exposure
   - Hazardous materials
   - Hazardous substance
   - Health hazard
   - Hormesis
   - Impact
   - Infectious dose
   - Lethal dose (LD_{50})
   - Natural hazards
   - Natural history of disease
   - Ordinal scale
   - Proximate cause of disease
   - Routes of human exposure
   - Sendai Framework for Disaster Risk Reduction
   - Technological hazards
2. Compare and contrast disaster hazards with health hazards.
3. Recognize health hazards commonly associated with the following 20 disaster hazards:
   - Cold weather
   - Cyclone

- Drought
- Earthquake
- Epidemic
- Explosion
- Fire
- Flood
- Hazardous material release
- Heat wave
- Landslide
- Mass gathering
- Mining
- Poisoning
- Structural collapse
- Tornado and convective storm
- Transportation accident
- Tsunami
- Volcanic eruption
- Wildfire

4. Recognize the three routes of human exposures.
5. Identify two key clusters of disaster consequences that affect health.
6. Identify the following parameters on a dose-response curve:
   - Maximum predicted mortality
   - Hazard dose
   - Hazard potency
   - Population vulnerability

DISASTER-RELATED HEALTH IMPACT

Disaster-related health effects result from hazardous exposures that cause a structural and/or functional abnormality that can lower the quality of life, contribute to a disabling illness, or lead to premature death.[1]

These adverse effects are often described as disaster **consequences,** and their severity is measured in terms of **impact**. Thus, consequence is a qualitative description of the adverse effect, while impact is a quantitative measure. Impact measures the net balance of outcomes resulting from a mismatch of human needs and resources available to meet those needs. (See Figure 4-1.)[2] Health impact is often expressed as the disease incidence rate resulting from exposure and **vulnerability** to a particular hazard. The impacts of health hazards are customarily assessed according to exposure and vulnerability—factors associated with the interaction between the environment and the host population, respectively, as follows[3,4]:

- Exposure (i.e., dose)
  - Potency of the hazard itself (e.g., toxicity, virulence, or potential energy)
  - Amount of hazard contacted over time (e.g., dose rate)
- Vulnerability (i.e., intrinsic risk and protective factors)
  - Susceptibility before disease onset
  - Severity of the disease after onset

DISASTER HAZARDS

In general, disaster hazards result in various social, technological, economic, environmental, and political consequences, including disease. Hazard characterization describes the adverse effects of exposure to the hazard. To summarize:

1. Hazards create consequences.
   - The characteristics of a hazard are expressed in terms of consequences.
2. Consequences result in losses.
   - The severity of losses is expressed in terms of impact.
3. Losses create needs.
   - The characteristics of needs are expressed in terms of capability.
4. Capabilities meet needs.
   - Capability availability over time is expressed in terms of capacity.

The **Sendai Framework for Disaster Reduction** recognizes two groups of hazards, natural and human-induced (i.e., technological or anthropogenic).[5] A disaster might also involve a combination of these hazards. For example, earthquake-related damages to the natural gas infrastructure often result in increased human exposure to fire hazards.

Disasters have traditionally been classified according to the causative hazard, commonly categorized as natural or technological. **Natural hazards** originate in nature—that is, they are biological, climatological, geophysical, and hydrometeorological phenomena. (See Table 4-2.)[6] **Technological hazards** are anthropogenic and originate from human technology (i.e., toxic, thermal, and kinetic phenomena) or activities (i.e., transportation, public gatherings, and industry). Thus, a hazard is defined within the context of the expected losses. Besides health, these losses may also include social, technological, economic, environmental, political, and cultural contexts. Table 5-1 lists 20 natural and technological hazards attributable to disasters during the past 60 years.

HEALTH HAZARDS

Disaster hazards differ from disaster-related **health hazards**. For example, a cyclone (i.e., a hurricane) is a disaster hazard that creates many health hazards, including high winds, storm surges, inland flooding, and landslides.

Table 5-1. Hazards Associated With Natural and Technological Disasters, 1961–2020

Natural Disasters	Technological Disasters
Cold waves and storms	Explosion
Cyclone (i.e., hurricane)	Fire
Drought	Hazardous material release
Earthquake	Mass gathering
Epidemic	Mining
Flood	Poisoning
Heat wave	Structural collapse
Landslide and avalanche	Transportation accident
Tornadoes and convective storms	
Tsunami	
Volcanic eruption	
Wildfire	

Biological health hazards are those microbiological organisms (i.e., bacteria, viruses, parasites, or fungi) known to cause infectious disease outbreaks and epidemics. Hazards that release energy or cause toxicity (i.e., mechanical, chemical, thermal, or radiological) are usually associated with injury. In some cases, environmental hazards (e.g., drought, floods, heat, and cold) cause injuries by restricting the essential requirements for life, such as water, food, oxygen, or temperature.

It is essential to differentiate between the broad categories of hazards that cause a disaster (i.e., a societal mismatch of needs and resources) and the specific health hazards that cause disaster-related disease. This difference is practical, since it is necessary to understand the proximate cause to attribute health effects and develop effective countermeasures accurately.

Compared with disaster hazards, health hazards represent agents or situations that when exposed to a human have the inherent capability to cause an adverse health outcome, resulting in morbidity and mortality. The World Health Organization has defined a health hazard as "a process, phenomenon or human activity that may cause loss of life, injury or other health impacts."[7]

For example, a tropical cyclone (i.e., a hurricane) is a meteorological hazard that frequently causes disasters. Cyclones produce health hazards that include high winds (that cause traumatic injuries and population displacement), inland flooding, and coastal storm surges that cause drowning. Table 5-2 lists individual health hazards associated with the incidence of disaster hazards.

Table 5-2. Health Hazards Associated With Individual Natural and Technological Disaster Hazards

Disaster Hazard	Health Hazards
Cold waves and storms	Motor vehicle accidents Heating and cooking stoves Portable power generators Increased physical exertion Cold ambient air temperatures Precipitation and wind
Cyclone (i.e., hurricane)	High winds Heating and cooking stoves Portable power generators Unsafe drinking water Floodwater Rooftop activity Power lines High ambient air temperature Insects, pets, and wild animals Traumatic stress Airborne particulates Poor sanitation and hygiene Toxic chemicals
Drought	Food insecurity Conflict Unsafe drinking water Poor sanitation and hygiene Waterborne pathogens Traumatic stress Violence and domestic abuse
Earthquake	Structural debris Structure fires Airborne particulates Entrapment Hazardous materials Traumatic stress Wound contamination Poor sanitation and hygiene
Epidemic	Pathogens of epidemic potential Health care overutilization
Flood	Debris cleanup Heating and cooking stoves Portable power generators Unsafe water Floodwater Power lines Traumatic stress Airborne particulates Poor sanitation and hygiene

(Continued)

Table 5-2. (Continued)

Disaster Hazard	Health Hazards
Heat wave	Endemic chronic disease High ambient air temperature
Landslide and avalanche	Falling debris Entrapment Airborne particulates Hazardous materials Wound contamination Poor sanitation and hygiene
Tornadoes and convective storms	High winds Ballistic projectiles Structural debris
Tsunami	Structural debris Floodwater Traumatic stress Wound contamination Poor sanitation and hygiene
Volcanic eruption	High ambient air temperature Blast projectiles Volcanic gas and debris Pyroclastic flows Lahars Tephra Chemical and radioactive substances
Wildfire	High ambient air temperature Fire Hot gases Airborne particulates Toxic chemicals
Explosion	Ballistic projectiles Structural debris Pressure wave Heat and/or fire Toxic chemicals Radioactive substances Violence
Fire	High ambient air temperature Fire Hot gases Airborne particulates Toxic chemicals

(Continued)

Table 5-2. (Continued)

Disaster Hazard	Health Hazards
Hazardous material release	Pressurized gas Airborne particulates Biological pathogens Toxic chemicals Radioactive substances
Mass gathering	Stampedes Fires Structural collapse Poor food safety High ambient air temperature Storms Violence
Mining	Structural collapse Entrapment Explosions Fires Air particulates Toxic chemicals
Poisoning	Adulterated commercial products Contaminated air, food, and/or water Toxic chemicals Radioactive substances
Structural collapse	Structural debris Fire Airborne particulates Entrapment Toxic chemicals
Transportation accident	Blunt and penetrating trauma Burns Drowning Toxic exposures Violence

HAZARDOUS EXPOSURES

Table 5-2 illustrates how various disaster hazards cascade to create an even more comprehensive array of health hazards. It also reveals how the resultant health hazards are not merely random or "acts of God" but instead occur as the result of predictable consequences (e.g., damage, losses, and health effects).

Concerning health, **hazardous substances** may be defined as *any disease-causing agent* that after releasing into the environment and upon exposure, ingestion, inhalation, or assimilation into any person will result in health risks, including death and disease, such as

- Behavioral abnormalities,
- Cancer,
- Genetic mutation,
- Physiological malfunctions, or
- Physiological deformations in such persons or their offspring.

Hazardous substances cause disease in the form of either infections or injuries. They can be infectious or noninfectious. Infectious, hazardous substances are typically referred to as **biohazardous materials** (i.e., **biohazards**). Noninfectious hazardous substances are often referred to as **hazardous materials** (or **hazmat**, for short). However, disaster-related hazards may occur in the absence of a disaster. The mere incidence of a hazard does not necessarily result in a disaster, per se. For example, a cyclone that travels across the ocean without striking an affected population is a hazard, not a disaster. Disasters (and their related health effects) occur when people become exposed to hazards.

Exposure is "contact with a hazard," which typically results in adverse outcomes. There are three commonly accepted **routes of human exposure**: inhalation, ingestion, and direct contact with the body. Concerning health, populations affected by disasters incur a risk of morbidity and mortality from the primary exposure to the hazard itself and other secondary hazardous exposures that are caused indirectly (largely due to the mismatch of needs and resources. (See Figure 5-1.)

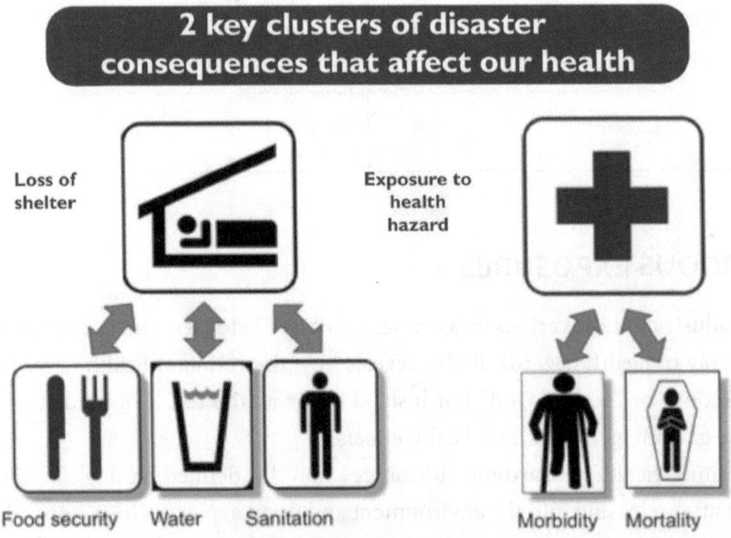

Figure 5-1. Direct and Indirect Health Consequences of Disaster Hazards

EXPOSURE DOSE

Assessing Exposure

Exposure science (e.g., analytical risk analysis and dose reconstruction) is a well-developed field of empirical investigation involving environmental health and medicine. Exposure assessment is the qualitative or quantitative evaluation of the likely contact with health hazards. This assessment consists in identifying and evaluating the human population exposed to a hazard, describing its composition and size, as well as identifying the type, magnitude, frequency, route, and duration of exposure.[8]

More specifically, exposure has been described as "contact made between a chemical, physical, or biological agent and the outer boundary of an organism. Exposure is quantified as the amount of an agent available at the exchange boundaries of the organism (e.g., skin, lungs, gut)."[6] Populations may also be exposed to a hazard without any adverse effect. Thus, the term *exposure* is not synonymous with the word *affected*.[9]

Exposure is calculated as a function of the dose rate of the hazard and the duration of exposure over time.[4] Dose rates are often expressed in magnitude (e.g., concentration) over time. In some cases, hazard magnitude can be measured directly in terms of concentration, reactivity, radioactivity, toxicity, infectivity, virulence, or transmissibility. In other cases, health hazards (e.g., wind, storm surge, and ground shaking) are described according to standardized hazard-specific indices and **ordinal scales** that reflect severity or "potency" (e.g., Enhanced Fujita, Saffir-Simpson, Modified Mercalli, respectively). For health, exposure is calculated as a function of hazard dose.

Dose is the amount of a substance (in this case, a hazardous substance) available for interactions with metabolic processes or biologically significant receptors after crossing the outer boundary of an organism.[8] Hazard dose associated with physical agents (involving a transfer of energy to the body; i.e., kinetic, nuclear, electromagnetic, chemical, and thermal energy) is calculated as a function of the hazard magnitude and the contact rate. Contact rates vary according to the route of exposure, be it respiratory rate, ingestion, or absorption.

For example, the chemical dose is calculated according to the concentration (mass/volume) and contact rate (mass/volume/time) multiplied by the duration of exposure (time).[10] The relative potency of a chemical dose is expressed as a **lethal dose (LD_{50})**, the amount of material given all at once, which causes the death of 50% of those exposed. LD_{50} is one way to measure the short-term acute toxicity of potentially hazardous material. Many biological processes are considered **hormetic**, since the effects of a given acute dose may differ from the effects of an equal fractionated dose. For example, 100 mSv of radiation received over five years would be expected to have different effects than received once as an acute dose over a short period.

By comparison, the dose of microbiological hazards (pathogenic bacteria and viruses) is expressed as an **infectious dose**, the amount of pathogen (measured in the number of microorganisms) required to cause an infection in the host.[4]

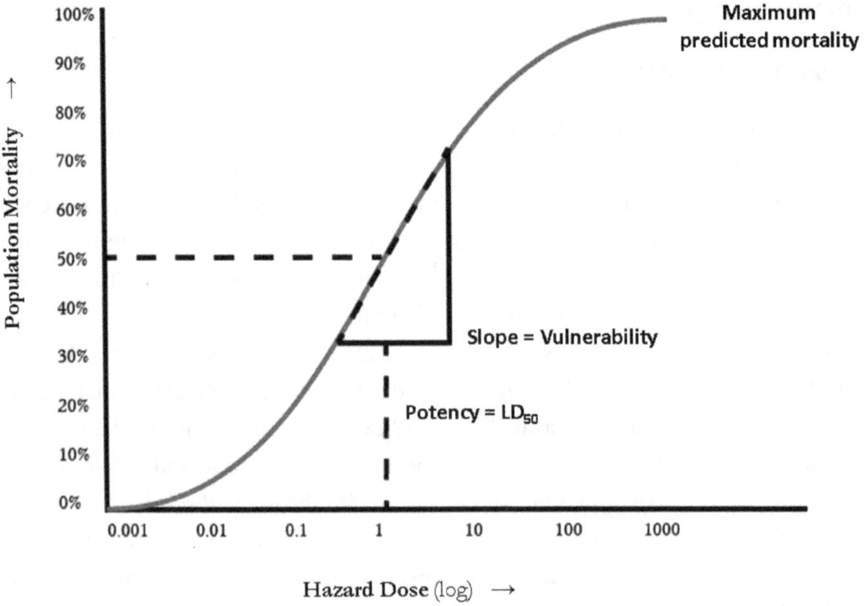

Figure 5-2. Example of the Logistic Function for a Disaster Hazard Dose-Response Curve

Dose-response assessments are used to study the relationship between the magnitude of a dose and a specific biological response (e.g., a health effect). Populations may also be exposed to a hazard without any adverse effect. Thus, the term *exposure* is not synonymous with the word *affected*.[9] The response can be expressed as a measured incidence or change in level or as the probability of a shift in incidence level within a population.

The dose-response curve is a graphic representation of the relationship between a dose and the proportion of subjects demonstrating specific biologically significant changes. (See Figure 5.2.)

The initial growth stage is approximately exponential (geometric); then, as saturation begins, the growth slows to linear (arithmetic), and at maturity growth stops.

Key parameters of the dose-response curve include the maximum expected effect after exposure (e.g., % of predicted mortality); the "rise" in mortality over the "run" in dose (i.e., population vulnerability to the hazard); and factors related to the relative "potency" of the hazard itself. In general, for disaster hazards, the risk of mortality and vulnerability begins relatively low and then at some point increases exponentially before plateauing at a maximum hazard dosage where predicted mortality reaches a maximum. Populations' vulnerability is decreased by protective actions that lessen the steepness of the dose-response curve—that is, that decrease the mortality per given dose. In general, healthy populations with access to resources, and thus with capacity for resilience, are less vulnerable to disaster-related health hazards. According to this function, the $\int(LD_{50})$ = maximum mortality/1+ $e^{\text{-Vulnerability } x \text{ (Exposure Dose} - LD_{50})}$.

Now let us consider the exposure dose for health hazards related to disasters. For example, in the case of high winds related to cyclones, tornadoes, and convective storms, increases at the low end of the dosage scale (e.g., sustained wind speed of 0–50 mph) are expected to have a minimal health impact. However, as wind speeds increase from 50 mph to 100 mph, some persons (those with higher vulnerability) may become adversely affected. By contrast, above 100 mph even small increases in wind speed may be expected to result in exponentially larger mortality rates among most persons exposed. And, at some point, a maximum degree of mortality will occur. Beyond this top level, even exponential increases in hazard dose do not result in additional deaths.

THE CAUSES AND EFFECTS OF HAZARDOUS EXPOSURES

Along with exposures as the proximate cause of disaster-related disease, distal causes of disaster-related disease (i.e., risk factors) in both directions also influence disaster-related health outcomes—both before and after exposure occurs. Those intermediate steps involve the mechanism of injury, exacerbation of chronic disease, or transmission of infections as the etiology of disease. Upstream determinants of health are considered components of a causal pathway of disease. Downstream determinants of health are regarded as components of the **natural history of disease**.

As the proximate cause of disaster-related disease, hazardous exposures initiate a change from wellness to illness. (See Figure 3-1.) Exposures may be considered a tipping point or the threshold event of an aggregate risk that has grown over time within the causal pathway. The causal pathway of disease considers the intermediate steps between the root cause (i.e., the hazard) and the etiology of the disease. At the same time, the natural history of a disease considers the intermediate steps between the etiology and the outcome of the disease.

TOPICS FOR DISCUSSION

1. Select one disaster hazard and describe the following terms related to that hazard:
   - Health hazards
   - Routes of exposure
   - The relationship between hazard dose and population mortality
   - Vulnerability
2. Compare the units for measuring a hazardous exposure dose related to
   - Liquids,
   - Gases,
   - Radiation, and
   - Viruses.

REFERENCES

1. Sherwin R. What is an adverse health effect? *Environ Health Perspect.* 1983;52:177–182.
2. Keim M. *Disaster Planning: A Practical Guide to Effective Health Outcomes.* Cambridge, UK: Cambridge University Press; 2021.
3. Frost WH. Some conceptions of epidemics in general. *Am J Epidemiol.* 1976;103(2):141–151.
4. World Health Organization; Food and Agriculture Organization of the United Nations. *Hazard Characterization for Pathogens in Food and Water: Guidelines.* Geneva, Switzerland: World Health Organization/United Nations FAO; 2003.
5. United Nations Office for Disaster Risk Reduction (UNDRR). *Sendai Framework for Disaster Reduction, 2015–2030.* New York, NY: United Nations; 2015.
6. Keim M. Environmental disasters. In: Frumkin H, ed. *Environmental Health: From Global to Local.* 3rd ed. San Francisco CA: Wiley & Sons; 2016.
7. World Health Organization (WHO). WHO international classification of diseases and related health problems. ICD-10. 2016. Available at: http://apps.who.int/classifications/icd10/browse/2016/en. Accessed November 27, 2022.
8. Environmental Protection Agency (EPA). Integrated Risk Information System (IRIS) glossary. 2017. Updated November 14, 2022. Available at: https://www.epa.gov/iris. Accessed November 27, 2022.
9. Center for Research on the Epidemiology of Disasters (CRED). EM-DAT: the OFDA/CRED international disaster database. 2009. Available at: www.emdat.be. Accessed November 27, 2022.
10. Keim ME. Environmental disaster. In: Frumkin H, ed. *Environmental Health: From Global to Local.* San Francisco, CA: Wiley & Sons; 2010:843–875.

6

Natural Disasters

LEARNING OBJECTIVES

Upon completion, the reader will be able to

1. Define the following terms and phrases:
    - Cold wave
    - Convective storm
    - Cyclone
    - Drought
    - Early warning system (EWS)
    - Earthquake
    - Effusive eruption
    - Endemic
    - Epidemic
    - Eruption cloud
    - Explosive eruption
    - Flood
    - Forest fire
    - Heat index
    - Heatwave
    - Hurricane
    - Lahar
    - Land fire
    - Landslide
    - Mass movement
    - Outbreak
    - Pandemic
    - Pyroclastic flow
    - Ring of Fire
    - Sediment flow
    - Slope failure
    - Storm surge
    - Subduction zone
    - Tectonic plate

- Tephra
- Tornado
- Tropical cyclone
- Tsunami
- Typhoon
- Volcanic eruption
- Wildfire
- Wildland
- Winter storm

2. Describe the following characteristics of individual natural disasters:
    - Causative hazard(s)
    - Speed of onset and duration
    - Consequences
    - Scale

NATURAL HAZARDS

Natural hazards are disaster-causing phenomena that originate in nature. These hazards cause various emergencies, disasters, and even catastrophes. They often result in loss of life, injury or other health impacts, property damage, loss of livelihoods and services, social and economic disruption, or environmental damage.[1]

This chapter defines individual natural disaster hazards and describes the primary causes of these phenomena and their timing, consequences, and scale.[1]

Cold Weather

Definition

Cold waves and winter storms cause cold weather disasters. **Cold waves** are weather phenomena distinguished by a rapid cooling of the air. Cold waves are characterized by the rate at which the temperature falls and its minimum. Winter storms are characterized by cold ambient temperatures accompanied by wind and precipitation.

Speed of Onset and Duration

A cold wave is a rapid fall in temperature within 24 hours.[2] It is measured in terms of the departure from average temperatures and exacerbated by windy conditions that create a wind chill effect. Most cold waves and winter storms occur throughout one-to-several days (usually associated with a warning), but their impacts are often felt for weeks and months afterward.

Consequences

The location of some cold wave disasters may at times appear somewhat counterintuitive. For example, cold waves have caused disaster-related deaths in places like Bangladesh, India; Mexico; and Egypt.[3] Cold waves have also been associated with the La Niña effect of lowering regional temperatures.

Like cold waves, winter storms are associated with low ambient temperatures. But winter storms can also immobilize an entire region, disrupting power, water, transportation, communications, health care, and even emergency services.[4]

Heavy accumulations of snow and ice can disrupt communications and power for days. This loss of power during winter commonly results in unheated homes that are more prone to water pipe ruptures, unsafe cooking and heating practices, and failure of telephone service. Winter storms such as blizzards can also disrupt air, ground, and sea transportation.

Scale

During the past 60 years, 381 cold weather disasters have been reported worldwide that caused an average of 73 deaths per incident. Of these cold weather disasters, 80% were associated with cold waves compared with winter storms.[3]

Cold waves typically involve large geographical areas. The geographical reach of winter storms is commonly less than that of cold waves. However, some storms (e.g., blizzards) can affect a large area. These events can affect entire geographical regions (e.g., North America) and involve multiple nations.

The Winter Storm Severity Index measures the potential impacts of winter storms on a 6-point scale in terms of wind, temperature, and precipitation.[5]

Cyclone

Definition

Storms include convective storms (i.e., thunderstorms and tornadoes) and cyclones. Cyclones are characterized by the storm's cyclonic rotation—a circular movement imparted by a planet's rotation.[2] A closed area of winds rotating in a circle is a cyclone. For Earth, the Coriolis effect causes cyclones to rotate in a counterclockwise direction in the Northern Hemisphere and clockwise in the Southern Hemisphere. Tropical cyclones are also called hurricanes, cyclones, and typhoons, depending on their geographical location. They are referred to as **hurricanes** in the North Atlantic, the Caribbean, the Gulf of Mexico, the eastern North Pacific, and the west coast of Mexico; as **typhoons** in the western Pacific; and as **cyclones** in the Indian Ocean and Australasia.[6]

Cyclones can occur in low, middle, and high latitudes. Tropical cyclones are low-pressure weather systems that develop over the warm waters of the oceans (typically between the latitudes of 30° N and 30° S).[2] Extratropical cyclones occur in middle and high latitudes.

Speed of Onset and Duration

Tropical cyclones typically affect individual populations throughout one-to-several days, depending on the magnitude and speed of the storm. Full recovery from large-scale, severe incidents can take years, even decades. Slow-moving storms associated with high precipitation tend to cause more inland flooding that can take weeks to resolve.

Consequences

Tropical cyclones create secondary hazards, including tornadoes, inland flooding, landslides, high wind conditions, and storm surge. Storm surge is a rise and onshore surge of seawater caused by high winds and the surface pressure drop near the storm center.[2] The surge's magnitude depends on the cyclone's size, intensity, and movement; the shape of the coastline, underwater topography; and the ocean tides.

Scale

During the past 60 years, there were 2,157 cyclone disasters reported worldwide that caused an average of 543 deaths per incident.[3]

Like winter storms, tropical cyclones can immobilize an entire region, disrupting power, water, transportation, communications, health care, and even emergency services.[7–9] One tropical cyclone can significantly affect millions of people.[3]

Cyclone severity is measured by the Saffir-Simpson scale that estimates potential property damage on a 5-point scale, according to wind velocity. While all tropical cyclones produce life-threatening winds, those rated Category 3 and higher are often called major storms. These storms can cause catastrophic wind damage and significant loss of life.

Drought

Definition

Drought is a period of abnormally dry weather sufficiently long enough to cause a serious hydrological imbalance.[2] Put simply, a drought is a period of drier-than-normal conditions that results in water-related problems.

Drought is relative to the local norm and may occur as a shortage of precipitation during the growing season resulting in crop damage. This is known as agricultural drought. Or it may occur during the winter runoff and percolation season, thereby affecting water supplies. This is known as hydrological drought.[2]

Speed of Onset and Duration

Droughts are slow-onset disasters that result from a long-term change in historically normal weather patterns. Droughts are common and of long duration, and the end of drought can occur as gradually as it began. A drought's exact beginning and end are notoriously difficult to determine and often require a specialized early warning system to identify.[10] Months or years can pass before people recognize that a drought is occurring. The effects of a drought on stream flow and reservoirs may not be recognized for weeks or months. Water levels in wells might not reflect a shortage of rainfall for a year or more after a drought begins.

Consequences

Counterintuitively, very few people suffer from thirst or dehydration during a drought, even in low-resource countries. Drought-related impacts are associated with poor governance, economic failure, food insecurity, substandard public health practices, unsafe water, migration, and social strife.[10,11] Accordingly, most drought-related morbidity and mortality occur in low-resource countries.

Drought-related impacts tend to be most severe in low-resource nations where food insecurity, poverty, conflict, poor public health practices, and the high burden of disease act synergistically to amplify health risks.[10,11] In low-resource countries, drought is often associated with displacement, epidemics, malnutrition, and conflict. In resource-rich nations, the impact of drought is primarily driven by economic stressors.[12] Besides increasing the likelihood of food insecurity and famine, a drought can have catastrophic effects on crop production, national economies, and individual livelihood.[12]

Scale

During the past 60 years, there were 727 drought disasters reported worldwide that caused an average of 38,126 deaths per incident.[3]

Droughts can be characteristically massive incidents, known to affect vast geographical areas and vast numbers of people. For example, in 2015, a single drought affected an estimated 330 million persons.[3]

Drought severity can be measured using the Palmer Drought Severity Index (PDSI). PDSI is calculated based on precipitation and temperature data, as well as the locally available water content of the soil.[13]

Earthquake

Definition

Earthquake is a term used to describe the radiated seismic energy and ground shaking caused by the sudden slip of a geological fault, volcanic activity, or other sudden stress changes in the earth.[14]

A fault is a fracture of the earth's crust along which separate blocks move relative to each other parallel to the fracture. A slip is the relative displacement of formerly adjacent points on opposite sides of a fault, measured on the fault surface.[14]

In addition to slips, earthquakes can result from volcanic eruptions or the subterranean movement of magma. Small human-generated earthquakes have also been reported to be caused by massive explosions, the release of a large body of water striking a dam, and underground injection associated with fracking.[15]

Most earthquake disasters occur along the boundaries of tectonic plates that actively move against each other to create, capture, and release seismic energy. (See Figure 6-1.) The majority of the world's earthquakes occur along the Pacific plate. The plate has been called the **Ring of Fire** because of the frequent seismic and volcanic activity along its boundary.

A significant exception is a border between the Pacific and North American plates. In this area, plates do not subduct but rather move sideways past each other. This type of boundary generates earthquakes as tension in the earth's crust builds up and is released.

Most of the world's earthquakes, volcanic eruptions, and tsunamis originate along the boundary of the Pacific plate. A similar band of relatively high seismic activity, known as

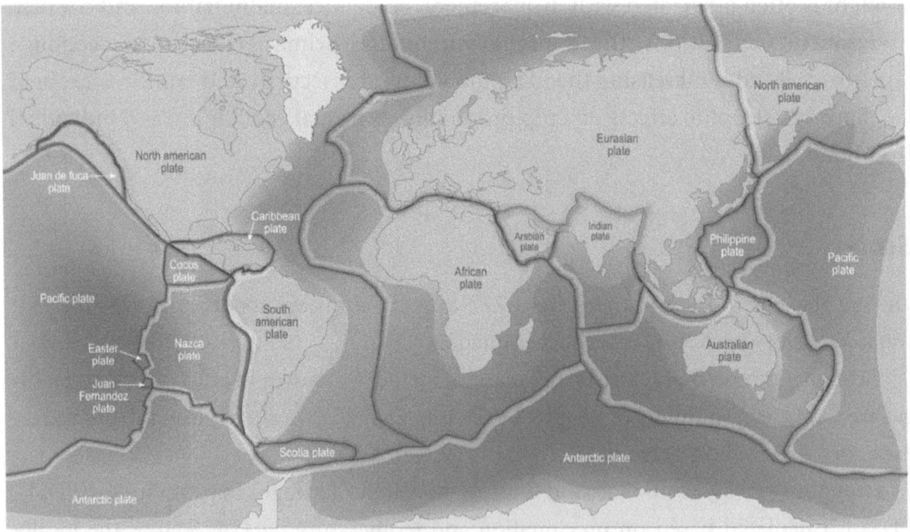

Figure 6-1. Tectonic Plates of the Earth's Crust

the Belt of Fire, is located in the Mediterranean region of the northern African plate.[15] Along these areas plates overlap at convergent boundaries called subduction zones. Earthquakes occur when these boundaries suddenly slip against each other. That is, one tectonic plate is pushed down (i.e., subducted) by another above. As rock is further subducted, it also melts and becomes magma, giving rise to volcanoes.

Speed of Onset and Duration

Earthquakes are the quintessential rapid-onset disaster that often occurs with little or no warning. Strong ground shaking typically lasts less than a minute. Readjustments after a fault slip cause aftershocks that can occur intermittently for weeks or months.

Consequences

Earthquakes represent one of the most violent natural disasters in terms of the severity and scale of destruction. Earthquakes can result in very severe and widespread damage to the built environment and critical infrastructure of affected populations. This critical infrastructure often includes extensive damage to crucial systems like communications, transportation, energy, commerce, and health care.

Earthquakes typically cause many injuries and extensive population displacement (and its associated loss of shelter, water, food, sanitation, hygiene, and personal safety). Earthquakes disrupt ground transportation, damage airports, and render significant transportation routes (e.g., roads, rail, subways, ports) impassable. Earthquakes also create secondary disaster hazards like fires and explosions, hazardous material releases, and landslides. One of the deadliest secondary disasters associated with an earthquake is the tsunami generated by a submarine earthquake.

Scale

During the past 60 years, there were 1,153 earthquake disasters reported worldwide that caused an average of 1,362 deaths per incident.[3]

Earthquakes can immobilize an entire city or region, disrupting finance, power, water, commerce, transportation, communications, health care, and even emergency services. The 2008 Sichuan earthquake, for example, is estimated to have affected 46 million people.[3]

There are multiple scales available to measure earthquake activity. Earthquake severity is often reported according to two scales. The Modified Mercalli Intensity (MMI) scale is a 12-point seismic scale used to estimate potential damage. It does not have a mathematical basis; instead, it is a ranking based on observed effects. Compared with measuring the effects of the earthquake, the Richter scale is logarithmic and represents the total amount of energy released by the earthquake.[16] Thus, while the Mercalli scale describes the intensity of an earthquake based on its observed effects, the 10-point Richter scale describes the earthquake's overall magnitude by measuring the seismic waves that cause the earthquake. The two scales have different applications and measurement techniques.

Epidemic

Definition

Biological hazards include those organisms that cause infectious diseases (e.g., bacteria, viruses, and fungi) and pests that cause infestations. Compared to other categories of disaster hazards, infectious disease is transmissible and, therefore, communicable from person to person.

Epidemics are increases in disease that often occur suddenly, with an increase above what is generally expected in that population in that area. The amount of a particular disease that is usually present (or expected) in a community is referred to as the endemic level of the disease.[16] *Endemic* refers to the constant presence and/or usual prevalence of a disease or infectious agent in a population within a geographic area. Outbreak carries the same definition of the epidemic but is often used for a more limited geographic area.[17] Finally, a **pandemic** is an epidemic spread over several countries or continents, affecting many people.[17] This book focuses on infectious disease disasters, specifically those historically associated with epidemics. This selection is both a pragmatic and normative one. Pragmatically, global disaster data is not yet specific enough to accurately differentiate between outbreaks and epidemics. In a normative sense (like armed conflict), pandemics represent a relatively unique set of social, technological, economic, environmental, and political circumstances that are better understood as a highly specialized disaster incident unto itself. And while many elements of pandemics are the same as epidemics, key differences warrant a separate discussion elsewhere.

Not all infectious disease has the potential to create an epidemic. Some pathogens have characteristics related to their route of exposure, ease of transmissibility, and virulence that increase the likelihood of increases in disease that often occur suddenly. During the past 60 years, epidemic disasters have reportedly involved less than 80 individual diseases and syndromes (many of which are likely referring to the same disease).[3]

Speed of Onset and Duration

Once exposed to an infectious disease pathogen, the incubation period frequently occurs within several days to several weeks. However, some infections may be more rapid or delayed in onset. The duration of an individual case of epidemic-related illness is usually measured in days to weeks. However, epidemics often last for months or years as transmission continues among the affected population.

Consequences

Epidemics are typically associated with large numbers of patient cases and deaths. This sudden increase in disease is often associated with a mismatch of acute needs and resources when health care systems become overwhelmed by the volume of patients. Besides causing overutilization of health care resources, epidemics can also have a significant economic impact involving international transportation, trade, and commerce. The impact on other critical infrastructure in the built environment is usually negligible. However, massive population displacements have been reported in association with epidemics, including that of over one-half million persons during an epidemic of bubonic plague in 1994.[3,18]

Scale

During the past 60 years, there were 1,467 epidemic disasters reported worldwide that caused an average of 429 deaths per incident.[3]

Epidemic disasters also vary widely in scale. Mismatches of needs and resources that result in an epidemic disaster depend on the sheer number of patients, the severity of illness, and the effectiveness of countermeasures. In 2017 the World Health Organization developed a tool to prioritize research and development for epidemic-prone diseases.[19] The intent was to identify those diseases that pose a public health risk because of their epidemic potential *and* for which there are insufficient countermeasures.[19] This list contains only viruses—one respiratory, five transmitted by direct contact, and one vectorborne.[20]

There is no standard scale or index for measuring the severity of an epidemic. A novel pandemic severity assessment framework has been proposed. The framework integrates a 7-point scale for clinical severity and a 5-point scale for viral transmissibility into one estimate.[21]

Flood

Definition

Floods are the "overflowing of the normal confines of a stream or other body of water or the accumulation of water over areas that are not normally submerged."[2]

Speed of Onset and Duration

Riverine (i.e., fluvial) flooding can occur as seasonal or flash floods.[22] Seasonal floods are typified by a gradual rise to the flood stage that may extend across large areas over a long duration. Because a relatively gradual accumulation usually causes seasonal floods, warning times are generally sufficient to allow the safe evacuation of nearby communities.

Flash floods are characterized by a short-duration, high-volume stream flow and usually occur within six hours of a rain event, after a dam or levy fails, or after the sudden release of water from an ice or debris jam. A brief warning and response time accompany them with the potential for a significant loss of life.[23]

Consequences

Floods have the potential to affect vast numbers of people. They are also relatively common as compared with other disaster hazards. Floods can result in very severe damage to critical infrastructure (e.g., water, power, hospitals). If the affected area is expansive enough, it can also disrupt major societal systems like communications, transportation, energy, commerce, and health care. The global consequence of floods is, therefore, enormous and widespread.

Floods typically cause a relatively low level of injuries but result in massive population displacement (along with an associated loss of shelter, water, food, sanitation, hygiene, and personal safety). Floods may also create secondary hazards like toxic mold, fires, hazardous material releases, and food insecurity. The number of deaths associated with flooding is closely related to the life-threatening characteristics of the flood (rapidly rising water, deep floodwaters, objects carried by the rapidly flowing water) and the victims' behavior.[22]

Floods' long duration and chronic nature are detrimental to mental health and wellness. The long-term effects of flooding on psychological health and chronic disease may be even more significant than on other illnesses or injuries. For many people, the emotional trauma continues long after the water has receded.[22]

Scale

Floods can be notoriously large in scale. For example, during 1961–2020, China's top five most-significant floods affected nearly 900 million people, averaging 180 million per event.[3] By comparison, the largest US flood during that same period occurred in eastern Iowa and affected 11 million.[3]

Heat Wave

Definition

A **heat wave** is a period of abnormally hot and humid weather.[2] Like cold waves, heat waves are relative to the local norm. Heat waves, therefore, represent a significant departure from normal seasonal temperatures. The comfort criteria for heat waves in any region depend on acclimation to the usual conditions.

Speed of Onset and Duration

A heat wave as such should last at least one day, but conventionally it lasts from several days to several weeks.[2] Heat waves are typically seasonal, with most incidents occurring during summer.

Consequences

Heat waves are known to cause extensive impacts on human morbidity and mortality while leaving infrastructure largely undamaged. Besides causing overutilization of health care resources, heat waves can also result in power outages that further exacerbate heat illness by disrupting cooling and ventilation. Power shortages can also affect transportation, communication, and health care systems. Heat waves can expose outdoor workers to extreme heat when working in hot environments, especially putting those in tropical low-middle-income countries at increased risk.[24] Heat waves have also been associated with secondary disasters, including air pollution and wildfires.[3,25]

Scale

During the past 60 years, 209 heat wave disasters were reported worldwide that caused an average of 804 deaths per incident.[3] Heat waves can affect an entire city or even a region. In 2003 one incident resulted in tens of thousands of excess deaths throughout Italy, France, Spain, and Germany. In 2010 one heat wave affected millions of persons throughout western Russia, including Moscow.

Several scales have been offered to describe the severity of heat waves. The heat index (i.e., apparent temperature) is widely used. It approximates how hot it "feels" for ambient air temperature and relative humidity. Simply put, relative humidity measures the water vapor in the air. Generally, higher values at the same temperature feel warmer and more stressful because of less evaporative cooling when people perspire.[2]

An excess heat factor, commonly referred to as an EHF, has been proposed as an index for relating heat wave intensity and severity. The factor is based on a three-day-averaged daily mean temperature.[26]

Landslide

Definition

Mass movement (also called mass wasting) is the down-slope movement of loose soil and rock particles resulting from the force of gravity. Mass movements are part of a continuum of erosional processes between long-term weathering and short-term stream transport and occur continuously on all slopes. Some mass movements act very slowly, and others occur very suddenly.[27]

The abrupt down-slope movement of bedrock, loose soil, and rock particles is called a **landslide**. Landslides include two general categories: slope failures and sediment flows. Slope failures are sudden failures of a slope resulting in the transport of debris downhill by sliding, rolling, falling, or slumping. Sediment flows involve materials that flow downhill when mixed with water or air.[27]

Speed of Onset and Duration

Slope failures involving falls and slides (of rock, soil, or debris) occur suddenly and travel at a very high velocity, some exceeding speeds of 250 miles (400 km) per hour. (See Table 6-1.)

The velocity of mud and grain flows typically range from one-half mile (~1 km) to 60 miles (~100 km) per hour. Avalanches and streams can also travel very fast, exceeding 60 miles (~100 km) an hour. By comparison, earth flows and debris flow often move at less than one-half mile (1 km) per hour, while solifluction and creep travel less than one inch (2 cm) each year. In summary, slope failures have the same velocity as a high-speed train. Avalanches and streams can travel as fast as a car, and earth and debris flows can travel as fast as a bicycle. Creep and solifluction move slower than a snail.

Falls, slides, and slumps are various forms of slope failure that differ according to steepness.

Avalanches are masses of snow, ice, and rocks. The earth flows are mainly composed of sand, gravel, and stones. Mudflows, by comparison, contain water, and debris flows include trees, cars, small buildings, and other anthropogenic material.[28]

Consequences

Landslide disasters are relatively violent events associated with a high degree of destruction that is relatively focal in location. Landslides can severely damage critical infrastructure (e.g., water, power, and hospital facilities). However, this destruction is rarely expansive enough to intensively disrupt major societal systems like communications, transportation, energy, commerce, and health care.

Table 6-1. Composition and Velocity of Mass Movements (i.e., Landslides)

↑ Increasing velocity	Slope Failure	Granular Flows	Slurry Flows	Comparative Speed
	Falls	Avalanche	Streams	High-speed rail
	Slides	Grain flow	Mudflow	Automobile
	Slumps	Earth flow	Debris flow	Bicycle
	Creep		Solifluction	Snail

Increasing % of water →

Landslides typically cause injuries along with population displacement and the loss of shelter, water, food, sanitation, hygiene, and personal safety. Landslides also create secondary disaster hazards like fires and explosions, hazardous material releases, and floods.

Scale

During the past 60 years, there were 769 landslide disasters reported worldwide that caused an average of 68 deaths per incident.[3]

Most individual landslide incidents are well localized; however, it is typical for multiple scattered debris flows to occur after heavy rains on steep terrain, given certain geological conditions. In one example, more than 250 landslides were triggered in the Federated States of Micronesia by rainfall from one tropical storm. Slumps and debris flow created during nearly 20 inches of rain in less than 24 hours caused 43 fatalities and the destruction or damage of 231 structures, including homes, schools, community centers, and medical dispensaries. Most failures began as slumps and transformed into debris flows, some traveling several hundred meters across coastal flatlands into populated areas.[29–31]

Many of these seasonal events create a recurrent risk associated with the wet season. The world's largest landslide disaster during the past century affected four million people.[3]

The destructiveness is measured regarding landslide intensity and related to the type of landslide, its propagation mechanism, and volume. This landslide intensity index is then used as an input for potential loss calculation.[32]

Tornadoes and Convective Storms

Definition

Storms are disturbed states of the earth's atmosphere, manifesting as temperature, humidity, pressure, wind velocity, cloud cover, lightning, and precipitation.[2]

A **tornado** is a rapidly rotating column of air extending vertically from the surface to the base of a cloud, often with a near-surface circulating debris/dust when over land or spray when over water. A funnel cloud is often (but not always) visible and may partly or wholly extend from the cloud base to the ground.[2]

Convective movement (i.e., warmer parts moving up and cooler parts moving down) in the atmosphere is also known to create **convective storms** (i.e., thunderstorms). Convective storms are generally accompanied by lightning and thunder, usually with strong gusts of wind, heavy rain, and sometimes with hail. Thunderstorm severity is measured according to (1) the nature of the lightning and thunder, (2) the type and intensity of the precipitation, (3) the speed of gusts and sustained winds, (4) the cloud appearance, and (5) the effect on surface temperature.[2]

Speed of Onset and Duration

Whereas convective storms commonly develop over hours, tornadoes are acute onset disasters that develop within a few minutes and limit advance warning effectiveness. Both types of storms most commonly occur within a relatively short period, seldom exceeding several hours in duration. Slow-moving storms associated with high precipitation tend to cause more inland flooding that can take weeks to resolve. Full recovery from localized, severe wind damage can take months to years.

Consequences

Convective storms create secondary hazards, including lightning, wildfires, inland flooding, landslides, and high wind conditions. Along with more limited warning times, the higher wind speeds of tornadoes often result in a destructive swath with multiple injuries. These incidents typically result in a relatively low number of injuries, as well as localized population displacement, and its associated loss of shelter, water, food, sanitation, hygiene, and personal safety.

Scale

During the past 60 years, there were 1,956 storm-related disasters reported worldwide that caused an average of 29 deaths per incident.[3]

Storms range in size from meters to a few kilometers (e.g., tornadoes), to a few-to-several-hundred kilometers (convective systems), and many hundreds of kilometers (extratropical cyclones).

Tornado severity is measured according to wind speeds using a standard index known as the Enhanced Fujita scale. This scale is based on estimated wind speeds and related damage (taking into consideration how most structures are designed).[33]

Tsunami

Definition

The Japanese word *tsunami* translates in English to "harbor wave." A **tsunami** is a series of ocean waves generated by any disturbance that displaces a large water mass.[34] About 90%–95% of tsunamis are caused by large earthquakes (usually Richter magnitude 6.5 or greater); the remainder is primarily the result of volcanic eruptions (e.g., the 1883 eruption of Mount Krakatoa) or landslides (e.g., the 1998 Papua New Guinea tsunami generated by a submarine landslide).[34] There are also composite events, such as the 1946 subduction earthquake in the Aleutian Islands that triggered a landslide-generated tsunami killing 159 in Hawai'i.[35] Prehistoric geological evidence has implicated meteorites or comet impacts as a rare cause of tsunamis.[36,37]

Subduction zones are faults in the earth's crust where one tectonic plate overrides another. Subduction movement along this fault typically produces the vertical land movement necessary to generate a tsunami. In addition, the original earthquake must occur at relatively shallow depths (<31 mi or 50 km) underground to efficiently transfer ground energy to the water above. Subduction earthquakes can impart a vertical displacement on the earth's surface that is hundreds of miles long and displace billions of tons of water. Earthquakes that produce essentially horizontal movement do not typically generate tsunamis.[37]

Tsunamis have occurred in all the oceans. About 90%–95% of the world's tsunamis have occurred in the Pacific Ocean because of its relatively large size and bordering the Ring of Fire, which comprises major tectonic subduction fault zones. Transpacific tsunamis are caused by earthquakes located at these subduction zones and occur about once a decade.[38]

Transocean tsunamis are typically caused by large earthquakes whose ruptures extend hundreds of kilometers. These tsunamis spread outward in all directions from the point of origin.[39] By comparison, tsunamis triggered by submarine landslides produce a relatively narrow radiation pattern, resulting in a focused beam of energy that could also reach far afield.[35]

Speed of Onset and Duration

Once generated, tsunami speed depends on the depth of the ocean. In the deep ocean, a tsunami can move as fast as a jet plane, over 500 mph (~800 kph), and the wavelength (distance from crest to crest) may be hundreds of miles.[40]

The energy of a tsunamis is spread throughout such a large volume in deep water and has such a long wavelength between crests that tsunamis may be only a few feet (<1 m) high in mid-ocean, making them capable of passing under ocean-going ships with little disturbance or detection. The physical dynamics of the fluid pressure wave also allow it to travel great distances with very little energy loss.[41]

The effect of water depth on wave speed causes individual waves to slow down as they approach shallow water. This creates higher waves and faster currents as the tsunami reach land.[42]

The last stage is inundation, in which a tsunami may run ashore. As a tsunami enters shallow water near coastal shorelines, it slows to 20 to 30 mph (~30–50 kph). Vertical run-up typically takes two to three meters to cause damage along the shoreline. Horizontal inundation, if unchecked by typography, can penetrate up to 10 miles (16 km) inland.[43]

As the tsunami enters shallow water near coastlines, the kinetic energy previously spread throughout the large volume of deep ocean water becomes concentrated in much smaller water, resulting in a tremendous destructive potential as it inundates the land.

Successive crests may arrive at the shore at period intervals of every 10–45 minutes. A single tsunami event may comprise up to 12 wave crests.[42] Before inundation of the wave crest, the sea often appears to recede for an unusually far distance.

Consequences

Tsunamis are highly destructive hazards that cause general and severe damage. The effects of tsunamis on coastal areas are characterized by a maximum destructive force occurring near the water's edge. Low-lying coastal regions, peninsulas, and coral atolls have also increased the destruction's severity. Damage farther inland is also potentially severe even though the force of the wave is diminished as floating debris then batters the inland structures.

Scale

During the past 60 years, there were 42 tsunami disasters reported worldwide that caused an average of 6,254 deaths per incident.[3]

A novel tsunami intensity scale has been proposed. This new 12-point tsunami intensity scale aligns with the 12-grade (Modified Mercalli) seismic intensity scale. The new scale measures tsunami intensity based on its effects on humans, nature, and the built environment, including vessels of variable size, buildings, and other engineered constructions.[44]

Volcanic Eruption

Definition

Volcanoes are openings or vents where molten rock, gases, small rocks, and steam erupt onto the earth's surface.[45] Molten rock beneath the surface of the earth is called magma. Magma that has erupted to the surface of the earth and maintains its integrity as a fluid mass is called lava. The gases and ash emitted during an eruption are referred to as tephra. Sometimes, a very hot (typically 1500°F / 800°C) mixture of rock, gas, and ash "travels rapidly (tens of meters per second) away from a volcanic vent or collapsing flow front."[45]

Like avalanches and stream flows, pyroclastic flows can also travel very fast, exceeding 60 miles (~100 km) an hour.

Volcanic eruptions can be effusive or explosive.[46,47] Effusive eruptions characteristically pour out lava flows and build broad lava domes. For an effusive eruption, magma must be porous enough to expel gas bubbles. If the magma cannot off-gas, it will erupt explosively. Explosive eruptions are characterized by violent magma fragmentation as it reaches the earth's surface. These eruptions produce mainly ash, pumice, and fragmental ballistic debris (unlike an effusive eruption). Mixtures of water (e.g., molten snow, rainfall, or a crater lake) and volcanic debris that move rapidly downhill are called lahars.[47,48]

Like mudflows, the velocity of a lahar is highly variable according to the topography and can range from one-half mile (~1 km) to 60 miles (~100 km) per hour. However, lahars have also been frequently described as traveling farther than typical mudflows.

Explosive eruptions create an "eruption column, the ascending, vertical part of the mass of erupting debris and volcanic gas that rises directly above a volcanic vent." An eruption cloud contains tephra and gases that travel downwind of an erupting volcano.[47]

Speed of Onset and Duration

The onset of a volcanic eruption can vary remarkably from minutes to days. The rate of eruption can also influence how explosive an eruption is. If magma ascends slowly from deep within the crust, the dissolved gases can escape nonviolently over time. But when the eruption rate is rapid, the dissolved gases escape all at once, like an opened carbonated beverage, and the eruption is more explosive. Most explosive eruptions occur as an acute onset event with a recognizable warning possible when earthquake swarms known to occur as underground magma become more active and eruptive.

Once at the surface, effusive lava moves on level ground at a relatively slow speed (~800 ft/250 m) per hour. However, lava may travel as fast as 30 mph (~50 kph) on steep slopes.[45]

Volcanic eruptions can last a few days, months, or even years. Mount Stromboli, off the coast of Italy, has been undergoing continuous volcanic eruptions since at least the seventh century BC.[45]

Consequences

Explosive eruptions are responsible for most volcano disasters. This impact not only includes a direct effect on health but also can involve disruption of commerce, transportation, and agriculture.[47]

Effusive eruptions often result in relatively well-localized population displacement due to environmental hazards like lava encroachment, fires, and air contaminants. By comparison, explosive eruptions are often associated with a range of potential secondary disaster hazards, including lava flows, pyroclastic flows, lahars and floods, blasts and projectiles, earthquakes and tsunamis, tephra fallout, acid rain, and gas emissions.[47] Most of the kinetic consequences of explosive eruptions are relatively well localized compared with other natural disasters. The geographical area affected by lava, pyroclastic flows, blasts, projectiles, and gas emissions is most often located near the volcano.

However, lahars are known to travel long distances from the volcano to affect populations that would otherwise not consider the proximity of such a hazard.[47]

The reach of toxic tephra fallout and acid rain is even more extensive, enabling tephra and acid rain to contaminate air, water sources, and agriculture for long distances downwind. It is common for such emissions to extend far across multiple international borders, affecting navigation, transportation, and commerce. Extensive tephra fallout also frequently results in large population displacements.

Scale

During the past 60 years, there were 225 volcano disasters reported worldwide that caused an average of 474 deaths per incident.[3]

Volcanic eruptions are most common near boundaries of the earth's tectonic plates, where subduction zones create pressure capable of melting rock and producing magma. Notably, 75% of the world's volcanoes are located along the so-called Ring of Fire surrounding the Pacific tectonic plate.[3]

Like landslides, volcanic eruptions are relatively violent events associated with a high degree of destruction that is pretty localized. However, some impacts of volcanoes (e.g., tephra fallout) also have the potential to extend well beyond national boundaries and affect an entire region.

The Volcanic Explosivity Index (VEI) is a scale that describes the size of explosive volcanic eruptions based on magnitude and intensity. The 8-point scale is generally analogous to the Richter and other logarithmic scales.[49]

Wildfire

Definition

Wildfire is defined as an "unplanned fire burning in natural (wildland) areas such as forests, shrub lands, grasslands, or prairies" and peatland.[50,51] This contrasts with the practice of planned or prescribed fires. During the past 60 years, forest fires accounted for two-thirds (67%) of wildfires and were 2.5 times more common than land fires (27%).[3]

Speed of Onset and Duration

Depending on environmental conditions, wildfires can start within hours and spread rapidly within a day. Depending on the location and resources available, it is possible to contain most wildfires within one week in the United States. However, wildfires can also burn for weeks or months. The largest wildfire in world history also had the most prolonged duration. One single fire in 1950 burned approximately three million acres (1.2 million ha) of forest and lasted for five months.[3]

Consequences

Wildfires often pose a characteristic logistical challenge related to the wilderness in which they occur. Wildlands are areas where development is essentially nonexistent (except for roads, railroads, power lines, and similar transportation facilities).

Because of the relative isolation and lack of infrastructure in wildlands, wildfires that result in evacuations do not typically result in the long-term displacement of large populations. During the past 60 years, 1% of persons affected by wildfires were also reported homeless.[3] However, some populations and locations are at higher risk of being trapped by wildfire. Forest fires occurring near highly populated cities are also of concern, since they add to the impacts of high urban pollution levels and can also affect navigation and transportation.

Scale

During the past 60 years, there were 445 wildfire disasters reported worldwide that caused an average of 15 deaths per incident.[3]

The geographical scale of the individual fire is often dwarfed by the extent of air pollution created by wildfire smoke. The adverse effect on air quality can have an enormous impact, extending throughout an entire world region. The term *South Asia haze* has been coined to describe the fire-related transboundary air pollution that recurrently results from burning biomass. First reported in the 1970s, this phenomenon has affected Indonesia, Malaysia, Singapore, Thailand, and Brunei. It has also been reported to affect the Philippines, Thailand, Vietnam, Cambodia, and countries outside the region.[51]

A widely used measure of fire intensity is known as fireline intensity, which is the rate of heat transfer per length of fire line. This measure represents the radiant energy release in the flaming front.[52]

Fireline intensity measures how likely a given fire is to start and how difficult it will be to stop. Fire severity measurements can vary depending on the local environment. Fire severity is often measured according to tree mortality, canopy loss, or bole and crown scorch. These measures are often interpreted as a proxy for fire intensity. Fire severity measures for forests are not applicable to grass, shrub, and peatlands.[52]

TOPICS FOR DISCUSSION

1. The World Bank said there are no natural disasters because disasters are not natural. Discuss the dual meaning of the English word *natural* and how the meanings apply here.
2. Provide an example of a natural disaster and then answer the following questions:
   - How does a natural disaster differ from a technological one?
   - In what ways are they the same?

REFERENCES

1. United Nations Office for Disaster Risk Reduction (UNDRR). Terminology on disaster risk reduction. 2022. Available at: https://www.undrr.org/terminology. Accessed November 27, 2022.
2. American Society of Meteorology. Glossary of meteorology. 2020. Available at: https://glossary.ametsoc.org/wiki/Welcome. Accessed November 27, 2022.
3. Center for Research on the Epidemiology of Disasters (CRED). EM-DAT: the international disaster database. 2022; Available at: www.emdat.be. Accessed November 27, 20222.
4. National Weather Service. The varying types of winter weather. 2020. Available at: https://www.weather.gov/rlx/wintvar. Accessed November 27, 2022.
5. Weather Prediction Center. Winter Storm Severity Index. 2022. Available at: https://www.wpc.ncep.noaa.gov/wwd/wssi/wssi.php. Accessed November 27, 2022.
6. Keim M. Cyclones, tsunamis, and human health: the key role of preparedness. *Oceanography*. 2006;19(2):40–49.
7. Doocy S, Dick A, Daniels A, Kirsch T. The human impact of tropical cyclones: a historical review of events 1980–2009 and systematic literature review. *PLoS Curr*. 2013;5.
8. Mosley L, Sharp D, Singh S. Effects of a tropical cyclone on the drinking-water quality of a remote Pacific island. *Disasters*. 2004;28(4):405–417.
9. Fussell E, Lowe S. The impact of housing displacement on the mental health of low-income parents after Hurricane Katrina. *Soc Sci Med*. 2014;113:137–144.
10. Stanke C, Kerac M, Prudhomme C, Medlock J, Murray V. Health effects of drought: a systematic review of the evidence. *PLoS Curr*. 2013;5.
11. Davis L. Famines and droughts. In: *Natural Disasters*. New York, NY: Checkmark Books; 2008:105–136.
12. Wilhite D. *Drought Mitigation Technologies in the United States: With Future Policy Recommendations*. Lincoln, NE: International Drought Information Center; 1993.
13. Environmental Protection Agency (EPA). Climate change indicators: drought 2020. Available at: https://www.epa.gov/climate-indicators/climate-change-indicators-drought. Accessed November 27, 2022.
14. US Geological Survey (USGS). Earthquake Hazards Program. 2022. Available at: https://www.usgs.gov/glossary/earthquake-hazards-program#E. Accessed December 17, 2022.
15. Keim M. Environmental disasters. In: Frumkin H, ed. *Environmental Health: From Global to Local*. San Francisco, CA: Wiley & Sons; 2010:843–875.
16. Bayram J, Zuabi S, McCord C, Sherak R, Hsu E, Kelen G. Disaster metrics: evaluation of de Boer's Disaster Severity Scale (DSS) applied to earthquakes. *Prehosp Disaster Med*. 2015;30(1):22–27.
17. Centers for Disease Control and Prevention (CDC). Epidemic disease occurrence. Lesson 1: introduction to epidemiology. 2022. Archived. Available at: https://www.cdc.gov/csels/dsepd/ss1978/lesson1/section11.html. Accessed November 28, 2022.
18. Garrett L. *Betrayal of Trust*. New York, NY: Hyperion; 2000.
19. World Health Organization (WHO). *The R&D Blueprint for Action to Prevent Epidemics*. Geneva, Switzerland: World Health Organization; 2017.

20. World Health Organization (WHO). Top epidemic prone diseases without sufficient counter-measures. 2018. Available at: https://www.preventionweb.net/news/top-epidemic-prone-diseases-without-sufficient-counter-measures. Accessed November 28, 2022.
21. Reed C, Biggerstaff M, Finelli L, et al. Novel framework for assessing epidemiologic effects of influenza epidemics and pandemics. *Emerg Infect Dis*. 2013;19(1):85–91.
22. Keim M. Floods. In: Koenig K, Schultz C, eds. *Disaster Medicine: Comprehensive Principles and Practices*. New York, NY: Cambridge University Press; 2010:529–542.
23. Schmidt W, Skala M, Donelon I, Donnell H. Morbidity surveillance following the Midwest flood—Missouri, 1993. *MMWR*. 1993;42:797–798.
24. Xiang J, Bi P. Health impacts of workplace heat exposure: an epidemiological review. *Ind Health*. 2014;52(2):91–101.
25. Arbuthnott K, Hajat S. The health effects of hotter summers and heat waves in the population of the United Kingdom: a review of the evidence. *Environ Health*. 2017;16:119.
26. Nairn J, Fawcett R. The excess heat factor: a metric for heatwave intensity and its use in classifying heatwave severity. *Int J Environ Res Public Health*. 2014;12(1):227–53.
27. Nelson S. *Mass Movements*. New Orleans, LA: Tulane University; 2015.
28. Varnes D. *Slope Movement Types and Processes*. Transportation Research Board Special Report 176. 1978.
29. Harp E, Reid M, Michael J. *Hazard Analysis of Landslides Triggered by Typhoon Chataĺan on July 2, 2002, in Chuuk State, Federated States of Micronesia*. Washington, DC: US Geological Survey; 2004.
30. Sanchez C, Lee T, Young S, Batts D, Benjamin J, Malilay J. Risk factors for mortality during the 2002 landslides in Chuuk, Federated States of Micronesia. *Disasters*. 2009;33(4):705–720.
31. UN Office for the Coordination of Humanitarian Affairs (OCHA). *Tropical Storm Chata'an, Federated States of Micronesia*. New York, NY: United Nations; July 16 2004.
32. Lorenzo S, Bianchinib S, Franceschinib R, et al. Satellite interferometric data for landslide intensity evaluation in mountainous regions. *Int J Appl Earth Observ Geoinf*. 2020;87.
33. National Weather Service. *The Enhance Fujita (EF) Scale*. Norman, OK: National Oceanic and Atmospheric Administration; 2022.
34. Boyarsky I, Shneiderman A. Natural and hybrid disasters: causes, effects and management. *Top Emerg Med*. 2002;24(3):1–25.
35. Fryer G, Watts P, Lincoln F. Source of the great tsunami of 1 April 1946: a landslide in the upper Aleutian forearc. *Marine Geol*. 2004;203(3–4):201–218.
36. McMurtry G, Watts P, Fryer G, Smith J, Imamura F. Giant landslides, mega-tsunamis and paleo-sea level in the Hawaiian Islands. *Marine Geol*. 2004;203:219–233.
37. Bolt BA. *Earthquakes: A Primer*. San Francisco, CA: WH Freeman and Company; 1978.
38. McCarty D. Tsunamis. In: Hogan D, Burstein J, eds. *Disaster Medicine*. Philadelphia, PA: Lippincott William and Wilkins; 2002:229–234.
39. Perez E, Thompson P. Natural hazards causes and effects. *Prehosp Disaster Med*. 2005;10(1): 66–70.
40. National Oceanic and Atmospheric Administration (NOAA). Tsunamis. Resource collections. 2018. Available at: https://www.noaa.gov/education/resource-collections/ocean-coasts/tsunamis. Accessed November 28, 2022.

41. Keim M. The public health impact of tsunami disasters. *Am J Disaster Med.* 2011;6(6): 341–349.
42. González FI. Tsunami. *Sci Am.* 1999;280(5):57–65.
43. Guha-Sapir D, van Panhuis W. *The Andaman Nicobar Earthquake and Tsunami, 2004: Impact on Diseases in Indonesia.* Brussels, Belgium: Centre for Research on the Epidemiology of Disasters; 2005.
44. Papadopoulos G, Imamura F. A proposal for a new tsunami intensity scale. Paper presented at: 20th International Tsunami Conference; 2001; Seattle, WA.
45. US Geological Survey (USGS). About volcanoes. 2022. Available at: https://www.usgs.gov/programs/VHP/about-volcanoes. Accessed November 28, 2022.
46. Doocy S, Daniels A, Dooling S, Gorokhovich Y. The human impact of volcanoes: a historical review of events 1900–2009 and systematic literature review. *PLoS Curr.* 2013;5.
47. Baxter P. Volcanoes. In: Noji E, ed. *Public Health Consequences of Disasters.* New York, NY: Oxford Univerisity Press; 1997:179–205.
48. Noji E. Public Health Issues in Disasters. *Crit Care Med.* 2005;33(suppl 1):29–33.
49. National Park Service. Volcanic Explosivity Index (VEI). 2022. Available at: https://www.nps.gov/subjects/volcanoes/volcanic-explosivity-index.htm. Accessed November 28, 2022.
50. Stein S, Menakis J, Carr M, et al. *Wildfire, Wildlands, and People: Understanding and Preparing for Wildfire in the Wildland-Urban Interface—a Forests on the Edge Report.* Gen. Tech. Rep. RMRS-GTR-299. Fort Collins, CO: US Department of Agriculture; 2013:36.
51. Ramakreshnan L, Aghamohammadi N, Fong C, et al. Haze and health impacts in ASEAN countries: a systematic review. *Environ Sci Pollut Res.* 2017;25(3).
52. Kelly J. Fire. In: Jorgenson S, That B, eds. *Encyclopedia of Ecology.* Cambridge, MA: Academic Press; 2008.

7

Technological Disasters

LEARNING OBJECTIVES

Upon completion, the reader will be able to

1. Define the following technological disasters:
   - Collapse
   - Explosion
   - Fire
   - Hazmat
   - Industrial
   - Mass gathering
   - Mining
   - Poisoning
   - Transportation
2. Compare the onset, duration, consequences, and scale of the following technological disasters:
   - Collapse
   - Explosion
   - Fire
   - Hazmat
   - Industrial
   - Mass gathering
   - Mining
   - Poisoning
   - Transportation

TECHNOLOGICAL HAZARDS

Technological hazards are disaster-causing phenomena generated by human activity (i.e., anthropogenic). Technological hazards often result in loss of life, injury or other health impacts, property damage, loss of livelihoods and services, social and economic disruption, or environmental damage. Like natural hazards, these human-made hazards also cause various emergencies, disasters, and even catastrophes.

Table 7-1. The Onset, Duration, and Consequences of Individual Technological Disasters

Disaster	Onset of Disaster	Duration of Response	Major Consequences
Collapse	seconds to minutes	days to weeks	health and infrastructure
Explosion	seconds to minutes	days to weeks	health and infrastructure
Fire	seconds to minutes	days to weeks	health and infrastructure
Hazmat	seconds to months	days to years	health and infrastructure
Industrial	seconds to months	days to years	health and infrastructure
Mass gathering	minutes to hours	hours to weeks	mostly health
Mining	seconds to minutes	days to weeks	health and infrastructure
Poisoning	hours to days	days to weeks	mostly health
Transportation	seconds to minutes	days to weeks	health and infrastructure

This chapter defines individual technological disaster hazards and describes their proximate causes, timing, consequences, and scale. Table 7-1 summarizes individual technological disasters' onset, duration, and consequences. Figure 7-1 compares the relative ranking of individual technological disasters in terms of the maximum number of fatalities per event.

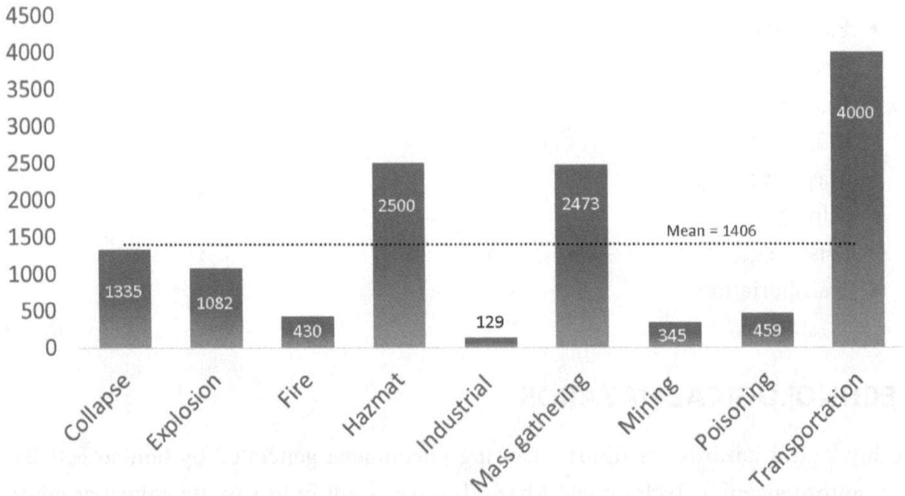

Figure 7-1. Maximum Number of Deaths Reported for Individual Technological Disasters, 1961–2020

DISASTERS CAUSED BY TECHNOLOGICAL HAZARDS

Collapse

Definition

Structural collapse occurs when internal load-bearing elements fail, resulting in the collapse of a structure.[1] Collapses may be internal or external in origin. When internal structural elements fail, a building will collapse, and exterior walls will be pulled into the falling structure. This may be caused by construction activity, excessive loads, seismic activity, or fire. Alternatively, the building may collapse in an outward direction if the structural failure is caused by an explosion or natural forces such as wind.[1] Collapse disasters are typically associated with kinetic hazards but may also involve toxic and thermal hazards.

Causes

Collapse disasters have been associated with a wide variety of structures, including balconies, basements, buildings, bridges, canals, churches, commercial centers, dams, docks, elevators, escalators, factories, hospitals, hotels, homes, houses of worship, nightclubs, nuclear sites, office buildings, platforms, power stations, reservoirs, roads, roofs, schools, septic tanks, swimming pools, training centers, tunnels, walls, and water tanks.[2]

Speed of Onset and Duration

Like landslides, structural collapse disasters typically occur as acute onset events. Collapse often occurs within seconds to minutes once the threshold for structural failure is exceeded. This can be caused by large forces such as excessive weight, explosions, extreme weather, and seismicity. Alternatively, collapses may occur covertly and go unrecognized (or ignored) over time because of substandard construction practices, improper maintenance, or long-term structural stresses resulting from habitation, weathering, aging, and overutilization.

Consequences

Collapse disasters are like earthquakes in terms of the severity of the destruction. The main difference is one of scale. Structural failures often result in mass casualty incidents involving a relatively large number of deaths and injuries. Collapses can damage critical infrastructures like communications, transportation, energy, commerce, and health care facilities. Structural collapses can disrupt air, sea, and ground transportation, damage airports, and render major transportation routes (e.g., roads, rail, subways, ports) impassable.

Along with traumatic injuries, collapses can cause a relatively focal population displacement. Collapses also create secondary disaster hazards like fires and explosions, floods, hazardous material releases, and power failures.

Scale

During the past 60 years, there were 342 collapse disasters reported worldwide that caused an average of 47 ± 12 (95% CI) deaths per incident and a moderate range of 1 to 1,335 deaths per disaster, as compared with other technological disasters. (See Table 8-1.) Most of these collapse disasters involved building failures.[2] Figure 8-1 illustrates how the maximum number of deaths caused by individual collapse disasters is close to the mean for all technological disasters (60-year mean = 1,406 deaths/event).[2]

While the impacts may be far-reaching, in most collapse disasters the physical damage occurs within a specific location and does not involve an entire city or region. In general, the effects of most collapse disasters occur near the structure involved. The impacts of internal collapses tend to be more localized than external collapse causes. Internal collapses tend to result in a dense debris field with a relatively small footprint, whereas external collapses result in a less dense and more scattered debris field.[1]

Explosion

Definition

The American Chemical Society defines an explosion as the rapid expansion of gases and the release of energy.[3] Many explosions occur when gases are exposed to a source of ignition (e.g., fire, sparks, static electricity) or an increase in pressure. Explosions can also be caused by chemical reactions when two or more incompatible substances are combined. Some chemicals explode when exposed to air or water. Explosions can also occur because of natural hazards (e.g., volcanic eruptions). This chapter focuses on technological disasters, including explosions that occur because of human activity.

Causes

Human-generated disasters can involve chemical, mechanical, or nuclear explosions.[4,5] Chemical explosions (e.g., dynamite) are caused by chemical reactions that produce large amounts of hot gas, which expands rapidly and creates a destructive pressure wave blast effect. Mechanical explosions occur when an expanding gas encounters a physical barrier that consequently ruptures, releasing highly pressurized gas (e.g., a boiling liquid–expanding vapor explosion, or BLEVE). The explosion is created when the barrier is breached. Nuclear explosions are caused by nuclear fusion or fission reactions resulting in a nuclear detonation (e.g., thermonuclear weapons).

Explosives are materials that combust or decompose quickly, creating large amounts of gas. Explosive materials are classified as high explosives and low explosives. The main difference between these two categories is the velocity of detonation. High explosives detonate at a rate greater than the speed of sound (i.e., supersonic), whereas low explosives burn very rapidly but subsonically. The supersonic shock wave of high explosives creates an expanding blast effect.[5]

During the past 60 years, explosion disasters have occurred at a wide range of locations, including the following examples: ammunition storage sites, buildings, chemical plants, cinemas, coal mines, factories, fireworks, grain silos, hospitals, hotels, landfills, markets, military installations, mines, oil pipelines, natural gas infrastructure, power plants, restaurants, stores, tanks, and warehouses.[2]

Speed of Onset and Duration

Explosions have a characteristically very rapid onset. Detonation often occurs within milliseconds, triggering a subsequent explosion that lasts only a few seconds. This rapidity of onset provides minimal opportunity for warning or protective actions to occur. Once an explosion occurs, the resultant emergency response often lasts for days to weeks.

Consequences

Explosions create three primary hazards, including a blast effect, a ballistic effect, and a thermal effect. A high-pressure shockwave creates the blast effect. The ballistic effect occurs when the debris is thrown into the air. And the thermal effect occurs when waves of light and heat are generated.[4,5]

Explosions have also been associated with various secondary hazards, including toxic spills and releases, combustion and fires, spontaneous secondary explosions, structural collapse, and secondary attacks on emergency responders. Explosions often cause the release of hazardous materials or structure fires. Large explosions in the open environment can also cause the spontaneous combustion of multiple car fuel tanks.[6] Finally, targeting emergency responders with secondary explosive devices has become a frequent tactic associated with intentional explosive disasters.[6]

Explosion disasters are somewhat like collapse disasters in terms of the potential severity of localized destruction that is possible. Explosions can disrupt air, sea, and ground transportation, damage airports, and render major transportation routes (e.g., roads, rail, subways, ports) impassable. Explosions commonly result in mass casualty incidents and can damage critical infrastructures like communications, transportation, energy, commerce, and health care facilities.

Scale

During the past 60 years, there were 926 explosion disasters reported worldwide that caused an average of 40 ± 5 (95% CI) deaths per incident, with a relatively moderate range from 1 to 1,082 deaths per disaster, as compared with other technological disaster hazards.[2] (See Figure 7-1.)

The scale of explosion disasters is influenced by the size of the explosion itself, the medium in which the explosion occurs, the distance from the center, and the presence of an enclosed space. Low explosives are associated with a minor explosion, while high explosives have the potential to damage a larger area.[5] By comparison, nuclear detonations can destroy an entire city. Underwater explosions transfer energy more efficiently as compared with air as a medium. Enclosed spaces also increase air pressure waves, as they are constrained and reflected within physical barriers.[4]

In general, the effects of these disasters are concentrated near where the explosion occurred. Debris fields are less dense and more scattered as the distance from the explosion increases.[7]

Fire

Definition

All fires are categorized as either wildfire or urban fire.[8,9] Both categories have been responsible for large, dangerous, and destructive disasters. Wildfire is discussed along with other natural disasters in Chapter 6. This chapter focuses on urban fire disasters. These **fire disasters** are typically associated with thermal hazards but may also involve toxic and kinetic hazards (e.g., smoke inhalation and structural collapse).

Causes

Although fires can start from numerous causes, urban fire disasters are often the result of other hazards such as storms, droughts, transportation accidents, hazardous material spills, criminal activity (arson), or conflict.

Many urban fire disasters result from a point source ignition and then spread as a front. However, an extraordinarily intense and relatively unique version of large-scale urban fire occurs when multiple ignition sources (e.g., firebombing) or the entire city is ignited at once (e.g., nuclear detonation). Extreme temperatures and high-velocity fire winds were reported in each of these fires. Firestorms, and violent atmospheric convection caused by a large continuous area of intense fire, also occur during these events.[10–12]

Speed of Onset and Duration

Most urban fire disasters are relatively acute incidents with an onset measurable in minutes to hours. Once ignited, some urban fires continue to smolder and burn for days. And fire in the rubble of collapsed buildings may also burn more slowly.

This contrasts with intense large-scale, high-intensity urban fires that start within minutes and can exhaust most urban-area fuel in a few hours.

Nuclear detonations differ from other urban fires that spread from a point or along a front in that vast areas are known to ignite simultaneously.[11,12]

Consequences

Disastrous urban fires have occurred throughout history. In most of these fires, there were few casualties, although property damage was extensive. Even the so-called Great Chicago Fire killed only 300 persons while it destroyed tens of thousands of structures in the city.[2]

Fires that spread from a limited number of ignition points tend to facilitate population evacuations and result in a lower overall impact. The consequences of this type of point source urban fire occur in stark contrast to the phenomenon of large-scale intense urban fires, such as those caused by incendiary and nuclear weapons. The resultant intense fire often coalesces to burn all combustible fuel completely and nearly simultaneously throughout an entire city. These conditions generate winds up to 90 miles (145 km) per hour. All buildings in the city burn nearly simultaneously. These high-intensity urban fires are associated with much higher levels of losses as compared to urban fires originating from a single point source.[10–12]

Scale

Scale is essential for differentiating the magnitude and severity of urban fire disasters. During 1961–2020, there were 919 urban fire disasters reported worldwide that caused an average of 35 ± 4 (95% CI) deaths per incident, with a relatively low range from 0 to 430 deaths per event, compared with other technological disasters.[2] (See Table 8-1.) Urban fires occur primarily in cities or towns with the potential to spread to adjoining structures rapidly. These fires damage and destroy homes, schools, commercial buildings, and vehicles. Small structural fires generally do not have an enormous impact on an area but rather increase the cost of insurance and other means of risk sharing (e.g., public fire services).

In comparison to a spreading point-source or fire front, there are many historical examples of extreme and unusual conditions that occur when large urban areas burn simultaneously, High-intensity, urban fire disasters have engulfed entire cities (e.g., Hamburg in 1943) and have also occurred in multiple cities at once (e.g., Japan in 1945).

Urban fires caused by nuclear detonations have also caused high-intensity citywide fires resulting in extensive damage over large areas.[10–12]

Hazardous Materials

Definition

The US Department of Transportation and the International Air Transportation Association define hazardous materials (i.e., "hazmat") as articles or substances that can pose a risk to health, safety, property, or the environment. Under this definition, hazardous materials are classified into nine general categories: explosives, gases, flammable liquids, solids, oxidizers, organic peroxides, poisons, infectious substances, radioactive materials, corrosives, and miscellaneous.[13] These hazardous materials may also be categorized as biological, chemical, and radiological hazards.

For our analysis, EM-DAT data related to chemical releases were combined with corresponding data for radiation releases to create a third category of hazardous material disasters (including biological hazards associated with biosafety and biosecurity).

Causes

Hazardous material (hazmat) disasters are caused by exposures to hazardous materials, including chemical, biological, and radiological materials. Not all hazardous materials can create an abrupt and severe disruption of society and widespread losses, as in a disaster. Over the past 60 years, events associated with chemical hazards have involved ammonia, various acids, benzene, chlorine, cyanide, formaldehyde, gasoline, insecticides, LPG, mine tailings, nitrogen oxide, petroleum, phenol, phosphorus chlorides, propane, sulfur oxides, and vinyl chloride.[2] During this same time, a total of eight known radiation disasters were reported to have occurred in Brazil, China, Japan, the former Soviet Union, and the United States.[2]

Hazmat disasters have also resulted from accidental and intentional releases of human-made biological hazards. For example, anthrax bioweapons were released accidentally in 1979 in the former USSR and, again, intentionally in 2001 in the United States.

Accidental releases have also involved laboratory-acquired infections and laboratory releases of lethal pathogens, containment failures in or during transport of deadly pathogens, incidents of exposure of lethal pathogens to laboratory personnel, improper disposal of contaminated waste, or the escape of laboratory animals.[14]

Many of these outbreaks were associated with biological agents that CDC has identified as high risk for use as a bioweapon (e.g., Category A) and other diseases of epidemic and pandemic potential. Reports have described laboratory-acquired infections involving anthrax, brucellosis, dengue fever, Ebola fever, influenza, plague, Marburg fever, SARS, SARS-COV-2, smallpox, West Nile, and Zika.[2,14]

Excluding the 1979 and 2001 anthrax incidents, nearly all these laboratory biosafety incidents resulted in one or two known cases. However, reporting laboratory-associated infections has been largely voluntary (with enormous liabilities attached). Consequently, it is difficult to determine the number of worldwide technological and biological disasters or the specific risks for workers.

It is also essential to consider the lack of specificity of global data related to individual technological disasters, including all hazardous materials. Anthropogenic biological hazards also represent a critical knowledge gap in this regard. In broader terms, there is also likely significant overlap between reports of hazardous material disasters and those caused by other natural and technological hazards. For example, industrial disasters, such as those involving explosions, fires, mining, poisoning, and transportation, often involve hazardous materials. While this classification may lack specificity, these criteria do appear sensitive enough to detect when many of these phenomena occur. The challenge appears more related to reporting than to classification.

Speed of Onset and Duration

The release of hazardous material can be overt or insidious in its onset. Depending on the agent, the beginning of hazardous material disasters can occur from that of an instant (e.g., the 1999 Tokaimura radiation release) to hours (e.g., the 1984 Bhopal chemical disaster) to days (e.g., the 1979 Sverdlovsk anthrax release) to years (e.g., the Times Beach dioxin release in the 1960s–1980s).[2]

Hazardous material disasters may also be acute or chronic in duration. Although less dramatic than a major explosion, environmental contamination from industrial pollution has resulted in health and environmental problems of immense proportions.[15]

There were at least four significant human-made biological disasters during 1961–2020. A 1967 event involving laboratory exposure to the Marburg virus resulted in 32 cases of hemorrhagic fever in Germany.[16] In 1971 there were 10 persons infected by smallpox at an Aral Sea weapons facility.[17]

A 1979 accidental aerial release of anthrax reportedly killed over 100 persons in the former USSR.[18] In 2001 anthrax spores were intentionally mailed to political figures and news organizations in the United States, resulting in 22 infections.[19]

Consequences

Hazardous material releases have the potential for far-reaching consequences that extend over decades. Hazardous material releases involving chemical and radioactive hazards can affect critical infrastructures like communications, transportation, energy, commerce, and health care facilities. These events may also disrupt air, sea, and ground transportation, damage airports, and render major transportation routes (e.g., roads, rail, subways, ports) impassable. The duration of this exclusionary zone can range from a few days (e.g., train derailment) to many years (e.g., nuclear power reactor breach). Hazardous materials also have the potential to create relatively focal population displacement. However, this displacement can extend for decades, even centuries. Chemical and radiological disasters can also create secondary disaster hazards like fires and explosions, poisoning, and power failures.

Just like natural epidemics, human-made epidemics (i.e., biological warfare agents) can cause large numbers of patient cases and deaths. This sudden increase in disease can result in a mismatch of acute needs and resources when health care systems become overwhelmed by the volume of patients. Deliberate epidemics could also enormously affect international politics, economics, transportation, trade, and commerce. The impact on the built environment is expectedly negligible.

Scale

According to the EM-DAT database, during 1961–2020 there were 187 hazmat disasters reported worldwide, with 179 (96%) of these incidents caused by chemical hazards and 8 caused by radiation hazards. In addition, at least four major outbreaks of infectious diseases were directly associated with human activity. The average number of deaths per incident was 57 ± 79 (95% CI), and the total number of deaths ranged from 1 to 2,500 per event—moderate compared with other technological disasters.[2] (See Table 8-1.)

Hazardous material disasters are like fire and explosion disasters in that the scale of hazmat disasters is influenced by the size of the release, the medium into which it occurs, the distance from the source, and the presence of an enclosed space.

Hazardous materials incidents are categorized as Level I, II, or III depending on the severity of the incident. Criteria include the following:

- Characteristics of the material
- Nature of its release
- Assets affected (e.g., populations, ecosystems, waterways, transportation)
- Extent of multiagency and multijurisdictional involvement
- Evacuations, injuries, or fatalities
- Capability (e.g., technical expertise and equipment) needed to mitigate the incident safely
- Duration of the incident[20]

In general, the effects of these disasters are concentrated nearest to the location of the hazmat incident. However, like volcanoes and wildfires, hazardous material disasters also have the potential to affect the air quality and respiratory health of thousands of persons. Atmospheric releases can create a toxic plume of respirable substances that occur downwind from the release site or through another route of exposure (ingestion or direct contact). Thus, there is often a significant risk for the secondary spread of hazardous materials via wind, water, personnel, equipment, food, explosions, and combustion.

Although there is no standard scale or index for measuring the severity of an epidemic, natural or human-made, a novel framework has been proposed for natural pandemics.[21]

Industrial

Definition

Industrial disasters are phenomena associated with human activities involving processing raw materials and manufacturing goods, often in plants or factories.[15,22]

Causes

While most disasters are classified according to the causative hazard, this classification according to environmental circumstances is also helpful in understanding where technological hazards are more likely to occur. For example, industrial disasters, like mine disasters and mass gathering disasters, involve specific environmental circumstances that have the potential to create a mass casualty incident. Industrial disasters may be associated with kinetic, thermal, or toxic hazards such as explosions, fires, and releases, respectively.[22]

In this dataset, most industrial disasters specifically reported as involving structural collapse, explosions, fires, hazardous material releases, mining, and transportation are included elsewhere under each specific hazard category.[2]

Speed of Onset and Duration

The onset of an industrial disaster can be obvious or insidious. Depending on the agent, the onset of an industrial disaster can vary widely from seconds to years. Industrial disasters can also be acute or chronic in duration. Industrial accidents may occur as abrupt releases of hazardous materials, structural failures, explosions, combustions, or irradiation. However, industrial disasters may also occur over time. Industrial exposures resulting in a disaster may occur under less evident and dramatic occupational circumstances.[15]

Consequences

Industrial disasters are related to manufacturing or processing activities that can result in explosions, toxic exposures, environmental contamination, fires, or structural collapse. Significant events often attract global attention and are known to create long-term economic impacts (e.g., Bhopal). Industrial disasters can occur at the site of fixed locations (e.g., processing, manufacturing, and storage facilities) or during the transportation of industrial materials (e.g., train derailment). Toxic chemicals are more strongly associated with worker injury, whereas flammables are more strongly associated with property damage.[22]

Industrial disasters can also involve critical infrastructures like communications, transportation, energy, commerce, and health care facilities. Industrial disasters can disrupt transportation or render major transportation routes (e.g., roads, rail, subways, ports) impassable.

Scale

During 1961–2020, there were 31 events reported as industrial disasters, with an average of 28 ± 11 (95% CI) deaths per event, a low range of 8 to 129 deaths per disaster.[2]

(See Table 8-1.) The largest industrial disaster during these 60 years occurred in 2006. It involved what appeared to be the intentional dumping of over 550 tons (~500 metric tons) of toxic waste in Abidjan, one of the biggest cities in West Africa. This incident involved at least 18 separate point-source releases around the city and is estimated to have affected over 100,000 people.[23] And while hazardous waste was of industrial origin, this instance of dumping hazardous waste in a low-resource nation appears to have been a deliberate act (unfortunately, not uncommon worldwide).

Mass Gathering

Definition

A gathering is an assembly of people, usually held for a specific purpose. Gatherings regularly occur in various settings involving entertainment, politics, religion, and sports. Public gatherings may be relatively small or large (i.e., mass gatherings).

Mass gathering has been defined as an occasion where the number of people attending is sufficient to strain the resources of the entity hosting the event.[24,25] Thus, mass gatherings are expressed in relative terms of their ability to cause a mismatch of needs and resources—that is, a disaster—compared with an arbitrary threshold or census. This approach recognizes that disasters have been reported to occur at both small and large public gatherings. Thus, perhaps a more accurate definition of mass gathering disasters acknowledges the potential for mass casualties rather than massive crowds.

Causes

Like other disasters based on a specific environment, mass gathering disasters may be caused by a range of kinetic, thermal, or toxic hazards. Mass gatherings typically occur at locations that will accommodate a large group of people (e.g., houses of worship, arenas, stadiums, arenas, streets, and open land). Mass gatherings may occur in a fixed location (e.g., sporting events) or involve the movement of crowds (e.g., parades and protests). Causes of disasters related to public gatherings have been reported to include extreme weather, fire, stampedes, structural collapse, and violence.[2]

Speed of Onset and Duration

Most public gatherings occur at a prescheduled time; however, some may occur spontaneously. Most disasters associated with gatherings have an abrupt onset, occurring over minutes to hours. Outbreaks of infectious disease associated with gatherings have been reported to last for weeks after a large gathering—indeed, long after the attendees return home.[26]

Consequences

While relatively few mass gathering disasters have occurred during the past 60 years (n = 80), these incidents appear to be associated with a relatively high degree of fatality (163 deaths) per event compared with other technological disasters.[2]

Most of the consequences of public gathering disasters involve the management of casualties and medical needs that occur during the event and their impact on the local health care system. However, minimal research focuses on the effects of mass gatherings, including health services, such as ambulance services and hospitals.[27]

Most disasters (excluding infectious disease outbreaks) occur onsite at the mass gathering location. They do not routinely extend to other sectors such as commerce, communications, or transportation (perhaps other than traffic congestion). And while many impacts are immediately apparent, some long-term effects of a public gathering disaster can also include significant social, economic, or geopolitical repercussions (e.g., the 1972 Olympic Games).

Scale

During 1961–2020, there were 80 public gathering disasters reported worldwide that caused an average of 73 ± 58 (95% CI) deaths per incident, with a relatively high range of deaths per incident (e.g., 1–2,236/event), as compared with other technological disasters.[2] (See Table 8-1.)

While the scale of the event is an important determinant, disasters resulting in mass casualty incidents have been reported to occur at both small and large public gatherings. For example, mass casualty events have been reported in religious gatherings ranging from one church building to an international pilgrimage. Entertainment-related incidents have included nightclubs as well as large-scale music concerts. Political protests of any size can quickly erupt into violence.[2] Violence during sporting events has been reported to spill out into the community afterward. Disease outbreaks have also been reported to extend well beyond the duration of the gathering itself.

Mining

Definition

Mining involves activities that produce, extract, leach, and refine mineral resources.[28] Mining disasters are defined by the relatively hazardous occupational environment in which they are often known to occur.

Causes

Like mass gathering disasters, which are also based on a specific environment, mine disasters may be associated with a range of kinetic, thermal, or toxic hazards.

During 1961–2020, the most significant portion (42%) of all mining disasters occurred at coal mines, with 85% located in China. Gold mining was the second most common type of mining disaster, associated with 24% of all mine disasters worldwide. Other types of mining involved copper, diamond, gypsum, iron, jade, lead, marble, sand, stone, tin, and uranium.[2]

Speed of Onset and Duration

Most mine disasters are acute in onset, occurring seconds to minutes and lasting days to weeks. Like geological mass movements, most structural collapse disasters occur as acute onset events. Mine disasters associated with structural failures and collapse often occur within minutes once the threshold for structural failure is exceeded. This can be triggered or exacerbated by excavation, extraction, explosions, extreme weather, and seismicity. Alternatively, some mine disasters may occur covertly (e.g., gas poisonings) and go unrecognized over time because of substandard safety practices, improper maintenance, and inadequate occupational health protections (e.g., personal protective equipment).

Consequences

Mine disasters are like earthquakes regarding the rapidity and severity of destruction but differ remarkably according to geographical scale. Mine disasters can result in mass casualty incidents but rarely damage critical societal infrastructures like communications, transportation, energy, commerce, and health care facilities. Along with traumatic injuries, some mine disasters have caused relatively focal population displacement as a result of environmental contamination. Mine disasters also create secondary disaster hazards like fires, explosions, and hazardous material released into the air, soil, and groundwater.[2,28]

Mine disasters have been associated with structural failures and tunnel collapses, mass movements, toxic exposures, explosions, fires, environmental contamination, and entrapment of workers.[2] As in industrial disasters, employees are the most reported victims. Nearly all mine disasters reported during that period occurred in what were at the time rapidly industrializing countries.

In many such situations less elaborate measures for protecting the environment, human health, and safety are essential in economic negotiations for these nations. This bargaining disadvantage has often led to the unfair international division of risk.[29–31] This relative powerlessness of low-resource nations to protect their workers from harm has been described as a "socio-political amplification of risk."[29]

Scale

During 1961–2020, there were 173 events reported as mine disasters with an average of 33 ± 7 (95% CI) deaths per event, with a relatively low range (e.g., 10–345) of fatalities per event.[2] (See Table 8-1.) The largest mine disaster during these 60 years occurred in 1991 as a consequence of flooding in Vietnam.[2]

As in collapse disasters and other localized events, the physical damage caused during a mine disaster often occurs within a specific location. It does not involve an entire city or region. However, disasters have been reported to extend well beyond mine locations, often occurring as slurry flows of mine tailings or groundwater contamination. One mine-related spill of cyanide contaminated rivers in Romania, Serbia, Hungary, and Bulgaria during 2000.[2] In general, though, the effects of most mine disasters occur near the mine involved.

Poisoning

Definition

Poisoning is the harmful effect that occurs when a toxic substance is swallowed, inhaled, or comes in contact with an affected person.[32]

Causes

Poisonings typically involve toxic substances. Sources of these poisons include animal venom, chemicals, food, fungi, pharmaceuticals, plants, and radioactive substances. But not all poisonous substances have the potential to cause a disaster resulting in mass casualties. Most poisoning disasters are associated with the mass distribution of a contaminated product or commodity (e.g., food, water, alcohol, cooking oil, or medicines).[2] During 1961–2020, for example, 29% of poisoning disasters were reported as food poisoning and 21% involved an alcohol.[2]

Speed of Onset and Duration

The onset of a poisoning disaster may vary according to the specific substance involved, its means of distribution, and its route of exposure. While most individual cases of poisoning can be expected to last for a few hours (e.g., gas intoxication) to a few days (e.g., bacterial food poisoning), poisoning disasters may also continue to propagate for months (e.g., adulterated milk in China in 2008) and to create long-term health effects that last years (e.g., lead-contaminated drinking water in Flint, Michigan, in 2014).[2]

Consequences

Like epidemics, poisoning disasters result in large numbers of patient cases and deaths with negligible impact on other critical infrastructure in the built environment. However, poisonings often occur on a much smaller scale than epidemics.

Poisonings rarely result in an acute mismatch of health care needs and resources caused by volume of patients. Poisonings most often occur as disease cluster outbreaks attributable to a common hazard or exposure.

Poisonings (e.g., product tampering) have been reported to affect consumer sales but have not significantly affected international transportation, trade, and commerce.

Scale

During 1961–2020, there were 126 poisoning disasters reported worldwide with an average of 50 ± 16 (95% CI) deaths per event, with a relatively low (1–459) range of deaths per event.[2] (See Table 8-1.) The largest poisoning disaster during this 60-year period was estimated to have affected over one-half million people.[2]

Transportation

Definition

Transportation disasters have been defined as disasters associated with mechanized modes of transport: road, rail, marine, and air.[33] These four subsets involve (1) motor vehicles on roads, tracks, and cables; (2) trains; (3) boats, fishing vessels, ferries, submarines, passenger ships, crafts carrying migrants, and tankers; and (4) airplanes, helicopters, airships, and balloons.[2]

Causes

Transportation disasters may be associated with a range of kinetic, thermal, and/or toxic hazards and can occur as the result of a collisions, engineering flaws, mechanical failure, weather, fires, explosions, and/or human behavior.[2,33] The 1912 sinking of the *Titanic* is an example of a widely recognized transportation disaster. However, a more recent 1987 ferry disaster involved two ships and killed nearly twice as many people as the *Titanic* disaster.[2]

Speed of Onset and Duration

The onset of a transportation disaster can occur within seconds (e.g., an exploding aircraft) to hours (e.g., a sinking ship). And while most emergency response activities typically last for days (e.g., train derailment), some response efforts (e.g., marine search and rescue) may continue for weeks.

Consequences

Transportation disasters can result in secondary explosions, toxic exposures, environmental contamination, fires, or structural collapse.[2,33] Large events often attract global attention and are known to create long-term economic and geopolitical impacts (e.g., the 2001 World Trade Center bombing).

Transportation disasters can also involve critical infrastructures such as communications, transportation, energy, commerce, and health care facilities. Transportation disasters can also disrupt transportation or render major transportation routes (e.g., roads, rail, subways, ports) impassable.[33]

Scale

During 1961–2020, there were 5,707 transportation disasters reported worldwide with an average of 40 ± 2 (95% CI) deaths per event, and a very high range of 1 to 4,000 deaths per event, as compared with other technological disasters.[2] (See Table 8-1.) The largest transportation disaster reported during that time occurred in the Philippines in 1987 and involved the sinking of a passenger ferry after it collided with an oil tanker. Out of over 4,000 passengers and crew, only 24 (0.5%) survived.[2,33]

TOPICS FOR DISCUSSION

1. Provide an example of the socio-political amplification of disaster risk. Justify your response.
2. Provide an example of an intentional technological disaster and then answer the following questions:
   - How does an intentional event differ from an unintentional one?
   - In what ways are they the same?
3. Brainstorm reasons why mass gatherings can result in a dangerous environment compared with other technological hazards.

REFERENCES

1. Occupational Safety and Health Administration (OSHA). Structural collapse guide. Emergency preparedness guides. 2022. Available at: https://www.osha.gov/emergency-preparedness/guides/structural-collapse. Accessed November 29, 2022.
2. Center for Research on the Epidemiology of Disasters (CRED). EM-DAT: the international disaster database. 2022. Available at: www.emdat.be. Accessed April 10, 2019.
3. Giroux RM. The definition of explosion. *Chem Engin News*. 2013. Available at: https://cen.acs.org/articles/91/i36/Definition-Explosion.html. Accessed November 29, 2022.
4. Federal Emergency Management Agency (FEMA). *Primer for Design of Commercial Buildings to Mitigate Terrorist Attacks*. Washington, DC: Federal Emergency Management Agency; 2003:2.1–4.5.
5. Federal Emergency Management Agency (FEMA). *Reference Manual to Mitigate Potential Terrorist Attacks Against Buildings*. Washingtopn, DC: Federal Emergency Management Agency; 2011:3.2–3.91.
6. Shapovalov VM, Samokhvalov IM. Blasting damage in human-made disasters and terrorist attacks. Article in Russian. *Voen Med Zh*. 2012;333(1):25–33.
7. Neel N. Explosive analysis. Explosives. 2022. Available at: https://www.asteetrace.org/explosives. Accessed November 29, 2022.
8. Shusterman D, Kaplan JZ, Canabarro C. Immediate health effects of an urban wildfire. *West J Med*. 1993;158(2):133–138.
9. Stein S, Menakis J, Carr M, et al. *Wildfire, Wildlands, and People: Understanding and Preparing for Wildfire in the Wildland-Urban Interface—a Forests on the Edge Report*. Gen. Tech. Rep. RMRS-GTR-299. Fort Collins, CO: US Department of Agriculture; 2013:36.
10. Glossary of fire terminology. 2022. Available at: https://www.fs.fed.us/nwacfire/home/terminology.html. Accessed June 17, 2022.
11. Frantz RR. Firestorms and wildfires In: Hogan D, Burstein J, eds. *Disaster Medicine*. Philadelphia, PA: Lippincott Williams & Wilkins; 2002:194–201.
12. Brode HL, Small RD. A review of the physics of large urban fires. In: Solomon F, Marston R, eds. *The Medical Implications of Nuclear War*. Washington, DC: National Academies Press; 1986.
13. Pipeline and Hazardous Materials Safety Administration, US Dept of Transportation. Federal hazmat law. 2021:5–8. Available at: https://www.phmsa.dot.gov/sites/phmsa.dot.gov/files/2021-09/Hazmat%20Law%20Overview_September-2021_0.pdf. Accessed November 22, 2022.
14. Gillum D, Krishnan P, Byers K. A searchable laboratory-acquired infection database. *Appl Biosafety*. 2016;21(4):203–207.
15. Lillibridge S. Industrial disasters. In: Noji E, ed. *The Public Health Consequences of Disasters*. New York, NY: Oxford University Press; 1997:354–369.
16. Centers for Disease Control (CDC). History of Marburg virus disease (MVD) outbreaks. Diseases and conditions. 2022. Available at: https://www.cdc.gov/vhf/marburg/outbreaks/chronology.html. Accessed November 29, 2022.
17. Pala C. Anthrax island. In: *New York Times Magazine*. New York, NY: New York Times; 2003.

18. Meselson M, Guillemin J, Hugh-Jones M, et al. The Sverdlovsk anthrax outbreak of 1979. *Science*. 1994;266(5188):1202–1208.
19. Centers for Disease Control (CDC). Update: investigation of anthrax associated with intentional exposure and interim public health guidelines, October 2001. *MMWR*. 2001;50(41): 889–908.
20. National Fire Protection Association. *Standard on Emergency Services Incident Management System and Command Safety*. Quincy, MA: National Fire Protection Association; 2020.
21. Reed C, Finelli L, Koonin L, et al. Novel framework for assessing epidemiologic effects of influenza epidemics and pandemics. *Emerg Infect Dis*. 2013;19(1):85–91.
22. Bertazzi PA. Industrial disasters and epidemiology: a review of recent experiences. *Scand J Work Environ Health*. 1989;15(2):85–100.
23. Minton J. Minton Report re: caustic tank washings, Abidjan, Ivory Coast. *The Guardian*. October 16, 2009, 2006:1–8.
24. World Health Organization (WHO). Public health for mass gatherings: key considerations. 2015. Available at: https://www.who.int/publications/i/item/public-health-for-mass-gatherings-key-considerations. Accessed November 22, 2022.
25. Tsouros AD, Efstathiou PA. *Mass Gatherings and Public Health: The Experience of the Athens 2004 Olympic Games*. Geneva, Switzerland: World Health Organization; 2007.
26. Lee L, Ostroff S, McGee H, et al. An outbreak of shigellosis at an outdoor music festival. *Am J Epidemiol*. 1991;133(6):608–615.
27. Ranse J, Hutton A, Keene T, et al. Health service impact from mass gatherings: a systematic literature review. *Prehosp Disaster Med*. 2017;32(1):71–77.
28. Thrush P. *A Dictionary of Mining, Mineral and Related Terms*. Washington, DC: US Bureau of Mines; 1968.
29. de Souza Porto MF, de Freitas CM. Major chemical accidents in industrializing countries: the socio-political amplification of risk. *Risk Anal*. 1996;16(1):19–29.
30. Brown HS. Development of environment interactions in the export of hazardous technologies: a comparative study of three multinational affiliates in developing countries. *Technol Forecasting Soc Change*. 1993;43:125–155.
31. Glickman T, Golding D, Terry K. *Fatal Hazardous Materials Accidents in Industry: Domestic and Foreign Experience from 1945 to 1991*. Washington, DC: Center for Risk Management; 1993.
32. O'Malley G, O'Malley R. Overview of poisoning. In: *Merck Manual*. Rahway, NJ: Merck Publishing Group; 2022.
33. Bjornstig U, Forsberg R. Transportation disasters. In: Koenig K, Schultz C, eds. *Disaster Medicine: Comprehensive Principles and Practices*. New York, NY: Cambridge University Press; 2010:253–274.

III. THE ETIOLOGY OF DISASTER-RELATED DISEASE

8

Causes of Disaster-Related Disease

LEARNING OBJECTIVES

Upon completion, the reader will be able to

1. Define the following term:
    - Disaster-related disease
2. List the three categories of disaster-related disease.
3. Recognize health effects commonly associated with the following disaster hazards:
    - Cold weather
    - Cyclone
    - Drought
    - Earthquake
    - Epidemic
    - Explosion
    - Fire
    - Flood
    - Hazardous material release
    - Heat wave
    - Landslide
    - Mass gathering
    - Mining
    - Poisoning
    - Structural collapse
    - Tornado and convective storm
    - Transportation accident
    - Tsunami
    - Volcanic eruption
    - Wildfire
4. Recognize that many disasters have similar patterns of disease.

DEFINING DISASTER-RELATED DISEASE

When discussing the definition of **disaster-related disease**, it is essential to recognize its context within emergency operations. During an emergency response, resources (like epidemiological investigations) are often characteristically triaged according to the incident's acuity, urgency, and scale. Usually, there is limited capacity available for in-depth studies that would identify subclinical disease cases, along with cases that are otherwise undiagnosed because of an absence of care. Under these conditions few opportunities exist for public health researchers not only to investigate the continuum of conditions that patients recognize as ranging from wellness to illness but also to learn how this definition of illness may change over time.

So, while it is difficult to perform an accurate long-term trend analysis when these emergency incidents are rarely studied systematically over time, it is also reasonable to posit that such studies involving disaster-related disease would likely identify significant levels of subclinical and otherwise undiagnosed/untreated clinical pathology (regardless of whether they recognize the health effect as a medical issue or seek clinical care). This chapter focuses on those most reported disaster-related diseases, recognizing that a wide range of health effects likely remain underrecognized by the patient, underdiagnosed by the clinician, and underreported by epidemiological investigations and surveillance systems.

Disaster-related disease includes communicable disease, non-communicable disease, and injuries. Most diseases related to biological disasters involve epidemics of communicable disease, compared with other types of natural and technological disasters that mainly cause injuries. Nearly all types of natural and technological disasters have been associated with the new onset and exacerbations of noncommunicable disease.

HAZARDOUS EXPOSURE AS THE PROXIMATE CAUSE OF DISASTER-RELATED DISEASE

Disease occurs as a result of exposure to causal agents (i.e., health hazards). Figure 8-1 depicts the inception of disease as a result of exposure to causal agents (i.e., health hazards). This exposure initiates a pathological process that may occur within just a few minutes (e.g., major hemorrhage) or over many years (e.g., cancer). Incidents are here represented as either "upstream" (occurring before exposure) or "downstream" (occurring after the exposure). Accordingly, upstream health interventions seek to lower disease incidence compared with downstream interventions, which aim to reduce disease prevalence.

Along with exposures as the proximate cause of disaster-related disease, more distal "causes of the cause"—that is, determinants of health (DoH)—also influence disaster-related health outcomes, and they do so both before and after the causative exposure occurs. Individuals experience upstream and downstream DoH within an ecosocial

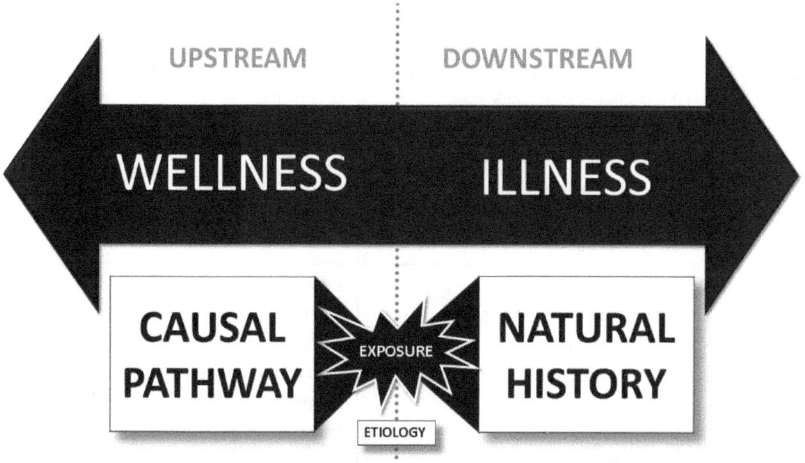

Figure 8-1. Relationship Between the Causal Pathway, Etiology, and Natural History of a Disease

context (recall the process-person-context-tone model). Let us consider upstream DoH as a causal pathway of disease and downstream DoH as components of the natural history of disease. Those intermediate steps involve the mechanism of injury, exacerbation of the chronic disease, or transmission of infections as the etiology of disease. (See Figure 8-1.) The etiology of individual disaster-related diseases can vary remarkably according to the causative hazard. By contrast, the causal pathways and natural history of many disaster-related diseases occur as symmetrical "mirror images" in reverse order of each other.

Health outcomes are influenced by many of the same factors regardless of the disaster hazard.

DISASTER HAZARDS, HEALTH HAZARDS, AND HEALTH EFFECTS

As introduced in Chapter 5, hazardous exposures are the proximate cause of disaster-related disease. Most disaster-related disease occurs in the form of infections or physical and psychological injury sustained through (1) exposure to biological or environmental hazards such as pathogens, water, wind, fire, smoke, debris, or heat; or (2) an absence of a life-sustaining requirement (e.g., air, food, and water). Indirect health effects also occur secondary to displacement and loss of health-sustaining services that can, under certain circumstances, result in outbreaks of infectious disease or exacerbations of chronic disease.

Table 8-1 lists disaster-related health effects according to their corresponding health and disaster hazards.[1-260]

Table 8-1. Disaster Hazards, Health Hazards, and Their Corresponding Health Effects

Disaster Hazard	Health Hazards	Health Effects
Cold waves and storms	Heating and cooking stoves Portable power generators Increased physical exertion Cold ambient air temperatures Precipitation and wind Pathogens Traumatic stress	Carbon monoxide poisoning[1] Cold injuries[1,2] Exacerbation of chronic disease[1,3-7] Hypothermia[1,2] Respiratory infections[4,6,8,9] Stress and mental illness[3]
Cyclone (i.e., hurricane)	High winds Heating and cooking stoves Portable power generators Unsafe drinking water Floodwater Rooftop activity Power lines Insects, pets, and wild animals Traumatic stress Airborne particulates Poor sanitation and hygiene Toxic chemicals Pathogens	Asthma[10,11] Blunt and penetrating trauma[12] Burns[12] Carbon monoxide poisoning[12] Diarrheal illness[12-15] Drowning[12,16] Electrocution[12] Inhalational injury[12] Stress and mental illness[12,17-19] Mold allergy[11,20] Poisoning[12,21] Respiratory infections[20] Skin infections[12] Stings, bites, and envenomation[12]
Drought	Food insecurity Conflict Unsafe drinking water Poor sanitation and hygiene Pathogens Traumatic stress Violence and domestic abuse	Blunt and penetrating trauma[22,23] Diarrheal illness[24] Malnutrition[25-27] Respiratory infections[28,29] Stress and mental illness[18,30-32]
Earthquake	Structural debris Structure fires Airborne particulates Entrapment Hazardous materials Traumatic stress Wound contamination Pathogens Poor sanitation and hygiene	Asphyxia[33] Blunt and penetrating trauma [33-35] Burns[33,35] Crush injury and renal failure[33] Exacerbations of chronic disease[33,36] Hypothermia[33] Inhalational injury[33] Poisonings[33] Wound infections[37] Respiratory infections[37] Stress and mental illness[33,38-42]
Epidemic	Pathogens of epidemic potential Health care overutilization	Communicable disease[261,43-48] Noncommunicable disease[44]
Flood	Debris cleanup Heating and cooking stoves Portable power generators	Blunt and penetrating trauma[49,50] Burns[50] Carbon monoxide poisoning[49,51]

(Continued)

Table 8-1. (Continued)

Disaster Hazard	Health Hazards	Health Effects
Flood (*cont.*)	Unsafe drinking water Floodwater Power lines Traumatic stress Airborne particulates Pathogens Poor sanitation and hygiene	Diarrheal illness[49,50,52] Drowning[49] Electrocution[49,50] Exacerbation of chronic disease[49,53] Inhalational injury[50,54] Poisoning[49,50] Mold allergy[50] Respiratory infections[49] Skin infections[49,55,56] Stings, bites, and envenomation[49,50] Stress and mental illness[49,50,57-59]
Heat wave	Endemic chronic disease High ambient air temperature	Dehydration[60] Exacerbations of chronic disease[3, 61-68] Mortality[69-73] Heat illness[62,71,74-77] Renal failure[65,78,79] Stress and mental illness[65]
Landslide	Falling debris Entrapment Hazardous materials Wound contamination Poor sanitation and hygiene	Asphyxia[80-83] Blunt and penetrating trauma[80,81,83,84] Crush injury and renal failure[85,86] Drowning[80] Wound infections[80]
Tornadoes and convective storms	Ballistic projectiles Structural debris Wound contamination	Blunt and penetrating trauma[87-92] Skin and respiratory infections[93,94] Stress and mental illness[90,95-101] Wound infections[87,102]
Tsunami	Structural debris Airborne particulates Inundation Entrapment Traumatic stress Hazardous materials Wound contamination Pathogens Poor sanitation and hygiene	Blunt and penetrating trauma[103-106] Crush injury and renal failure[107] Drowning Exacerbations of chronic disease[108-111] Pregnancy complication[112] Respiratory and skin infections[104,113-117] Stress and mental illness[108,118-123] Wound infections[104]
Volcanic eruption	Blast projectiles Volcanic gas and debris Pyroclastic flows Lahars Tephra Chemical and radioactive substances	Asphyxia[124] Asthma[125-129] Blunt trauma and burns[124,130] Exacerbations of chronic disease[125,126,128] Inhalational injury[124,125,131-133] Neurodegenerative disease[134,135] Pregnancy complication[136] Stress and mental illness[128,137]

(*Continued*)

Table 8-1. (Continued)

Disaster Hazard	Health Hazards	Health Effects
Wildfire	High ambient air temperature Fire Airborne particulates Toxic chemicals	Asthma[138,139] Blunt trauma and burns [140] Cancer[141,142] Exacerbations of chronic disease[139,143-145] Heat illness[141,146] Inhalational injury[140] Pregnancy complications[147,148] Poisoning[149,150] Stress and mental illness[151-153]
Explosion	Ballistic projectiles Structural debris Pressure wave Heat or fire Hazardous materials	Blunt and penetrating trauma[154-159] Burns[155,160-162] Eye injuries[163-165] Hollow organ injury[155,166-168] Inhalational injury[169] Poisoning[170-172] Stress and mental illness[173-176] Traumatic brain injury[177-180]
Fire	High ambient air temperature Fire Hot gases Airborne particulates Toxic chemicals	Burns[181,182] Exacerbations of chronic disease[182] Inhalational injury[182,183] Poisoning[182,184,185] Stress and mental illness[182,186,187]
Hazardous material release	Pressurized gas Airborne particulates Pathogens Toxic chemicals Radioactive substances	Bunt and penetrating trauma[172,188] Burns[189,190] Cancer[191-193] Eye injuries[194] Inhalational injury[194-197] Outbreaks[198,199] Poisoning[195,196,200] Pregnancy complication[201,202] Stress and mental illness[203-207]
Mass gathering	Stampedes Fires Structural collapse Food contamination Pathogens High ambient air temperature Toxic chemicals Violence	Asphyxia[208,209] Blunt trauma[208-210] Burns[208,211-213] Foodborne illness[211] Heat illness[214,215] Poisoning[212] Sexual assault[212,216]
Mining	Structural collapses Entrapment Explosions Fires Airborne particulates Toxic chemicals	Blunt and penetrating trauma[217-220] Burns[217] Electrocution[217] Inhalational injury[183,221] Poisoning[217,222,223]

(*Continued*)

Table 8-1. (Continued)

Disaster Hazard	Health Hazards	Health Effects
Poisoning	Adulterated commercial products Contaminated food or water Toxic chemicals Radioactive substances	Cancer[224] Inhalational injury[197] Poisoning[225-237] Pregnancy complcations[238] Stress and mental illness[207,239]
Structural collapse	Structural debris Fire Airborne particulates Entrapment Toxic chemicals	Asphyxia[240,241] Blunt and penetrating trauma[242-245] Burns[244] Cancer[246,247] Exacerbations of chronic disease[244] Inhalational injury[244,246,248] Poisoning[246,248]
Transportation accident	Downing Crashes and derailment Explosions Fires Sinking Hazardous material release Violence	Blunt and penetrating trauma[249-253] Burns[254-257] Drowning[258] Stress and mental illness[252,259,260]

SUMMARY OF DISASTER-RELATED HEALTH EFFECTS

In general, it is safe to conclude that disaster-related health effects have a predictable etiology when considered in terms of the causative hazard. These same health effects also have a predictable causal pathway and natural history.

Diseases that are predictable are also preventable.

In summary, 20 types of natural and technological disasters have been most frequently reported associated with a surprisingly limited number of adverse health outcomes. The health outcomes listed in Table 8-1 are summarized in Table 8-2 according to disease category.

Note that many of the disasters have similar patterns of disease. For example, injuries are the leading cause of death in all natural disasters (excluding pandemics) and all technological disasters (including conflict). Disasters that result in displacement also appear to involve pathology related to post-traumatic stress, communicable disease, food insecurity, conflict, shelter, and security. Disasters resulting in power loss (cold and storms) often reported electrocutions, burns, and carbon monoxide poisoning. Those related to toxic chemicals were often associated with poisonings and burns. Disasters involving

Table 8-2. Adverse Health Outcomes Associated with Disasters

Communicable Disease	Noncommunicable (Chronic) Disease	Injury
Foodborne illness	Anxiety and stress	Asphyxia
Gastrointestinal infections	Birth defects	Blunt trauma
Respiratory infections	Chronic respiratory disease	Burns
Skin infections	Cancer	Carbon monoxide poisoning
Waterborne illness	Cardiovascular disease	Cold injuries
Wound infections	Diabetes	Crush injury
	Hypertension	Dehydration
	Mental illness	Drowning
		Electrocution
		Eye injuries
		Heat illness
		Hollow organ injury
		Inhalational injury
		Malnutrition
		Mold allergy
		Penetrating trauma
		Poisoning
		Pregnancy complications
		Renal failure
		Sexual assault
		Stings, bites, and envenomation

falling debris (e.g., earthquakes, landslides, and structural collapses) reported casualties involving severe multisystem trauma, crush injury, rhabdomyolysis, and subsequent renal failure. Most storm-related injuries (such as nail puncture wounds, lacerations, falls, burns, electrocutions, and carbon monoxide poisonings) are sustained during the disaster recovery cleanup phase.

For geophysical disasters, the leading causes of death are burns, asphyxia, and other blunt and penetrating trauma. For hydrometeorological disasters such as cyclones and floods, the leading cause of mortality is drowning. The main cause of death in tornadoes and landslides is a traumatic injury sustained during disaster impact. The leading causes of death caused by heat waves are heat illness and exacerbations of chronic respiratory and cardiovascular disease. Drought-related deaths are generally mediated by agricultural, economic, and health effects such as malnutrition, poverty, poor sanitation and hygiene, unsafe water, infectious disease, and conflict. The leading causes of death during wildfires are burns and smoke inhalation injuries. The public health impact of wildfires may include burn injuries, exacerbations of chronic obstructive pulmonary disease and asthma, and temporary population displacement that results in a need for humanitarian assistance.

Infectious disease epidemics following natural disasters are rare and differ according to the affected nation's economic development level. Geophysical disasters are seldom associated with epidemics of communicable disease.[261] Hydrometeorological disasters are uncommonly associated with epidemics of communicable disease. However, outbreaks of endemic diseases have been known to occur, particularly in low-income settings where risk factors include contamination of water and overcrowding leading to transmission of disease. Behavioral health effects are among the most debilitating long-term outcomes of environmental disasters.

Most technological disasters result in injuries that reflect the specific character of the health hazard. Disasters associated with mining, structural collapse, explosions, and transportation accidents tend to create mass casualties with many severely injured patients. Explosions and fires expectedly result in traumatic injuries, whereas hazardous material releases and poisoning events are also commonly associated with intoxications. Like mass casualty events, mass gatherings have also been associated with foodborne outbreaks.

ETIOLOGY OF DISASTER-RELATED DISEASE

Appendix A contains a series of tables that detail the health hazards, health effects, and associated etiologies of disaster hazards. (See Appendix A: Tables A-1 to A-20.) In summary, these tables illustrate how detailed knowledge regarding the etiology of disaster-related disease can also be used to inform interventions intended to identify and disrupt the causal pathway and the natural history of the disease.

TOPICS FOR DISCUSSION

1. Using Appendix A, select one natural hazard and one technological hazard and then do the following:
   - List disaster-related health effects for each hazard.
   - List the corresponding etiology for each health effect.

REFERENCES

1. Cattamanchi S, Curcio A. winter storm. In: Ciottone G, ed. *Disaster Medicine*. 2nd ed. Philadelphia, PA: Elsevier; 2016:592–597.
2. Kilbourne E. Cold environments. In: Noji E, ed. *Public Health Consequences of Disasters*. New York, NY: Oxford University Press; 1997:270–286.
3. Rocklov J, Forsberg B, Ebi K, Bellander T. Susceptibility to mortality related to temperature and heat and cold wave duration in the population of Stockholm County, Sweden. *Global Health Action*. 2014;7:22737.
4. Bunker A, Wildenhain J, Vandenbergh A, et al. Effects of air temperature on climate-sensitive mortality and morbidity outcomes in the elderly; a systematic review and meta-analysis of epidemiological evidence. *EBioMed*. 2016;6:258–268.
5. Ageev FT, Smirnova MD, Svirida ON, et al. Impact of a cold wave on disease course, hemodynamics, carbohydrate metabolism, and blood rheological properties in cardiac patents. Article in Russian. *Ter Arkh*. 2015;87(9):11–16.
6. Chen TH, Du XL, Chan W, Zhang K. Impacts of cold weather on emergency hospital admission in Texas, 2004–2013. *Environ Res*. 2019;169:139–146.
7. Tang ZY, Zhu QY, Xu LJ, et al. Artificial cold wave–induced cerebral infarction in rats with carotid atherosclerosis. *J Mol Neurosci*. 2012;47(2):278–285.
8. Chak Ho H, Chan TC, Xu Z, Huang C, Li C. Individual- and community-level shifts in mortality patterns during the January 2016 East Asia cold wave associated with a super El Niño event: empirical evidence in Hong Kong. *Sci Total Environ*. 2020;711:135050.
9. Chan EY, Goggins WB, Yue JS, Lee P. Hospital admissions as a function of temperature, other weather phenomena and pollution levels in an urban setting in China. *Bull World Health Organ*. 2013;91(8):576–584.
10. Grimsley LF, Chulada PC, Kennedy S, et al. Indoor environmental exposures for children with asthma enrolled in the HEAL study, post-Katrina New Orleans. *Environ Health Perspect*. 2012;120(11):1600–1606.
11. Park KJ, Moon JY, Ha JS, et al. Impacts of heavy rain and typhoon on allergic disease. *Osong Public Health Res Perspect*. 2013;4(3):140–145.
12. Malilay J. Tropical cyclones. In: Noji E, ed. *The Public Health Consequences of Disasters*. New York, NY: Oxford University Press; 1997:207–227.
13. Panda S, Pati KK, Bhattacharya MK, Koley H, Pahari S, Nair GB. Rapid situation & response assessment of diarrhoea outbreak in a coastal district following tropical cyclone AILA in India. *Indian J of Med Res*. 2011;133:395–400.
14. Guill CK, Shandera WX. The effects of Hurricane Mitch on a community in northern Honduras. *Prehosp Disaster Med*. 2001;16(3):166–171.
15. Mendoza MT, Roxas EA, Ginete JK, et al. Clinical profile of patients diagnosed with leptospirosis after a typhoon: a multicenter study. *Southeast Asian J Trop Med Public Health*. 2013;44(6):1021–1035.
16. Sergienko E. Hurricanes, cyclones, and typhoons. In: Ciottone G, Darling R, Anderson P, et al., eds. *Disaster Medicine*. 3rd ed. Philadelphia, PA: Mosby-Elsevier; 2006:475–478.

17. Harville EW, Xiong X, Smith BW, Pridjian G, Elkind-Hirsch K, Buekens P. Combined effects of Hurricane Katrina and Hurricane Gustav on the mental health of mothers of small children. *J Psychiatr Ment Health Nurs*. 2011;18(4):288–296.
18. Kolves K, Kolves KE, De Leo D. Natural disasters and suicidal behaviours: a systematic literature review. *J Affective Disord*. 2013;146(1):1–14.
19. Fussell E, Lowe SR. The impact of housing displacement on the mental health of low-income parents after Hurricane Katrina. *Soc Sci Med*. 2014;113:137–144.
20. Rando RJ, Lefante JJ, Freyder LM, Jones RN. Respiratory health effects associated with restoration work in post–Hurricane Katrina New Orleans. *J Environ Public Health*. 2012;2012:462478.
21. Sengul H, Santella N, Steinberg LJ, Cruz AM. Analysis of hazardous material releases due to natural hazards in the United States. *Disasters*. 2012;36(4):723–743.
22. Eriksson J, Adelman H, Borton J, et al. The international response to conflict and genocide: lessons from the Rwanda experience. 1996. Available at: www.oecd.org/countries/rwanda/50189495.pdf. Accessed November 26, 2022.
23. Selbya J, Dahib O, Fröhlich C, Hulmee M. Climate change and the Syrian civil war revisited. *Polit Geogr*. 2017;60:232–244.
24. Stanke C, Kerac M, Prudhomme C, Medlock J, Murray V. Health effects of drought: a systematic review of the evidence. *PLoS Curr*. 2013;5.
25. Kim JJ, Guha-Sapir D. Famines in Africa: is early warning early enough? *Global Health Action*. 2012;5.
26. Arlappa N, Venkaiah K, Brahmam GN. Severe drought and the vitamin A status of rural pre-school children in India. *Disasters*. 2011;35(3):577–586.
27. Davis L. Famines and droughts. In: *Natural Disasters*. New York, NY: Checkmark Books; 2008:105–136.
28. Smith LT, Aragao LE, Sabel CE, Nakaya T. Drought impacts on children's respiratory health in the Brazilian Amazon. *Sci Rep*. 2014;4:3726.
29. Bernstein AS, Rice MB. Lungs in a warming world: climate change and respiratory health. *Chest*. 2013;143(5):1455–1459.
30. Hanigan IC, Butler CD, Kokic PN, Hutchinson MF. Suicide and drought in New South Wales, Australia, 1970–2007. *PNAS*. 2012;109(35):13950–13955.
31. Rigby CW, Rosen A, Berry HL, Hart CR. If the land's sick, we're sick: the impact of prolonged drought on the social and emotional well-being of Aboriginal communities in rural New South Wales. *Australian J Rural Health*. 2011;19(5):249–254.
32. Carnie TL, Berry HL, Blinkhorn SA, Hart CR. In their own words: young people's mental health in drought-affected rural and remote NSW. *Australian J Rural Health*. 2011;19(5):244–248.
33. AlKhadi K. Earthquake. In: Ciottone G, ed. *Disaster Medicine*. Philadelphia, PA: Elsevier; 2016:572–574.
34. Raines A, Lees J, Fry W, Parks A, Tuggle D. Field amputation: response planning and legal considerations inspired by three separate amputations. *Ame J Disaster Med*. 2014;9(1):53–58.
35. Bolin R, Stanford L. *The Northridge Earthquake: Vulnerability and Disaster*. London, UK: Routledge; 2003.

36. Ogawa S, Ishiki M, Nako K, et al. Effects of the Great East Japan Earthquake and huge tsunami on glycaemic control and blood pressure in patients with diabetes mellitus. *BMJ Open.* 2012;2(2):e000830.
37. Schultz C. Earthquakes. In: Hogan D, Burstein J, eds. *Disaster Medicine.* Philadelphia, PA: Lippincott Williams & Wilkins; 2002:163–170.
38. Shiga H, Miyazawa T, Kinouchi Y, et al. Life-event stress induced by the Great East Japan Earthquake was associated with relapse in ulcerative colitis but not Crohn's disease: a retrospective cohort study. *BMJ Open.* 2013;3(2).
39. Moriyama K, Kaga M. Mental healthcare efforts for the public after the Great East Japan Earthquake: "Guide to Good Mental Health for Those Affected by Natural Disasters" published by the Cabinet Office. *Brain Dev.* 2013;35(3):201–208.
40. Valenti M, Masedu F, Mazza M, et al. A longitudinal study of quality of life of earthquake survivors in L'Aquila, Italy. *BMC Public Health.* 2013;13:1143.
41. Shultz JM, Forbes D, Wald D, et al. Trauma signature analysis of the great East Japan disaster: guidance for psychological consequences. *Disaster Med Public Health Prep.* 2013;7(2):201–214.
42. Sugiura H, Akahane M, Ohkusa Y, et al. Prevalence of insomnia among residents of Tokyo and Osaka after the great East Japan earthquake: a prospective study. *Interact J Med Res.* 2013;2(1):e2.
43. World Health Organization (WHO). Top epidemic-prone diseases without sufficient countermeasures. 2018. Available at: https://www.preventionweb.net/news/top-epidemic-prone-diseases-without-sufficient-counter-measures. Accessed November 26, 2022.
44. Frost WH. Some conceptions of epidemics in general. *Am J Epidemiol.* 1976;103(2):141–151.
45. Zell R. Global climate change and the emergence/re-emergence of infectious diseases. *Int J Med Microbiol.* 2004;293(suppl 37):16–26.
46. Centers for Disease Control and Prevention (CDC). Epidemic disease occurrence. Introduction to epidemiology. 2022. Available at: https://www.cdc.gov/csels/dsepd/ss1978/lesson1/section11.html. Accessed November 26, 2022.
47. Davis L. Plagues and epidemics. In: *Natural Disasters.* New York, NY: Checkmark Books; 2008:203–230.
48. Bompangue D, Giraudoux P, Piarroux M, et al. Cholera epidemics, war and disasters around Goma and Lake Kivu: an eight-year survey. *PLoS Negl Trop Dis.* 2009;3(5):e436.
49. Kim SH. Flood. In: Ciottone G, Darling R, Anderson P, et al., eds. *Disaster Medicine.* 3rd ed. Philadelphia, PA: Mosby-Elsevier; 2006:489–491.
50. Malilay J. Floods. In: Noji E, ed. *The Public Health Consequences of Disasters.* New York, NY: Oxford University Press; 1997:207–227.
51. Waite T, Murray V, Baker D. Carbon monoxide poisoning and flooding: changes in risk before, during and after flooding require appropriate public health interventions. *PLoS Curr.* 2014;6.
52. Chaturongkasumrit Y, Techaruvichit P, Takahashi H, Kimura B, Keeratipibul S. Microbiological evaluation of water during the 2011 flood crisis in Thailand. *Sci Total Environ.* 2013; 463–464:959–967.
53. Vanasse A, Cohen A, Courteau J, et al. Association between floods and acute cardiovascular diseases: a population-based cohort study using a geographic information system approach. *Int J Environ Res Public Health.* 2016;13(2):168.

54. Alderman K, Turner LR, Tong S. Floods and human health: a systematic review. *Environ Int.* 2012;47:37–47.
55. Tempark T, Lueangarun S, Chatproedprai S, Wananukul S. Flood-related skin diseases: a literature review. *Int J Dermatol.* 2013;52(10):1168–1176.
56. Diaz JH. Superficial and invasive infections following flooding disasters. *Am J Disaster Med.* 2014;9(3):171–181.
57. Bei B, Bryant C, Gilson KM, et al. A prospective study of the impact of floods on the mental and physical health of older adults. *Aging Ment Health.* 2013;17(8):992–1002.
58. Nahar N, Blomstedt Y, Wu B, Kandarina I, Trisnantoro L, Kinsman J. Increasing the provision of mental health care for vulnerable, disaster-affected people in Bangladesh. *BMC Public Health.* 2014;14(1):708.
59. Kolves K, Kolves KE, De Leo D. Natural disasters and suicidal behaviours: a systematic literature review. *J Affective Disord.* 2013;146(1):1–14.
60. Kettaneh A, Fardet L, Mario N, et al. The 2003 heat wave in France: hydratation status changes in older inpatients. *Eur J Epidemiol.* 2010;25(7):517–524.
61. Brunetti ND, Amoruso D, De Gennaro L, et al. Hot spot: impact of July 2011 heat wave in southern Italy (Apulia) on cardiovascular disease assessed by emergency medical service and telemedicine support. *Telemed J E Health.* 2014;20(3):272–281.
62. Bustinza R, Lebel G, Gosselin P, Bélanger D, Chebana F. Health impacts of the July 2010 heat wave in Québec, Canada. *BMC Public Health.* 2013;13:56–56.
63. Tian Z, Li S, Zhang J, Guo Y. The characteristic of heat wave effects on coronary heart disease mortality in Beijing, China: a time series study. *PloS One.* 2013;8(9):e77321.
64. Shaposhnikov D, Revich B, Bellander T, et al. Mortality related to air pollution with the Moscow heat wave and wildfire of 2010. *Epidemiol.* 2014;25(3):359–364.
65. Sherbakov T, Malig B, Guirguis K, Gershunov A, Basu R. Ambient temperature and added heat wave effects on hospitalizations in California from 1999 to 2009. *Environ Res.* 2018;160:83–90.
66. Zheng S, Wang M, Shang K, et al. A case-crossover analysis of heat wave and hospital emergency department visits for cardiovascular diseases in three hospitals in Beijing. Article in Chinese. *Wei Sheng Yan Jiu.* 2016;45(2):246–251.
67. Tian Z, Li S, Zhang J, Guo Y. The characteristic of heat wave effects on coronary heart disease mortality in Beijing, China: a time series study. *PloS One.* 2013;8(9):e77321.
68. Chen K, Bi J, Chen J, Chen X, Huang L, Zhou L. Influence of heat wave definitions to the added effect of heat waves on daily mortality in Nanjing, China. *Sci Total Environ.* 2015; 506-507:18–25.
69. Kue R, Dyer KS. The impact of heat waves on transport volumes in an urban emergency medical services system: a retrospective review. *Prehosp Disaster Med.* 2013;28(6):610–615.
70. Turner L, Connell D, Tong S. The effect of heat waves on ambulance attendances in Brisbane, Australia. *Prehosp Disaster Med.* 2013;28(5):482–487.
71. Sun X, Sun Q, Zhou X, et al. Heat wave impact on mortality in Pudong New Area, China in 2013. *Sci Total Environ.* 2014;493:789–794.
72. Yang J, Liu HZ, Ou CQ, et al. Impact of heat wave in 2005 on mortality in Guangzhou, China. *Biomed Environ Sci.* 2013;26(8):647–654.

73. D'Ippoliti D, Michelozzi P, Marino C, et al. The impact of heat waves on mortality in 9 European cities: results from the EuroHEAT project. *Environ Health*. 2010;9:37.
74. Azhar G, Mavalankar D, Nori Sarma A, et al. Heat-related mortality in India: excess all-cause mortality associated with the 2010 Ahmedabad heat wave. *PloS One*. 2014;9(3):e91831.
75. Ricco M. Air temperature exposure and agricultural occupational injuries in the Autonomous Province of Trento (2000–2013, North-Eastern Italy). *Int J Occup Med Environ Health*. 2018;31(3):317–331.
76. Josseran L, Fouillet A, Caillere N, et al. Assessment of a syndromic surveillance system based on morbidity data: results from the Oscour network during a heat wave. *PloS One*. 2010;5(8):e11984.
77. Hartz DA, Golden JS, Sister C, Chuang WC, Brazel AJ. Climate and heat-related emergencies in Chicago, Illinois (2003–2006). *Int J Biometeorol*. 2012;56(1):71–83.
78. Kim E, Kim H, Kim YC, Lee JP. Association between extreme temperature and kidney disease in South Korea, 2003–2013: Stratified by sex and age groups. *Sci Total Environ*. 2018;642:800–808.
79. Hausfater P, Megarbane B, Fabricatore L, et al. Serum sodium abnormalities during nonexertional heatstroke: incidence and prognostic values. *Am J Emerg Med*. 2012;30(5):741–748.
80. Pereira BM, Morales W, Cardoso RG, Fiorelli R, Fraga GP, Briggs SM. Lessons learned from a landslide catastrophe in Rio de Janeiro, Brazil. *Am J Disaster Med*. 2013;8(4):253–258.
81. Homma Y, Watari T, Baba T, et al. Injury patterns after the landslide disaster in Oshima, Tokyo, Japan on October 16, 2013. *Disaster Med Public Health Prep*. 2016;10(2):248–252.
82. Uddin T, Islam MT, Gosney JE. 2017 Bangladesh landslides: physical rehabilitation perspective. *Disabil Rehabil*. 2019:1–8.
83. Sanchez C, Lee TS, Young S, Batts D, Benjamin J, Malilay J. Risk factors for mortality during the 2002 landslides in Chuuk, Federated States of Micronesia. *Disasters*. 2009;33(4):705–720.
84. Keim M. Landslides. In: Ciottone G, Darling R, Anderson P, et al., eds. *Disaster Medicine*. 3rd ed. Philadelphia, PA: Mosby; 2006:509–513.
85. Sette P, Carlini M, Berti D, et al. Complex alpine extrication: case report of mountain and speleological rescue cooperation. *Wilderness Environ Med*. 2015;26(2):180–184.
86. Arango-Granados MC, Cruz Mendoza DF, Salcedo Cadavid AE, García Marin AF. Amputation in crush syndrome: a case report. *Int J Surg Case Rep*. 2020;72:346–350.
87. Jones MD, Pfaff J. Tornado. In: Ciottone G, Darling R, Anderson P, et al., eds. *Disaster Medicine*. 3rd ed. Philadelphia, PA: Mosby-Elsevier; 2006:484–488.
88. Regens JL, Mould N. Prevention and treatment of traumatic brain injury due to rapid-onset natural disasters. *Frontiers Public Health*. 2014;2:28.
89. Deng Q, Lv Y, Zhao F, Yu W, Dong J, Zhang L. Factors associated with injuries among tornado victims in Yancheng and Chifeng, China. *BMC Public Health*. 2019;19(1):1556.
90. Niederkrotenthaler T, Parker EM, Ovalle F, et al. Injuries and post-traumatic stress following historic tornados: Alabama, April 2011. *PloS One*. 2013;8(12):e83038.
91. Zhao F, Hu C, Xu Z, Deng Q, Wu Y, Zhang L. Injury patterns and memdical evacuation of patients in Chifeng tornado in China, August 11, 2017. *Disaster Med Public Health Prep*. 2019:1–6.
92. Chern JJ, Miller JH, Tubbs RS, et al. Massive pediatric neurosurgical injuries and lessons learned following a tornado disaster in Alabama. *J Neurosurg Pediatr*. 2011;8(6):588–592.

93. Neblett Fanfair R, Benedict K, Bos J, et al. Necrotizing cutaneous mucormycosis after a tornado in Joplin, Missouri, in 2011. *New Engl J Med*. 2012;367(23):2214–2225.
94. Mu GH, Li X, Hou SS, Lu ZQ, Deng YJ. Injury patterns and outcomes of victims after the 2016 Jiangsu tornado in China: a retrospective analysis of injuries treated at a teaching hospital. *Disaster Med Public Health Prep*. 2020;14(2):208–213.
95. Niederkrotenthaler T, Parker EM, Ovalle F, et al. Injuries and post-traumatic stress following historic tornados: Alabama, April 2011. *PloS One*. 2013;8(12):e83038.
96. Adams ZW, Sumner JA, Danielson CK, et al. Prevalence and predictors of PTSD and depression among adolescent victims of the spring 2011 tornado outbreak. *J Child Psychol Psychiatry*. 2014;55(9):1047–55.
97. Houston JB, Spialek ML, Stevens J, First J, Mieseler VL, Pfefferbaum B. 2011 Joplin, Missouri tornado experience, mental health reactions, and service utilization: cross-sectional assessments at approximately 6 months and 2.5 years post-event. *PLoS Curr*. 2015;7.
98. Danielson CK, Sumner JA, Adams ZW, et al. Adolescent substance use following a deadly US tornado outbreak: a population-based study of 2,000 families. *J Clin Child Adolesc Psychol*. 2017;46(5):732–745.
99. Xu W, Fu G, An Y, Yuan G, Ding X, Zhou Y. Mindfulness, posttraumatic stress symptoms, depression, and social functioning impairment in Chinese adolescents following a tornado: mediation of posttraumatic cognitive change. *Psychiatry Res*. 2018;259:345–349.
100. Xu W, Yuan G, Liu Z, Zhou Y, An Y. Prevalence and predictors of PTSD and depression among adolescent victims of the summer 2016 tornado in Yancheng City. *Arch Psychiatr Nurs*. 2018;32(5):777–781.
101. Resnick H, Zuromski KL, Galea S, et al. Prior interpersonal violence exposure and experiences during and after a disaster as predictors of posttraumatic stress disorder and depression among adolescent victims of the spring 2011 tornadoes. *J Interpers Violence*. 2020 Nov;35(23–24):5179–5197.
102. Cluster of rare fungal infections identified after tornado. *BMJ*. 2012;345:e8382.
103. Lastra TJ, Guzmán CG, Conejeros RC, Suárez VG, Chávez FO. Epidemiological profile of deaths after the 2010 earthquake in Chile. Article in Spanish. *Rev Med Chil*. 2012;140(6):732–739.
104. Guha-Sapir D, van Panhuis WG. Health impact of the 2004 Andaman Nicobar earthquake and tsunami in Indonesia. *Prehosp Disaster Med*. 2009;24(6):493–499.
105. Matsuzawa G, Sano H, Ohnuma H, et al. Patient trends in orthopedic traumas and related disorders after tsunami caused by the Great East Japan Earthquake: an experience in the primary referral medical center. *J Orthop Sci*. 2016;21(4):507–511.
106. Yamanda S, Kobayashi S, Hanagama M, et al. Two cases of tsunami dust pneumonia: organizing pneumonia caused by the inhalation of dried tsunami sludge after the 2011 Great East Japan Earthquake. *Intern Med*. 2016;55(24):3645–3653.
107. Nagamatsu S, Maekawa T, Ujike Y, Hashimoto S, Fuke N; Japanese Society of Intensive Care Medicine. The earthquake and tsunami—observations by Japanese physicians since the 11 March catastrophe. *Crit Care*. 2011;15(3):167.
108. Li X, Aida J, Hikichi H, Kondo K, Kawachi I. Association of postdisaster depression and posttraumatic stress disorder with mortality among older disaster survivors of the 2011 Great East Japan Earthquake and tsunami. *JAMA Netw Open*. 2019;2(12):e1917550.

109. Ishiura Y, Fujimura M, Yamamoto H, et al. Asthma exacerbations after the East Japan disaster. *J Med Invest.* 2013;60(1–2):61–65.
110. Nakamura M, Tanaka F, Nakajima S, et al. Comparison of the incidence of acute decompensated heart failure before and after the major tsunami in Northeast Japan. *Am J Cardiol.* 2012;110(12):1856–1860.
111. Morita T, Nomura S, Tsubokura M, et al. Excess mortality due to indirect health effects of the 2011 triple disaster in Fukushima, Japan: a retrospective observational study. *J Epidemiol Community Health.* 2017;71(10):974–980.
112. Schwab FD, Zettler EK, Moh A, Schotzau A, Gross U, Gunthert AR. Predictive factors for preterm delivery under rural conditions in post-tsunami Banda Aceh. *J Perinat Med.* 2016;44(5):511–515.
113. Shibata Y, Ojima T, Tomata Y, et al. Characteristics of pneumonia deaths after an earthquake and tsunami: an ecological study of 5.7 million participants in 131 municipalities, Japan. *BMJ Open.* 2016;6(2):e009190.
114. Ebisawa K, Yamada N, Okada S, et al. Combined Legionella and Escherichia coli lung infection after a tsunami disaster. *Intern Med.* 2011;50(19):2233–2236.
115. Kawakami Y, Tagami T, Kusakabe T, et al. Disseminated aspergillosis associated with tsunami lung. *Respir Care.* 2012;57(10):1674–1678.
116. Daito H, Suzuki M, Shiihara J, et al. Impact of the Tohoku earthquake and tsunami on pneumonia hospitalisations and mortality among adults in northern Miyagi, Japan: a multicentre observational study. *Thorax.* 2013;68(6):544–550.
117. Kawano T, Tsugawa Y, Nishiyama K, Morita H, Yamamura O, Hasegawa K. Shelter crowding and increased incidence of acute respiratory infection in evacuees following the Great Eastern Japan Earthquake and tsunami. *Epidemiol Infect.* 2016;144(4):787–795.
118. Kuwabara H, Araki T, Yamasaki S, Ando S, Kano Y, Kasai K. Regional differences in post-traumatic stress symptoms among children after the 2011 tsunami in Higashi-Matsushima, Japan. *Brain Dev.* 2015;37(1):130–136.
119. Isaranuwatchai W, Coyte PC, McKenzie K, Noh S. The 2004 tsunami and mental health in Thailand: a longitudinal analysis of one-and two-year post-disaster data. *Disasters.* 2017;41(1):150–170.
120. Sitdhiraksa N, Piyasil V, Pariwatcharakul P, et al. Association of adolescent substance use: behavioral problems and family background among school students in tsunami affected area in southern Thailand. *J Med Assoc Thai.* 2014;97(suppl 6):58–65.
121. Dyb G, Jensen TK, Nygaard E. Children's and parents' posttraumatic stress reactions after the 2004 tsunami. *Clin Child Psychol Psychiatry.* 2011;16(4):621–634.
122. Terayama T, Shigemura J, Kobayashi Y, et al. Mental health consequences for survivors of the 2011 Fukushima nuclear disaster: a systematic review. Part 2: emotional and behavioral consequences. *CNS Spectr.* 2020:1–13.
123. Irwanto, Faisal, Zulfa H. Posttraumatic stress disorder among indonesian children 5 years after the tsunami. *Southeast Asian J Trop Med Public Health.* 2015;46(5):918–923.
124. Doocy S, Daniels A, Dooling S, Gorokhovich Y. The human impact of volcanoes: a historical review of events 1900–2009 and systematic literature review. *PLoS Curr.* 2013;5.

125. Tam E, Miike R, Labrenz S, et al. Volcanic air pollution over the Island of Hawai'i: emissions, dispersal, and composition. Association with respiratory symptoms and lung function in Hawai'i Island school children. *Environ Int.* 2016;92-93:543–552.
126. Gudmundsson G. Respiratory health effects of volcanic ash with special reference to Iceland: a review. *Clin Respir J.* 2011;5(1):2–9.
127. Zabert I, Benitez S, Maldonado C, Uribe Evhevarría L, Zabert GE. Prevalence of asthma at-risk symptoms in adolescents exposed to volcanic ash, in two Patagonian cities. Article in Spanish. *Rev Fac Cien Med Univ Nac Cordoba.* 2020;77(2):61–67.
128. Carlsen HK, Hauksdottir A, Valdimarsdottir UA, et al. Health effects following the Eyjafjallajokull volcanic eruption: a cohort study. *BMJ Open.* 2012;2(6).
129. Cadelis G, Tourres R, Molinie J, Petit RH. Exacerbations of asthma in Guadeloupe (French West Indies) and volcanic eruption in Montserrat (70 km from Guadeloupe). Article in French. *Rev Mal Respir.* 2013;30(3):203–214.
130. Baxter PJ, Jenkins S, Seswandhana R, et al. Human survival in volcanic eruptions: thermal injuries in pyroclastic surges, their causes, prognosis and emergency management. *Burns.* 2017;43(5):1051–1069.
131. Trisnawati I, Budiono E, Sumardi, Setiadi A. traumatic inhalation due to Merapi volcanic ash. *Acta Med Indones.* 2015;47(3):238–243.
132. Camarinho R, Garcia PV, Choi H, Rodrigues AS. Chronic exposure to non-eruptive volcanic activity as cause of bronchiolar histomorphological alteration and inflammation in mice. *Environ Pollut.* 2019;253:864–871.
133. Jones T, Bérubé K. The bioreactivity of the sub-10 mum component of volcanic ash: Soufrieìre Hills volcano, Montserrat. *J Hazard Mat.* 2011;194:128–134.
134. Nguyen HT, Wijayanti LW, Kim K, Lee WK, Lee CH, Shin K. High prevalence of cognitive impairment among students near Mount Merapi: a case study. *J Exerc Rehabil.* 2018;14(4):573–580.
135. Giacoppo S, Galuppo M, Calabro RS, et al. Heavy metals and neurodegenerative diseases: an observational study. *Biol Trace Elem Res.* 2014;161(2):151–160.
136. Balsa AI, Caffera M, Bloomfield J. Exposures to particulate matter from the eruptions of the Puyehue volcano and birth outcomes in Montevideo, Uruguay. *Environ Health Perspect.* 2016;124(11):1816–1822.
137. Warsini S, Buettner P, Mills J, West C, Usher K. Post-traumatic stress disorder among survivors two years after the 2010 Mount Merapi volcano eruption: a survey study. *Nurs Health Sci.* 2015;17(2):173–180.
138. Gan RW, Liu J, Ford B, et al. The association between wildfire smoke exposure and asthma-specific medical care utilization in Oregon during the 2013 wildfire season. *J Expo Sci Environ Epidemiol.* 2020;30(4):618–628.
139. Reid CE, Considine EM, Watson GL, Telesca D, Pfister GG, Jerrett M. Associations between respiratory health and ozone and fine particulate matter during a wildfire event. *Environ Int.* 2019;129:291–298.
140. Schranz CI, Castillo EM, Vilke GM. The 2007 San Diego wildfire impact on the emergency department of the University of California, San Diego hospital system. *Prehosp Disaster Med.* 2010;25(5):472–476.

141. Glass DC, Del Monaco A, Pircher S, Vander Hoorn S, Sim MR. Mortality and cancer incidence among male volunteer Australian firefighters. *Occup Environ Med.* 2017;74(9): 628–638.
142. Navarro KM, Kleinman MT, Mackay CE, et al. Wildland firefighter smoke exposure and risk of lung cancer and cardiovascular disease mortality. *Environ Res.* 2019;173:462–468.
143. Alman BL, Pfister G, Hao H, et al. The association of wildfire smoke with respiratory and cardiovascular emergency department visits in Colorado in 2012: a case crossover study. *Environ Health.* 2016;15(1):64.
144. Stowell JD, Geng G, Saikawa E, et al. Associations of wildfire smoke $PM_{2.5}$ exposure with cardiorespiratory events in Colorado, 2011–2014. *Environ Int.* 2019;133(part A):105151.
145. DeFlorio-Barker S, Crooks J, Reyes J, Rappold AG. Cardiopulmonary effects of fine particulate matter exposure among older adults, during wildfire and non-wildfire periods, in the United States, 2008–2010. *Environ Health Perspect.* 2019;127(3):37006.
146. Raines J, Snow R, Nichols D, Aisbett B. Fluid intake, hydration, work physiology of wildfire fighters working in the heat over consecutive days. *Ann Occup Hyg.* 2015;59(5):554–565.
147. Holstius DM, Reid CE, Jesdale BM, Morello-Frosch R. Birth weight following pregnancy during the 2003 Southern California wildfires. *Environ Health Perspect.* 2012;120(9): 1340–1345.
148. O'Donnell MH, Behie AM. Effects of wildfire disaster exposure on male birth weight in an Australian population. *Evol Med Public Health.* 2015;2015(1):344–354.
149. Kim YH, Tong H, Daniels M, et al. Cardiopulmonary toxicity of peat wildfire particulate matter and the predictive utility of precision cut lung slices. *Part Fibre Toxicol.* 2014;11:29.
150. Santos LR, Alves-Correia M, Cámara M, et al. Multiple victims of carbon monoxide poisoning in the aftermath of a wildfire: a case series. *Acta Med Port.* 2018;31(3):146–151.
151. Papadatou D, Giannopoulou I, Bitsakou P, Bellali T, Talias MA, Tselepi K. Adolescents' reactions after a wildfire disaster in Greece. *J Trauma Stress.* 2012;25(1):57–63.
152. Brown MRG, Agyapong V, Greenshaw AJ, et al. After the Fort McMurray wildfire there are significant increases in mental health symptoms in grade 7–12 students compared to controls. *BMC Psychiatry.* 2019;19(1):18.
153. Marshall GN, Schell TL, Miles JN. All PTSD symptoms are highly associated with general distress: ramifications for the dysphoria symptom cluster. *J Abnorm Psychol.* 2010;119(1): 126–135.
154. McAlister CN, Marble AE, Murray TJ. The 1917 Halifax explosion: the first coordinated local civilian medical response to disaster in Canada. *Can J Surg.* 2017;60(6):372–374.
155. Romolo FS, Aromatario M, Bottoni E, Cappelletti S, Fiore PA, Ciallella C. Accidental death involving professional fireworks. *Forensic Sci Int.* 2014;234:e5–e9.
156. Sanghi A, Ambrose RPK. Analysis of the effect of prevailing weather conditions on the occurrence of grain dust explosions. *J Agric Safety Health.* 2016;22(3):187–197.
157. Ramasamy A, Hill AM, Hepper AE, Bull AM, Clasper JC. Blast mines: physics, injury mechanisms and vehicle protection. *J R Army Med Corps.* 2009;155(4):258–264.
158. Ramasamy A, Hill AM, Masouros S, Gibb I, Bull AM, Clasper JC. Blast-related fracture patterns: a forensic biomechanical approach. *J R Soc Interface.* 2011;8(58):689–698.

159. Karimi H, Montevalian A, Motabar AR, Safari R, Parvas MS, Vasigh M. Epidemiology of paediatric burns in Iran. *Ann Burns Fire Disasters*. 2012;25(3):115–120.
160. Qin FJ, Chen Z, Zhao YH, et al. Analysis of effects of discipline cooperation on rescue and treatment of severe mass burn patients involved in August 2nd Kunshan factory aluminum dust explosion accident. Article in Chinese. *Zhonghua Shao Shang Za Zhi*. 2018;34(6):349–353.
161. Shao F, Ren WJ, Meng WZ, Wang GZ, Wang TY. Burn wound bacteriological profiles, patient outcomes, and tangential excision timing: a prospective, observational study. *Ostomy Wound Manage*. 2018;64(9):28–36.
162. Roeder RA, Schulman CI. An overview of war-related thermal injuries. *J Craniofac Surg*. 2010;21(4):971–975.
163. Jiang H, Xue C, Gao Y, Wang Y. Analysis of ocular injury characteristics in survivors of the 8.12 Tianjin Port explosion, China. *J Ophthalmol*. 2019;2019:1360805.
164. Zhang Y, Zhang MN, Jiang CH, Qiu HY. Analysis on characteristics of ocular trauma caused by military affairs in soldiers. Article in Chinese. *Zhonghua Yan Ke Za Zhi*. 2011;47(10):920–926.
165. Kalayci M, Er S, Tahtabasi M. Bomb explosion: ocular effects of primary, secondary and tertiary mechanisms. *Clin Ophthalmol*. 2020;14:1145–1151.
166. Tian LQ, Guo ZH, Meng WZ, et al. The abnormalities of coagulation and fibrinolysis in acute lung injury caused by gas explosion. *Kaohsiung J Med Sci*. 2020;36(suppl 6).
167. Arch-Tirado E, Garnica-Escamilla MA, Delgado-Hernández A, Campos-Muñoz T, Rodríguez-Rodríguez L, Verduzco-Mendoza A. Acoustic trauma generated by exposure to gun powder. Article in Spanish. *Cir Cir*. 2014;82(5):528–536.
168. Peng LH, Guo GH. Advances in the research of blast lung injury. Article in Chinese. *Zhonghua Shao Shang Za Zhi*. 2016;32(3):156–159.
169. Zhang YH, Guo GH, Shen GL, et al. Analysis on treatment of extremely severe burn patients with severe inhalation injury in August 2nd Kunshan factory aluminum dust explosion accident. Article in Chinese. *Zhonghua Shao Shang Za Zhi*. 2018;34(7):455–458.
170. Liu W. An accident of trichlorosilane explosion. Article in Chinese. *Zhonghua Lao Dong Wei Sheng Zhi Ye Bing Za Zhi*. 2011;29(3):175.
171. O'Neill TB, Rawlins J, Rea S, Wood F. Complex chemical burns following a mass casualty chemical plant incident: how optimal planning and organisation can make a difference. *Burns*. 2012;38(5):713–718.
172. Xing Y, Chen S, Zhu S, Zhang Y, Lu J. Exploring risk factors contributing to the severity of hazardous material transportation accidents in China. *Int J of Environ Res Public Health*. 2020;17(4).
173. Hansen MB, Birkeland MS, Nissen A, Blix I, Solberg O, Heir T. Prevalence and course of symptom-defined PTSD in individuals directly or indirectly exposed to terror: a longitudinal study. *Psychiatry*. 2017;80(2):171–183.
174. Su YJ. Prevalence and predictors of posttraumatic stress disorder and depressive symptoms among burn survivors two years after the 2015 Formosa Fun Coast Water Park explosion in Taiwan. *Eur J Psychotraumatol*. 2018;9(1):1512263.

175. Su YJ, Chow CC. PTSD, depression and posttraumatic growth in young adult burn survivors: three-year follow-up of the 2015 Formosa Fun Coast Water Park explosion in Taiwan. *J Affect Disord.* 2020;274:239–246.
176. Williams G, O'Malley M. Surgical considerations in the management of combined radiation blast injury casualties caused by a radiological dirty bomb. *Injury.* 2010;41(9):943–947.
177. Kobeissy F, Mondello S, Tumer N, et al. Assessing neuro-systemic & behavioral components in the pathophysiology of blast-related brain injury. *Front Neurol.* 2013;4:186.
178. Perez-Arredondo A, Cazares-Ramirez E, Carrillo-Mora P, et al. Baclofen in the therapeutic of sequele of traumatic brain injury: spasticity. *Clin Neuropharmacol.* 2016;39(6):311–319.
179. Cernak I. Blast injuries and blast-induced neurotrauma: overview of pathophysiology and experimental knowledge models and findings. In: Cernak I, Kobeissy FH, eds. *Brain Neurotrauma: Molecular, Neuropsychological, and Rehabilitation Aspects.* Boca Raton, FL: CRC Press/Taylor & Francis; 2015:chap. 15.
180. Li BC, Li Y, Xu C, et al. Blast-induced traumatic brain injury of goats in confined space. *Neurol Res.* 2014;36(11):974–982.
181. Manning WA. *The World Trade Center Bombing: Report and Analysis.* USFA-TR-076. New York, NY: US Fire Administration, Dept of Homeland Security; 1993.
182. Sanderson L. Fires. In: Noji ER, ed. *The Public Health Consequences of Disasters.* New York, NY: Oxford University Press; 1997:373–396.
183. Geldner G, Koch EM, Gottwald-Hostalek U, et al. Report on a study of fires with smoke gas development: determination of blood cyanide levels, clinical signs and laboratory values in victims. *Der Anaesthesist.* 2013;62(8):609–616.
184. Dumestre D, Nickerson D. Use of cyanide antidotes in burn patients with suspected inhalation injuries in North America: a cross-sectional survey. *J Burn Care Res.* 2014;35(2):e112–e117.
185. Guidotti T. Acute cyanide poisoning in prehospital care: new challenges, new tools for intervention. *Prehosp Disaster Med.* 2006;21(2):s40–s48.
186. Laugharne J, van der Watt G, Van de Watt G, Janca A. After the fire: the mental health consequences of fire disasters. *Curr Opin Psychiatry.* 2011;24(1):72–77.
187. Trinh NH, Nadler DL, Shie V, et al. Psychological sequelae of the Station Nightclub fire: comparing survivors with and without physical injuries using a mixed-methods analysis. *PloS One.* 2014;9(12):e115013.
188. Sanderson L. Toxicologic disasters: natural and technologic. In: Sullivan J, Krieger G, eds. *Hazardous Materials Toxicology: Clinical Principles of Environmental Health.* Philadelphia, PA: Lippincott Williams & Wilkins; 1992.
189. Berry L, Perera TB. EMS, hazardous waste response. In: *StatPearls* [Internet]. Treasure Island, FL: StatPearls Publishing; 2020. Available at: https://www.ncbi.nlm.nih.gov/books/NBK482193. Accessed November 26, 2022.
190. Keim M, Humphrey A, Dreyfuss A. *Situation Assessment Report Involving the Hazardous Material Disaster Site at LaGuaira Port, Venezuela.* CDC Report to Office of Disaster Assistance, US Agency for International Development; 2000.
191. Choi KH, Park MS, Ha M, Hur JI, Cheong HK. Cancer incidence trend in the Hebei Spirit oil spill area, from 1999 to 2014: an ecological study. *Int J Environ Res Public Health.* 2018;15(5):1006.

192. Diaz JH. The legacy of the Gulf oil spill: analyzing acute public health effects and predicting chronic ones in Louisiana. *Am J Disaster Med.* 2011;6(1):5–22.
193. Hildur K, Templado C, Zock JP, et al. Follow-up genotoxic study: chromosome damage two and six years after exposure to the Prestige oil spill. *PloS One.* 2015;10(7):e0132413.
194. Rispens JR, Jones SA, Clemmons NS, et al. Anhydrous ammonia chemical release—Lake County, Illinois, April 2019. *MMWR.* 2020;69(4):109–113.
195. Culley JM, Richter J, Donevant S, Tavakoli A, Craig J, DiNardi S. Validating signs and symptoms from an actual mass casualty incident to characterize an irritant gas syndrome agent (IGSA) exposure: a first step in the development of a novel IGSA triage algorithm. *J Emerg Nurs.* 2017;43(4):333–338.
196. Melnikova N, Wu J, Yang A, Orr M. Acute chemical incidents with injured first responders, 2002–2012. *Disaster Med Public Health Prep.* 2018;12(2):211–221.
197. Grainge C, Rice P. Management of phosgene-induced acute lung injury. *Clin Toxicol* (Phila). 2010;48(6):497–508.
198. Meselson M, Guillemin J, Hugh-Jones M, et al. The Sverdlovsk anthrax outbreak of 1979 *Science.* 1994;266(5188):1202–1208.
199. Čobeljić M. Smallpox outbreak in Yugoslavia in 1972. *Vojnosanitetski Pregl.* 2004;61(5):569–573.
200. Michaels D, Howard J. Review of the OSHA-NIOSH response to the Deepwater Horizon oil spill: protecting the health and safety of cleanup workers. *PLoS Curr.* 2012;4:e4fa83b7576b7576e.
201. Harville EW, Shankar A, Zilversmit L, Buekens P. Self-reported oil spill exposure and pregnancy complications: the GROWH study. *Int J Environ Res Public Health.* 2017;14(7).
202. Harville EW, Shankar A, Zilversmit L, Buekens P. The Gulf oil spill, miscarriage, and infertility: the GROWH study. *Int Arch Occup Environ Health.* 2018;91(1):47–56.
203. Nugent N, Gaston SA, Perry J, Rung AL, Trapido EJ, Peters ES. PTSD symptom profiles among Louisiana women affected by the 2010 Deepwater Horizon oil spill: a latent profile analysis. *J Affect Disord.* 2019;250:289–297.
204. Généreux M, Maltais D, Petit G, Roy M. Monitoring adverse psychosocial outcomes one and two years after the Lac-Mégantic train derailment tragedy (Eastern Townships, Québec, Canada). *Prehosp Disaster Med.* 2019;34(3):251–259.
205. Osofsky JD, Osofsky HJ, Weems CF, Hansel TC, King LS. Effects of stress related to the Gulf oil spill on child and adolescent mental health. *J Pediatr Psychol.* 2016;41(1):65–72.
206. Bromet E. Mental health consequences of the Chernobyl disaster. *J Radiol Prot.* 2012; 32(1):N71–N75.
207. Collins D. Human responses to the threat of or exposure to ionizing radiation at Three Mile Island, Pennsylvania, and Goiania, Brazil. *Mil Med.* 2002(suppl 2);167:137–138.
208. Molloy MS, Sherif Z, Natin S, McDonnel J. Management of mass gatherings. In: Koenig K, Schultz C, eds. *Disaster Medicine: Comprehensive Principles and Practices.* New York, NY: Cambridge University Press; 2010:228–252.
209. Hsieh YH, Ngai KM, Burkle FM, Jr., Hsu EB. Epidemiological characteristics of human stampedes. *Disaster Med Public Health Prep.* 2009;3(4):217–223.
210. El Warea M, Sasso R, Bachir R, El Sayed M. Riots in Beirut: Description of the impact of a new type of mass casualty event on the emergency system in Lebanon. *Disaster Med Public Health Prep.* 2019;13(5-6):849–852.

211. Tsouros AD, Efstathiou PA, eds. *Mass Gatherings and Public Health: The Experience of the Athens 2004 Olympic Games*. World Health Organization Europe; 2007. Available at: https://www.researchgate.net/publication/233387448_Mass_Gatherings_and_Public_Health. Accessed November 26, 2022.

212. Turris SA, Lund A, Bowles RR. An analysis of mass casualty incidents in the setting of mass gatherings and special events. *Disaster Med Public Health Prep*. 2014:1–7.

213. Tavakoli H, Khashayar P, Amoli HA, et al. Firework-related injuries in Tehran's Persian Wednesday Eve Festival (Chaharshanbe Soori). *J Emerg Med*. 2011;40(3):340–345.

214. Brennan RJ, Keim ME, Sharp TW, et al. Medical and public health services at the 1996 Atlanta Olympic Games: an overview. *Med J Aust*. 1997;167(11–12):595–598.

215. Aleeban M, Mackey TK. Global health and visa policy reform to address dangers of Hajj during summer seasons. *Front Public Health*. 2016;4:280.

216. Andrews T. Riots, deaths, sexual assault: maybe Woodstock was always a nightmare. *Washington Post*. August 13, 2019.

217. Ozer E, Yilmaz R, Evcuman D, et al. Autopsy evaluation of coal mining deaths in the city of Zonguldak, Turkey. *Med Sci Monit*. 2014;20:438–443.

218. Jafari H, Jafari AJ, Nekoei-Moghadam M, Goharinezhad S. Morbidity and mortality from technological disasters in Iran: a narrative review. *J Educ Health Promot*. 2019;8:147.

219. Luo X, Lin F, Zhu S, et al. Mine landslide susceptibility assessment using IVM, ANN and SVM models considering the contribution of affecting factors. *PloS One*. 2019;14(4):e0215134.

220. Thrush P. *A Dictionary of Mining, Mineral and Related Terms*. Washington, DC: US Bureau of Mines; 1968.

221. Orecka B, Sikora L, Misiołek M, et al. The quality of voice in coal-miners after burn/inhalation injury due to methane explosion. Article in Polish. *Otolaryngol Pol*. 2012;66(2):102–108.

222. Bolaños-Álvarez Y, Alonso-Hernández CM, Morabito R, Díaz-Asencio M, Pinto V, Gómez-Batista M. Mercury contamination of riverine sediments in the vicinity of a mercury cell chlor-alkali plant in Sagua River, Cuba. *Chemosphere*. 2016;152:376–382.

223. Hall HI, Dhara R, Price-Green PA, Kaye W. Surveillance for emergency events involving hazardous substances—United States, 1990–1992 *MMWR*. 1994;43(SS-2):1–6.

224. Wang X, Liu G, Hu R, Zhang H, Zhang M, Zhang F. Distribution, sources, and health risk assessment of volatile organic compounds in Hefei City. *Arch Environ Contam Toxicol*. 2020;78(3):392–400.

225. James AK, Nehzati S, Dolgova NV, et al. Rethinking the Minamata tragedy: what mercury species was really responsible? *Environ Sci Technol*. 2020;54(5):2726–2733.

226. Kloske M, Witkiewicz Z. Novichoks—the A group of organophosphorus chemical warfare agents. *Chemosphere*. 2019;221:672–682.

227. Worek F, Wille T, Koller M, Thiermann H. Toxicology of organophosphorus compounds in view of an increasing terrorist threat. *Arch Toxicol*. 2016;90(9):2131–2145.

228. Sawano T, Kambe T, Seno Y, et al. High internal radiation exposure associated with low socio-economic status six years after the Fukushima nuclear disaster: a case report. *Medicine* (Baltimore). 2019;98(47):e17989.

229. Li Q, Song P, Wen J. Melamine and food safety: a 10 year review. *Curr Opin Food Sci*. 2019;30:79–84.

230. Hanna-Attisha M. Lead poisoning in the 21st century: the silent epidemic continues. *Am J Public Health*. 2018;108:1430.

231. Cruz M, Keim M, Schier J, Gonzalez R, Valencia A, Telfer J. Organizational and command aspects for coordinating the public health response to an outbreak of acute renal failure, Republic of Panama, 2006. *Prehosp Disaster Med*. 2011;26(3):217–223.

232. Campos AMS, Bucaretchi F, Fernandes LCR, Fernandes CB, Capitani EM, Beck ARM. Toxic exposures in children involving legally and illegally commercialized household sanitizers. *Rev Paul Pediatr*. 2017;35(1):11–17.

233. Li Y, Gao Y, Yu X, Peng J, Ma F, Nelson L. Tetramine poisoning in China: changes over a decade viewed through the media's eye. *BMC Public Health*. 2014;14:842.

234. Desel H. Mass poisoning events. Article in German. *Med Klin Intensivmed Notfmed*. 2015;110(1):15–20.

235. Deng X, Li G, Mei R, Sun S. Long term effects of tetramine poisoning: an observational study. *Clin Toxicol* (Phila). 2012;50(3):172–175.

236. Jaworowski Z. Observations on the Chernobyl disaster and LNT. *Dose-Response*. 2010;8(2):148–171.

237. Hatch M, Cardis E. Somatic health effects of Chernobyl: 30 years on. *Eur J Epidemiol*. 2017;32:1047–1054.

238. Park AS, Ritz B, Ling C, Cockburn M, Heck JE. Exposure to ambient dichloromethane in pregnancy and infancy from industrial sources and childhood cancers in California. *Int J Hyg Environ Health*. 2017;220(7):1133–1140.

239. Kruger D, Cupal S, Franzen S, et al. Toxic trauma: household water quality experiences predict posttraumatic stress disorder symptoms during the Flint, Michigan, water crisis. *J Community Psychol*. 2017;45(7):957–962.

240. Oshima T, Yoshikawa H, Ohtani M, Mimasaka S. Three cases of suprachoroidal hemorrhage associated with chest compression or asphyxiation and detected using postmortem computed tomography. *Leg Med* (Tokyo). 2015;17(3):188–191.

241. Colville-Ebeling B, Freeman M, Banner J, Lynnerup N. Autopsy practice in forensic pathology—evidence-based or experience-based? A review of autopsies performed on victims of traumatic asphyxia in a mass disaster. *J Forensic Leg Med*. 2014;22: 33–36.

242. US Occupatonal Safety and Health Administration. Structural collapse guide. Emergency preparedness guides. 2022. Available at: https://www.osha.gov/emergency-preparedness/guides/structural-collapse. Accessed December 5, 2022.

243. Ingrassia P, Geddo A, Lombardi F, Della Corte F. Events associated with structural collapse/crashing/crushing. In: Ciottone G, Darling R, Anderson P, et al., eds. *Disaster Medicine*. 3rd ed. Philadelphia, PA: Mosby-Elsevier; 2006:817–859.

244. Holtz TM, Leighton J, Balter S, Weiss D, Blank S, Weisfuse I. The public health response to the World Trade Center disaster. In: Levy BS, Sidel VS, eds. *Terrorism and Public Health*. New York, NY: Oxford University Press; 2003:19–48.

245. Boodram B, Torian L, Thomas P, et al. Rapid assessment of injuries among survivors of the terrorist attack on the World Trade Center—New York City, September 2001. *MMWR*. 2002;51(1):1–5.

246. Perritt KR, Herbert R, Levin SM, Moline J. Work-related injuries and illnesses reported by World Trade Center response workers and volunteers. *Prehosp Disaster Med.* 2011;26(6): 401–407.
247. Boffetta P, Hall C, Todd A, et al. Cancer risk among World Trade Center rescue and recovery workers: a review. *CA Cancer J Clin.* 2022;72(4):308–314.
248. Beusse R, Hatfield J, Fabirkiewicz S, et al. *EPA's Response to the World Trade Center Collapse: Challenges, Successes, and Areas of Improvement.* EPA Report No. 2003-P-00012. Environmental Protection Agency (EPA); 2003.
249. Postma IL, Weel H, Heetveld MJ, et al. Mass casualty triage after an airplane crash near Amsterdam. *Injury.* 2013;44(8):1061–1067.
250. Postma IL, Winkelhagen J, Bloemers FW, et al. February 2009 airplane crash at Amsterdam Schiphol Airport: an overview of injuries and patient distribution. *Prehosp Disaster Med.* 2011;26(4):299–304.
251. Centers for Disease Control and Prevention (CDC). Fatal and nonfatal injuries involving fishing vessel winches—southern shrimp fleet, United States, 2000–2011. *MMWR.* 2013;62(9):157–160.
252. Doohan I, Bjornstig U, Ostlund U, Saveman BI. Exploring injury panorama, consequences, and recovery among bus crash survivors: a mixed-methods research study. *Prehosp Disaster Med.* 2017;32(2):165–174.
253. Postma IL, Winkelhagen J, Bijlsma TS, Bloemers FW, Heetveld MJ, Goslings JC. Delayed diagnosis of injury in survivors of the February 2009 crash of flight TK 1951. *Injury.* 2012;43(12):2012–2017.
254. Goers M, Leidman E, Sultan AS, Hassan A, Bilukha O. Injury-related deaths before and during the Islamic State insurgency—Baghdad, Iraq, 2010–2015. *Confl Health.* 2020;14:8.
255. Morita S, Omata A, Yoshizaki C, Miura N, Inokuchi S. The fatal fire accident of the Japanese high-speed railway lines (Shinkansen). *Burns.* 2016;42(1):232–233.
256. Khodadadizadeh A, Jahangiri K, Khorasani-Zavareh D, Vazirinejad R. Epidemiology of vehicle fire fatalities of road traffic injuries in Kerman Province, Iran: a cross-sectional study. *Open Access Maced J Med Sci.* 2019;7(12):2036–2043.
257. Zakrevskii YN, Shevchenko AG, Peretechikov AV, Serdyuk VI, Arkhangelskii DA. Combined mechanical-cold and mechanical-burn injuries in patients injured in maritime disasters. Article in Russian. *Voen Med Zh.* 2015;336(6):34–40.
258. Lincoln JM, Lucas DL. Occupational fatalities in the United States commercial fishing industry, 2000–2009. *J Agromed.* 2010;15(4):343–350.
259. Doohan I, Gyllencreutz L, Bjornstig U, Saveman BI. Survivors' experiences of consequences and recovery five years after a major bus crash. *Scand J Caring Sci.* 2018;32(3):1179–1187.
260. Lenferink LIM, de Keijser J, Smid GE, Djelantik A, Boelen PA. Prolonged grief, depression, and posttraumatic stress in disaster-bereaved individuals: latent class analysis. *Eur J Psychotrauma.* 2017;8(1):1298311.
261. Floret N, Viel JF, Mauny F, Hoen B, Piarroux R. Negligible risk for epidemics after geophysical disasters. *Emerg Infect Dis.* 2006;12(4):543–548.

9

Upstream: Causal Pathways of Disaster-Related Disease

LEARNING OBJECTIVES

Upon completion, the reader will be able to

1. Define the following terms:
   - Assumptions
   - Candidate cause
   - Causal assessment
   - Causal pathway
   - Functional ability
   - Modifiable risk factor
2. Recognize candidate causes of disease according to six ecosocial levels as follows:
   - Macro: related to beliefs, attitudes, policies
   - Exo: related to societal resources
   - Meso: related to the environment
   - Micro: related to people
   - Individual: related to the person
   - Chrono: related to age and life stage
3. Recognize likely causes of disaster-related disease according to six ecosocial levels as follows:
   - Macro: related to beliefs, attitudes, policies
   - Exo: related to societal resources
   - Meso: related to the environment
   - Micro: related to people
   - Individual: related to the person
   - Chrono: related to age and life stage

THE CAUSES OF THE CAUSE

Many of the causes of excess morbidity and mortality are associated with social inequality. "Multiple intersecting causes and multiple forms of morbidity characterize social exclusion. The result is people with little hope or prospects and considerably shortened lives."[1] It is among these distal determinants of health (DoH) that pathways of causation first originate. Seated within the context of societal beliefs and attitudes are the undercurrents of public sentiment that create, sustain, tolerate, or ignore public opinion and policy. Here, the "causes of the cause" arise, some born out of a primitive need for social inclusion (or exclusion). This perception of "us" and "them" provides a familiar framework for adjudicating privilege, opportunity, equity, burden, and disease risk.

> "Us and them. And, in the end, we're only ordinary men."[2]
>
> –Roger Waters and Richard Wright

CAUSAL ASSESSMENT

According to an ecosocial model of health, disease is caused by the interaction of individual characteristics within ecological and social contexts. Causal assessments are used to determine the root causes of environmental exposures that may result in adverse health effects. No single method can accommodate the range and diversity of evidence available. CADDIS, the US government's Causal Analysis/Diagnosis Decision Information System, is one example of a system used for causal analysis and decision-making related to hazardous materials in the environment.[3]

Assessments begin by establishing a case definition for the health condition being assessed. Once defined, **candidate causes** are listed, and conceptual models are developed for each candidate cause. The data are then evaluated using fundamental methods that address simple situations with only one candidate cause. Thus, the most likely cause or causes are identified based on available evidence.

CAUSAL PATHWAYS

Causal pathways depict the intermediate steps between what may be multiple DoH and the proximate cause of disease. By contrast, after exposure has already occurred, the natural history of disease represents the intermediate steps between the proximate cause and the observed health outcome. Causal assessments often use flow diagrams to illustrate the steps involved in a causal pathway. Causal pathway diagrams represent **assumptions** about the relationship between exposures, outcomes, and covariates.[3]

CAUSAL PATHWAYS FOR DISASTER-RELATED DISEASE

Upstream Factors and the Causal Pathway

As discussed in Chapter 3, health is determined by a complex set of factors that include the proximate cause of hazardous exposures and the more distal upstream DoH that occur at the level of the **individual**, family, community, or society. (See Table 3-2.) Characteristics of the individual (e.g., demographic, psychological, physiological) often serve as both risk and protective factors for determining the likelihood of illness and disease. These upstream factors include a range of personal characteristics that make exposures, and thus resultant disease, more likely to occur.

In addition to personal factors, an individual's family, community, and societal context encompass crucial DoH. They include upstream factors such as social, technological, economic, environmental, cultural, and political influences that make exposures (and resultant disease) more likely to occur.

Some upstream risk and protective factors are modifiable (e.g., behavior), while others are not (e.g., age). Some are considered intrinsic to the individual (e.g., race), while others are acquired (e.g., education). The best opportunity for intervention exists among those DoH that may be modified or acquired. Figure 9-1 provides a listing of candidate causes commonly associated with disease development. All these factors are thought to influence the likelihood of hazardous exposure. In other words, all are considered potential DoH.

Societal beliefs and attitudes provide a broad context for policies that either increase or decrease the risk of exposure. These beliefs may be related to diversity, equity, environmental justice, and human rights and under the influence of economics, climate, interpersonal conflicts, and risk perceptions. The availability of societal resources also plays into the likelihood of hazardous exposure. Various potential resources provide better leverage for preventing hazards and exposures. Environmental factors, including the weather, season, topography, time of day, and built environment, are essential in

Macro	Exo	Meso	Micro	Individual
BELIEFS	RESOURCES	ENVIRONMENT	PEOPLE	PERSON
• Accessibility • Conflict • Culture • Equality • Equity • Food • Health • Human rights • Justice • Norms • Resources • Risk • Self	• Commercial • Economic • Environmental • Financial • Governmental • Human • Informational • Legal • Logistical • Medical • Organizational • Political • Social • Technological	• Built environment • Community • Healthcare facilities • Home • Incarceration • Markets • Natural environment • Neighborhood • Public safety • Workplace	• Advocates • Care providers • Coworkers • Criminals • Family and friends • Healthcare workers • Leaders • Media • Neighbors • Retailers • Patients • Police • Service providers • Teachers	• Age • Behavior • Ethnicity • Functional ability • Genetics • Health status • Race • Sex and gender • Education • Income/SES • Motivation • Occupation • Nutrition • Safety • Security

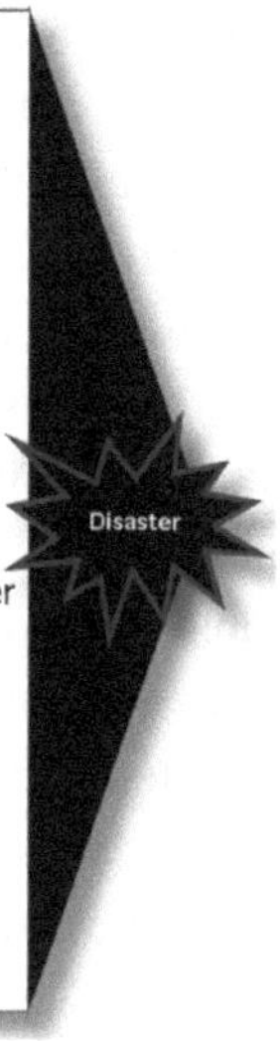

Figure 9-1. Upstream Factors Affecting Health Outcome

determining a person's risk for life-threatening exposures. In addition to this ecological environment, the social environment involving community services, social networks, and socioeconomic status is an important influence in avoiding exposure. More proximal to the individual, the close social network of a person's family, friends, coworkers, and community also provides practical and technical assistance, psychosocial support, and risk communication that directly assist the individual in avoiding exposure. And finally, the person's individual risk and protective factors also significantly influence the likelihood of exposure. Persons with limited functional abilities, for example, may not receive adequate warning or be able to evacuate hazardous areas. Behaviors may be protective or maladaptive. Race, ethnicity, sex, and age are significant predictors of hazardous exposure. A person's education and occupation may also influence the type or degree of exposure a person may incur. Thus, it may be said that exposures are determined by a wide variety of DoH that begin proximal to the individual and extend distally to include the population.

The Downstream Causal Pathway for Disaster-Related Disease

Upstream factors have an enormous impact on the likelihood of disaster-related disease. Some populations are more likely to experience disaster-related disease than others. This pattern is recurrent and pervasive enough to be entirely predictable. As the saying goes, Disasters seek out the poor and bind them in their poverty. Is this because disasters have some inherent hatred toward the disadvantaged? Is it because of some unspoken transgression or sin committed by the poor? Of course not. Disaster hazards predominantly affect resource-poor populations due to pre-determined risk factors that result in a much higher degree of exposure to these hazards than their more privileged counterparts. It is, therefore, not an effective health strategy to wait for such populations to become exposed and then treat the resultant disease, especially using the same health care systems that were previously underresourced and poorly accessible even before the disaster.

Upstream DoH are easily considered in terms of Bronfenbrenner's ecosocial model of health. In this approach, individual risk and protective factors are related to a person's functional ability, behavior, genetics, race, ethnicity, sex, or gender. These individual risk and protective factors also influence a person's life stage (e.g., newborn, infant, child, adolescent, adult, or elderly).

In addition to these individual factors related to the person, upstream DoH also include a range of contexts that influence health outcomes. This range extends from influences that are most proximal to the individual to other DoH that are more overarching and distal as follows:

- individual: related to the person
- micro: related to people in one's life

- meso: related to one's environment
- exo: related to resources available in one's society
- macro: related to beliefs, attitudes, culture, policies
- chrono: related to age and life stage

Let us consider an example of the influence of upstream DoH on heat wave disasters. Klinenberg's study of the 1995 Chicago heat wave that killed 700 people described how the physical and social isolation of the elderly, the institutional abandonment of poor neighborhoods, and the absence of public assistance programs contributed to the high fatality rates.[4] (See Figure 9-2.) These high fatality rates were exacerbated among isolated, poor, elderly black and Hispanic populations that lived in poorly ventilated, brick apartment buildings located within the heat islands of the inner city.[4]

According to an ecosocial model (see Table 3-2), risk factors for heat wave–related mortality were associated with individual DoH, including age, functional ability, behavior, race, and ethnicity. However, there is also good evidence that heat wave–related disease is also influenced by a person's domicile, family, friends, and neighborhood. The person's socioeconomic status and sense of community (or lack thereof) also affected health outcomes, as did the natural and built environment. In addition, the societal interaction between commercial, economic, and political factors further exacerbated the environmental conditions that resulted in health hazards. And finally, at the macro level, mortality occurred as a result of socio-political conflict related to culture, resources, and a changing climate.

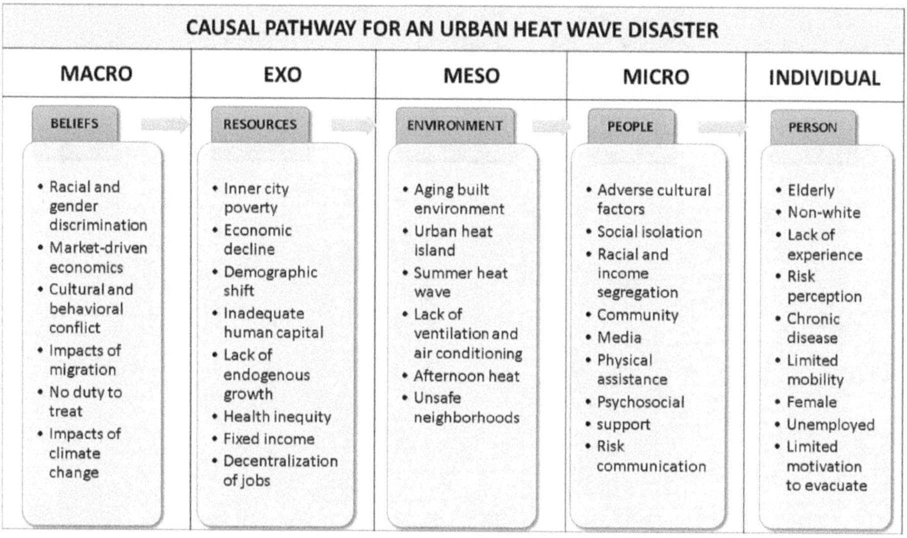

Source: Based on Klinenberg,[4] Teitz and Chapple,[5] and Bronfenbrenner.[6]

Figure 9-2. Example of the Development of Disaster-Related Disease, According to an Ecosocial Model

TOPICS FOR DISCUSSION

1. Select one natural disaster (other than a heat wave) and for it create a causal pathway that includes five levels of the ecosocial model (i.e., macro, exo, meso, micro, and individual).
2. Select one technological disaster and for it create a causal pathway that includes five levels of the ecosocial model (i.e., macro, exo, meso, micro, and individual).
3. Compare and contrast the causal pathways for natural and technological disasters.

REFERENCES

1. Marmot M. Inclusion health: addressing the causes of the causes. *Lancet.* 2017;391(10117): 186–188.
2. Waters R, Wright R. *Us and Them.* Pink Floyd. March 1, 1973. Available at: https://genius.com/Pink-floyd-us-and-them-lyrics. Accessed January 19, 2023.
3. US Environmental Protection Agency (EPA). Causal Analysis/Diagnosis Decision Information System (CADDIS). 2021. Available at: https://www.epa.gov/caddis. Accessed November 29, 2022.
4. Klinenberg E. *Heat Wave: A Social Autopsy of Disaster in Chicago.* 2nd ed. Chicago, IL: University of Chicago Press; 2015.
5. Teitz MB, Chapple K. The causes of inner-city poverty: eight hypotheses in search of reality. *J Policy Dev Res.* 1998;3(3):33–70.
6. Bronfenbrenner U. Ecological systems theory. In: Vasta R, ed. *Six Theories of Child Development: Revised Formulations and Current Issues.* London, UK: Jessica Kingsley Publishers; 1992: 187–249.

10

Downstream: The Natural History of Disaster-Related Disease

LEARNING OBJECTIVES

Upon completion, the reader will be able to

1. Define the following terms and phrases:
   - All-hazard approach
   - Epidemiology
   - Hierarchy of process control
2. Recognize wellness and illness in terms of upstream and downstream determinants that occur before and after hazardous exposures.
3. Recall five phases in the natural history of disease model.
4. Recognize three stages in the natural history of disease: upstream determinants, hazardous exposures, and downstream determinants.
5. Recognize the five tiers of Frieden's public health impact pyramid in terms of both impact and individual effort needed.
6. Recognize upstream determinants of health (DoH) according to five levels in an ecosocial model (i.e., macro, exo, meso, micro, and individual).
7. Recognize the downstream DoH according to five levels in an ecosocial model (i.e., macro, exo, meso, micro, and individual).

NATURAL HISTORY OF DISEASE

Progression of the Disease Process

Let's consider Schultz's "production of health" as a process for achieving wellness. The natural history of disease model consists of a succession of states or subprocesses and involves factors that may affect costs, quality, and length of life.[1,2]

Natural history is one of the major elements of descriptive epidemiology. It refers to the progression of the disease process in an individual over time in the absence of treatment. Understanding the natural history of disease is essential to recognizing opportunities for prevention across the spectrum of illness.

The natural history of disaster-related health outcomes is influenced by a range of factors that occur as a result of hazardous exposures. The course of illness is, therefore,

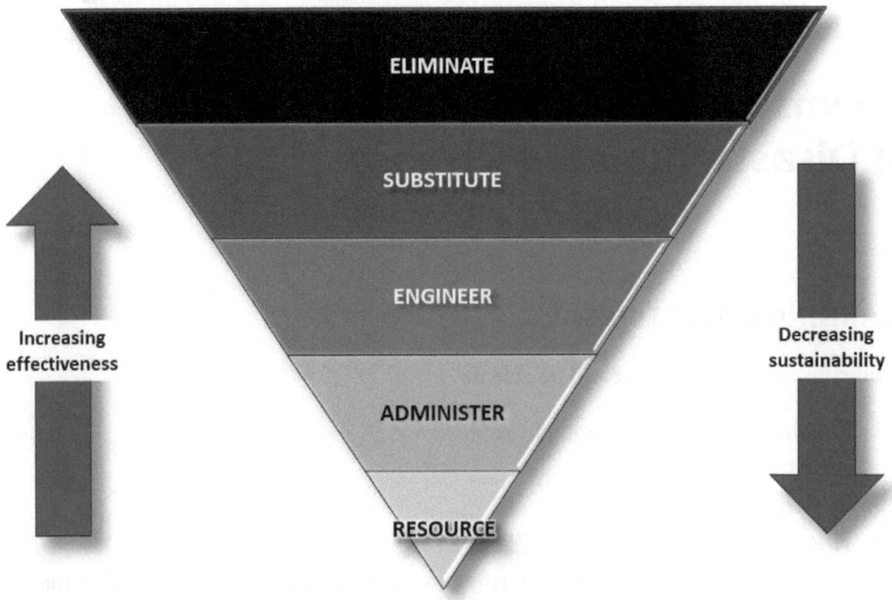

Source: Keim.[4] Adapted with permission of Cambridge University Press. © Cambridge University Press 2021.

Figure 10-1. The Hierarchy of Process Control

predictable for disaster-related disease. This predictability allows interventions to address not only those modifiable risk and protective factors related to the individual but also those DoH related to other people, places, resources, beliefs, and life stage. Understanding and recognizing the natural history of disaster-related disease allows modifications to occur upstream and downstream from disaster-related exposures. This comprehensive approach is based on a **process control hierarchy** that prioritizes processes—producing health over resourcing and maintenance of solutions.[3] (See Figure 10-1.)[4]

Figure 3-4 depicts the natural history of disease, the concept of disease as a process that unfolds over time in a series of steps.[5,6] This model considers the progression of a disease process as occurring in distinct stages. If left untreated, a disease will evolve through a series of stages that characterize its "natural course."[7]

The goal of public health and medicine is to discover the natural progression of a disease and to intervene as early as possible. The natural history is modified if an intervention is applied, producing a typical clinical course for the condition. Effective disease management requires not only the management of the immediate problem (downstream) but also the management of the patient's (upstream) DoH and proximate causes, or etiology. (See Figure 8-1.)

Figure 10-2 outlines a process that begins with a healthy individual being exposed to a pathogenic (e.g., biological, thermal, toxicological, or kinetic) hazard. The process

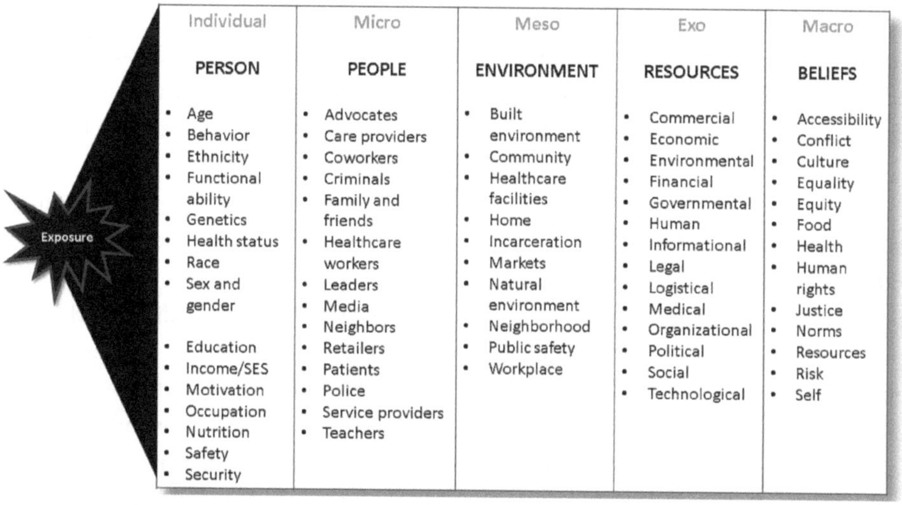

Figure 10-2. Downstream Factors Affecting Health Outcome

starts with exposure to or accumulating factors sufficient for the disease to begin in a susceptible host.

Occasionally, pathological changes may begin without apparent symptoms (i.e., subclinical disease). This stage of subclinical disease extending from the time of exposure to the onset of disease symptoms is referred to as the incubation period for infectious diseases and the latency period for chronic diseases and some injuries. Symptoms may appear after a delay that can vary from seconds (as with injury) to days (as with infections) to years (as with cancer). Patients may interpret their symptoms as indicating an illness and seek professional care.

Clinical disease begins when the patient recognizes the illness and seeks care for the symptoms. Once the diagnosis is made, health care providers seek to intervene downstream in the natural history of the disease through courses of treatment. This clinical course then results in one of the following health outcomes: recovery, ongoing impairment, disability, or death.

Downstream Factors in Disease Progression

In addition to upstream factors that occur beforehand are a range of factors that affect health outcomes after exposure. These downstream factors involve the individual's characteristics and ecosocial context. Some persons are more likely than others to become exposed. Once exposed, some individuals are less likely to recognize illness and seek care (for various reasons, including their family, social network, community, society, or belief system). In addition, some persons simply have less access to quality health care and other resources that will alleviate their illness once it occurs. Downstream interventions tend to focus on providing information or clinical care to this subset of disaster-affected individuals within the population. Figure 10-2 outlines the natural history of disease overlaid across an ecosocial model for health, the process-person-context time (PPCT) model.

This natural history of disease begins with hazardous exposure as the proximate cause or etiology. After exposure, the natural history of disease may be considered to occur within an ecosocial context. In other words, once exposure has occurred, the health outcome is subsequently influenced by a series of factors that begin with individual characteristics and extend to society's aspects (i.e., PPCT). The five columns in Figure 10-2 represent categories of the ecosocial context, ranging from the person to the overall culture. In the far-left column, examples of both intrinsic and acquired individual risk and protective factors are listed. Many of the social DoH are listed in column 2 at the micro level and extend throughout the meso, exo, and macro levels to become further affected by the environment, available resources, and guiding values and beliefs. The micro level represents the social support system available to the individual at risk; correspondingly, the meso level represents the environmental context within which subsequent diseases will occur, progress, and then be diagnosed and, ideally, treated, leading to recovery.

The fourth column of "exo" context represents those resources of society at large (i.e., capacity) that may become available to prevent the progression of (1) health to disease after an exposure or (2) disease to death or permanent disability. Finally, in the fifth "macro" column, we see the more extensive societal belief systems that influence national, local, and interpersonal policies. These beliefs can potentially affect the quality and accessibility of health care, even at the last moment. Thus, it can be said that in practice, the natural history of disease unfolds within the context of human experience. This human development experience is driven by social and ecological factors that extend from the individual to society and vice versa.

The health impact pyramid is used to illustrate how downstream interventions that address the individual (e.g., counseling, education, and clinical care) typically require more personal effort on the part of the individual and have less impact than upstream factors that address context over time (e.g., micro, meso, exo, and macro levels of interaction). In summary, the more a public health intervention depends on the actions of individuals, the less impact it may be expected to have on the entire population. (See Figure 10-3.)[8]

Causes of Disaster-Related Disease

Disaster-related disease is caused when susceptible populations are exposed to biological, climatological, geophysical, hydrological, and/or meteorological hazards that create biological, toxic, thermal, and/or kinetic health hazards. As is the case for all diseases,

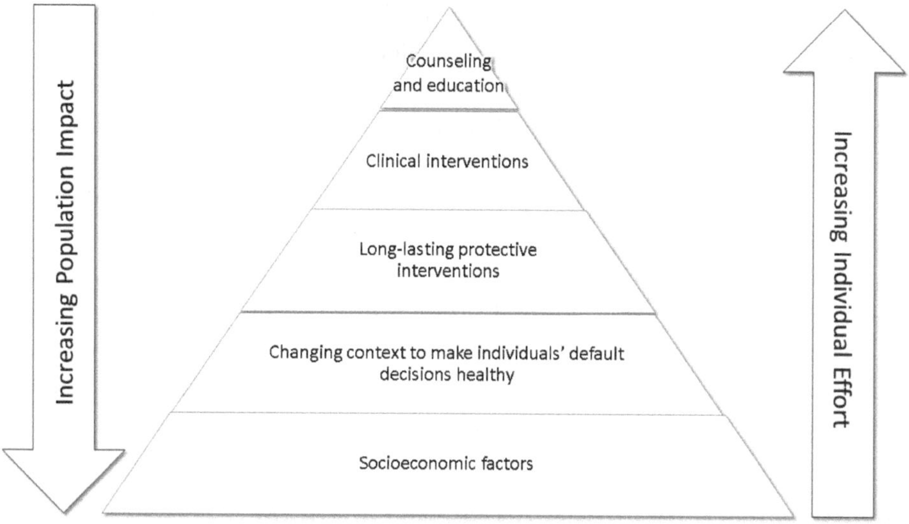

Source: Adapted from Frieden.[8]

Figure 10-3. The Health Impact Pyramid

disaster-related diseases do not occur randomly. The natural history of disaster-related diseases is therefore predictable.

In the case of disasters, otherwise healthy populations become exposed to disaster-related health hazards either directly or indirectly. Direct exposures involve proximity to the hazard itself. Indirect exposures occur because of population displacement or the loss of other critical resources that increase the possibility of secondary exposures. Once exposed, persons may or may not experience subclinical disease, and they may or may not be able to have their symptoms diagnosed and treated because of a lack of access to medical care. This high degree of variability necessitates a more complex and strategic approach to meeting disaster-related health care needs. For example, the **all-hazard approach** has been used to describe an all-inclusive strategy of preparing for downstream emergency response activities to the range of likely hazards.

By comparison, the natural history of disease model considers the progression of a disease process as occurring in distinct stages. In the case of disasters, the goal of the medical profession remains the same: to discover the natural progression of a disease and to intervene as early as possible. The opportunities to intervene in the natural history of disaster-related disease include upstream and downstream determinants. Effective management of disaster-related disease requires addressing the outcomes and the root causes.

The natural history of disaster-related disease varies according to the specific, individual disaster hazard. For example, biological disasters result from exposure to pathogenic organisms. This exposure may be unintentional (e.g., a natural outbreak or accidental release) or the result of a deliberate and malicious act (e.g., biowarfare). Victims first develop subclinical and clinical disease at variable rates according to the pathogen. Depending on the specific hazard (e.g., respiratory, neurological, or hematological), signs and symptoms may involve various body organ systems. The clinician's ability to diagnose and treat the patient efficiently and effectively also depends on the specific hazard and diagnostic capability. In addition to creating the course of illness in one individual person, communicable diseases may be transmitted during the subclinical and clinical phase, amplifying the hazard's impact on the entire population at risk.

While all types of disasters result in exacerbations of chronic disease, compared with biological disasters, the natural history of disease associated with other natural and technological disasters most often results in injury rather than infection. Excluding biological disasters, all other disaster-related diseases are caused by toxic, thermal, or kinetic health hazards that result mainly in traumatic or metabolic injury.

Downstream Factors Affecting Health Outcomes

Once exposed, disaster-affected populations are also affected by various downstream factors that affect health outcomes. Like all DoH, downstream DoH may also be considered in the ecosocial (PPCT) model. According to this model, individual risk and protective factors are related to a person's functional ability, behavior, genetics, race, ethnicity, sex, or gender. These individual risk and protective factors also influence a person's life stage (e.g., newborn, infant, child, adolescent, adult, or elderly). (See Figure 10-4.)

Let us now consider an example of the influence of downstream DoH on heat wave disasters, again using Klinenberg's social autopsy of the 1995 Chicago heat wave.

NATURAL HISTORY OF AN URBAN HEAT WAVE DISASTER				
INDIVIDUAL	**MICRO**	**MESO**	**EXO**	**MACRO**
PERSON	PEOPLE	ENVIRONMENT	RESOURCES	BELIEFS
• 70-year-old black female • History of diabetes and hypertension • Cannot climb stairs. • Social security and Medicare recipient • Anxious, fearful • Now-onset of stroke	• Lives in social isolation • Found by neighbors • Low-income black neighborhood • Limited community services • No physical assistance • No psychosocial support	• Lives in 3rd floor brick apartment • No ventilation • Inner city hospital with peak service utilization • Power outage and hospital operating on generator • Limited human resources • High crime neighborhood	• Inadequate medical access • Inadequate medical quality • Limited rehabilitative services • Limited resources for assisted living • Increased cost of living • Less resources in the future	• Age, racial and gender discrimination • Market-driven economics • Cultural conflict • Duty to treat • Altruism • Public service

Figure 10-4. Example of the Natural History of Disaster-Related Disease

This natural history begins with the person's characteristics after exposure to hazardous heat. Figure 10-4 represents a case involving a 70-year-old Black female with a history of chronic disease who has suffered a stroke caused by the heat wave. She cannot climb stairs but lives on the third floor of a poorly ventilated brick apartment and is therefore highly dependent on social interactions for her health. Her windows are kept closed and locked because of the high level of crime in her neighborhood. She lives in relative social isolation with limited community services and a lack of physical or psychosocial support. When neighbors find her, her stroke has progressed beyond a reversible stage. After waiting for volunteer emergency medical services to arrive, she is transported to the nearest public hospital. The hospital is overloaded by the significant surge of patients during a power outage. Once one physician makes a diagnosis, she is admitted to the hospital by another. Days later she is discharged to home with recommendations to follow up with her physician. Her neighbors pick her up at the hospital and help to carry her up the stairs to her apartment. Medicare is billed $20,000 for the cost of her hospitalization. Over the next six months, her diabetic control worsens. She worries about the future. Public policy does not change.

TOPICS FOR DISCUSSION

1. Compare the disease incubation period for severe infectious disease (e.g., COVID-19) to the latency period for severe injuries (e.g., skull fracture during an earthquake).
2. Compare windows of opportunity—that is, the length of time available for interventions to occur during the incubation period for infectious disease and the latency period for injury.
3. Describe what is meant by the health impact pyramid description of "changing the context to make an individual's default decisions healthy."
4. Describe what is meant by "the causes of the cause" of disaster-related disease.

REFERENCES

1. Dias S, Welton NJ, Sutton AJ, Ades AE. Evidence synthesis for decision making 5: the baseline natural history model. *Med Decis Making*. 2013;33(5):657–670.
2. Schultz J, Sullivan L, Galea S. *Public Health: An Introduction to the Science and Practice of Population Health*. New York, NY: Springer Publishing; 2021.
3. Bequette B. *Process Control: Modeling, Design, and Simulation*. Upper Saddle River, NJ: Prentice Hall; 2003.
4. Keim, M. *Disaster Planning: A Practical Guide for Effective Health Outcomes.* Cambridge UK: Cambridge University Press; 2021.
5. Keim M. Managing disaster-related health risk: a process for prevention. *Prehosp Disaster Med.* 2018;33(3):326–334.

6. Association of Faculties of Medicine of Canada. AFMC primer on population health. 2017. Available at: http://phprimer.afmc.ca/Glossary. Accessed November 28. 2022.
7. Jewell N. Natural history of diseases: statistical designs and issues. *Clinl Pharmacol Ther.* 2016;100(4):353–361.
8. Frieden T. A framework for public health action: the health impact pyramid. *Am J Public Health.* 2010;100(4):590–595.

IV. THE EPIDEMIOLOGY OF DISASTER-RELATED DISEASE

11

Public Health Consequences of Disasters

LEARNING OBJECTIVES

Upon completion, the reader will be able to

1. Define the following terms and phrases:
   - Household goods
   - Mass casualty incident (MCI)
   - Planning
   - Public health impact
   - Risk perception
   - Sanitation
   - Scenario
2. Recognize that most disaster hazards cause the same 16 public health consequences, differing mostly in scale.
3. Recognize use of capability-based planning to address 16 predictable public health consequences of disasters.

HEALTH CONSEQUENCES OF DISASTER HAZARDS

At-risk populations face a broad range of hazards with many possible scenarios.[1] While the hazards that cause disasters may vary greatly, fortunately the potential public health consequences and subsequent public health and medical needs of the population do not.[2,3] Regardless of the hazard, most disasters result in the same set of major public health consequences. This unpredictability is poorly suited to **scenario**-based approaches.

For example, warfare, chemical releases, floods, hurricanes, and earthquakes all displace people from their homes. These hazards require the same sheltering capability with only minor adjustments based on the rapidity of onset, scale, duration, location, and intensity.

Many disasters cause the same public health consequences regardless of the hazard.

The Public Health Impacts of Individual Natural Disasters

Table 11-1 summarizes various natural disasters' relative public health impacts.[4] This table generally illustrates how many of these disaster hazards cause the same 16 public

Table 11-1. The Relative Public Health Impact of Natural Disasters

Public Health Impact	Geophysical				Hydrometeorological					Climatological		Biological	
	Earthquake	Tsunami	Volcanic Eruption	Landslide	Tornado and Storm	Cyclone	Flood	Heat	Cold	Drought	Wildfire	Epidemic	Pandemic
Deaths	Many	Many	Few	Few	Few	Few to many	Few to many	Moderate to many	Few	Few to many	Few	Moderate to many	Many
Cases	Many	Moderate	Few	Few	Moderate	Moderate to many	Many	Moderate	Many	Many	Few	Many	Many
Loss of clean water	Local to broad	Local to broad	Local to broad	Local	Local	Local to broad	Local to broad	Local	Local	Broad	Local	Unlikely	Unlikely
Loss of shelter	Local to broad	Local to broad	Local to broad	Local	Local	Local to broad	Local to broad	Local	Local	Local to broad	Local	Unlikely	Unlikely
Loss of household goods	Local to broad	Local to broad	Local to broad	Local	Local	Local to broad	Local to broad	Unlikely	Unlikely	Local to broad	Local	Unlikely	Unlikely
Population displacement	Local to broad	Local to broad	Local to broad	Local	Local	Local to broad	Local to broad	Local	Local	Local to broad	Local	Unlikely	Unlikely
Loss of hygiene	Local to broad	Local to broad	Local to broad	Local	Local	Local to broad	Local to broad	Local		Broad	Local	Unlikely	Unlikely
Loss of sanitation	Local to broad	Local to broad	Local to broad	Local	Local	Local to broad	Local to broad	Local		Focal	Local	Unlikely	Unlikely
Loss of waste management	Local to broad	Local to broad	Local to broad	Local	Local	Local to broad	Local to broad	Unlikely		Focal	Local	Unlikely	Possible
Public risk perception	Moderate	Moderate	Low	Low	Low	Moderate	Low	Low	Low	Low to moderate	Low	Moderate	High

(Continued)

Table 11-1. (Continued)

Public Health Impact	Geophysical				Hydrometeorological					Climatological		Biological	
	Earthquake	Tsunami	Volcanic Eruption	Landslide	Tornado and Storm	Cyclone	Flood	Heat	Cold	Drought	Wildfire	Epidemic	Pandemic
Increased pests	Unlikely	Unlikely	Unlikely	Unlikely	Local to broad	Local to broad	Local to broad	Unlikely	Unlikely	Unlikely	Unlikely	Unlikely	Unlikely
Impact on health care system	Local to broad	Local to broad	Local to broad	Local	Local to broad	Local to broad	Local to broad	Local to broad	Local to broad	Broad	Local	Local	Broad
Worsening of chronic illnesses	Local to broad	Local to broad	Local to broad	Local	Local to broad	Local to broad	Local to broad	Local to broad		Broad	Local to broad	Local	Broad
Loss of electrical power	Local to broad	Local to broad	Local to broad	Local	Local to broad	Local to broad	Local to broad	Local		Local	Unlikely	Unlikely	Possible
Toxic exposures	Broad	Broad	Broad	Local	Broad	Broad	Broad	Unlikely	Broad	Broad	Broad	Unlikely	Unlikely
Food scarcity	Unlikely	Unlikely	Unlikely	Unlikely	Unlikely	Likely in deltas	Local to broad	Unlikely	Unlikely	Likely in poor nations	Unlikely	Unlikely	Possible

Source: Keim.[4] Adapted with permission of the publisher.

health consequences. In most cases, the difference is only one of scale. For example, all these hazards are associated with morbidity and mortality. However, volcanic eruptions tend to cause fewer cases and deaths than do tsunamis and pandemics.

Many natural disaster hazards can markedly affect the ability of the population to maintain and access adequate shelter, water, electricity, **sanitation**, hygiene, health care, nutrition, security, or public services to maintain their health during an incident. These factors have a significant influence on morbidity following a disaster. Displacement (and its associated losses of resources) can be a crucial contributor to a range of adverse health effects caused by environmental hazards compared with biological hazards. Incidents that result in the loss of electricity without displacement from home are often associated with poisonings as affected populations seek to heat, cook, or generate power using devices that emit carbon monoxide.

Public **risk perception** also varies according to a natural disaster. In general, the public tends to underestimate the risk of those disaster hazards with which they are most familiar.[1] As a result, many populations are less concerned about relatively common droughts, floods, and temperature extremes compared with less frequent (but perhaps more dramatic) earthquakes, tsunamis, and cyclones.

All natural disasters have some impact on the health care system, whether by direct damage or by overutilization caused by mass casualties or outbreaks. In addition, all-natural disasters tend to exacerbate preexisting conditions, such as a noncommunicable disease. It is also essential to recognize that many natural disasters result in toxic exposures. Earthquakes and floods have the potential to cause toxic exposures by causing a release of hazardous industrial materials. In addition, storms, floods, and cyclones are also known to cause contamination from household chemicals stored in homes.

Food scarcity is rare for most natural disasters, excluding drought incidents in low-resource countries, where it may be the primary concern. There have been reports of short- to intermediate-term food scarcity because of large cyclones and flood disasters in major river and delta regions. Food scarcity is also possible in the case of severe pandemics associated with high fatality rates affecting worker availability and distribution networks.

Earthquakes and tsunamis are characteristically associated with many deaths and injuries and have significant potential for large-scale population displacement. **Mass casualty incidents** typically overwhelm the resources of the already damaged local health care system. By comparison, volcanic eruptions, wildfires, and landslides tend to occur on a smaller scale, with an impact primarily associated with damages localized to the incident. However, volcanic and wildfire emissions can also have a far-reaching impact on the respiratory health of downwind populations.

In general, storms tend to have relatively low mortality associated with moderate morbidity. Cyclones and floods usually cause few injuries in high-resource countries. However, in low-resource nations these same incidents often cause many deaths.

Heat waves are notoriously deadly and have been associated with large numbers of deaths in Europe, North America, and Asia. Cold waves and winter storms are frequently associated with few deaths but many injuries, including carbon monoxide poisoning. Drought deaths typically occur in only low-resource countries. In high-resource countries, drought-related health effects tend to involve mental health and the indirect health impacts of economic losses.

Biological disasters may occur as an outbreak, epidemic, or pandemic. The pathogen's specific characteristics often determine the scale of the event. Not all communicable diseases have the potential to cause an epidemic. Even fewer pathogens can create a global pandemic. Epidemics are characteristically associated with a moderate or large number of deaths among specific populations. Pandemics, by comparison, typically cause a vast number of deaths worldwide. Either of these incidents can have a great impact on the health care system, which under the circumstances becomes overutilized and affects the workforce's availability.

The Public Health Impacts of Individual Technological Disasters

Table 11-2 summarizes various technological disasters' relative public health impacts.[4] Technological hazards cause the same 16 public health consequences as natural disasters, mainly varying in scale. Overall, mortality is moderate for most technological disasters, except for highly kinetic hazards like transportation accidents and explosions. Transportation accidents and hazardous material releases are often associated with more cases than other technological disasters. Population displacement varies depending on the individual technological hazard and is usually localized to areas relatively near the incident.

Explosions, fires, and hazardous material releases are responsible for most displacements associated with technological disasters. The impacts of technological disasters on public utilities, including power, water, and sewer, are also expectedly localized. Like natural disasters, technological disasters also exacerbate pre-existing chronic diseases such as cardiovascular disease, diabetes, respiratory disease, and mental illness.

Public perception of risk is characteristically high for nearly all technological disasters, excluding mass gatherings and structural collapses. Once again, the public tends to judge familiar environmental hazards less harshly.[1] Many technological hazards have the potential to cause toxic exposures. Food scarcity, however, is rarely associated with human-made technology. Instead, it is more commonly associated with socioeconomic disruption, conflict, and poor governance.

Considering individual hazards, poisonings and hazardous material releases are associated with average mortality and high morbidity levels. Poisonings are expectedly not

Table 11-2. The Relative Public Health Impact of Technological Disasters

Public Health Impact	Toxic		Thermal		Kinetic			
	Poisoning	Hazmat	Fire	Explosion	Transportation	Gathering	Mining	Collapse
Deaths	Moderate	Moderate	Moderate	Moderate to many	Many	Moderate	Moderate	Moderate
Cases	Moderate	Many	Few to moderate	Moderate	Many	Few to moderate	Few	Few to moderate
Loss of clean water	Unlikely	Local	Unlikely	Unlikely	Unlikely	Unlikely	Unlikely	Local
Loss of shelter	Unlikely	Local	Local	Local	Unlikely	Unlikely	Unlikely	Local
Loss of household goods	Unlikely	Local	Local	Local	Unlikely	Unlikely	Unlikely	Local
Population displacement	Unlikely	Local	Local	Local	Unlikely	Unlikely	Unlikely	Local
Loss of hygiene	Unlikely	Local	Local	Local	Unlikely	Unlikely	Unlikely	Local
Loss of sanitation	Unlikely	Local	Local	Local	Unlikely	Unlikely	Unlikely	Local
Loss of waste management	Unlikely	Local	Unlikely	Unlikely	Unlikely	Unlikely	Unlikely	Local
Public risk perception	High	High	High	High	High	Low	Moderate	Low
Increased pests	Unlikely	Unlikely	Unlikely	Unlikely	Unlikely	Unlikely	Unlikely	Unlikely
Impact on health care system	Local to broad	Local	Local	Local	Local	Local	Local	Local
Worsening of chronic illnesses	Unlikely	Local	Local to broad	Local	Unlikely	Local	Unlikely	Local
Loss of electrical power	Unlikely	Unlikely	Unlikely	Unlikely	Unlikely	Unlikely	Unlikely	Local
Toxic exposures	Many	Many	Moderate	Few to moderate	Few to moderate	Few	Few	Few to moderate
Food scarcity	Unlikely	Unlikely	Unlikely	Unlikely	Unlikely	Unlikely	Unlikely	Unlikely

Source: Keim.[4] Adapted with permission of the publisher.

commonly associated with displacement. Hazardous material releases, by contrast, frequently result in significant population displacements and cause many injuries. Fire disasters are associated with a moderate level of mortality and morbidity, whereas explosions are associated with a higher degree of mortality, and transportation accidents are related to high levels of morbidity and mortality. Surprisingly, mass gatherings are responsible for the highest mortality per event, with 163 deaths per disaster, followed by structural collapse (45 deaths/incident). Mining accidents have a high case fatality, usually resulting in more deaths than injuries. However, structural collapses cause more deaths overall.

In summary, nearly all disasters create the same public health needs, regardless of the causative hazard. As a result, almost all disasters require the same capabilities for public health emergency response. This capability-based approach represents one of the fundamental principles of emergency management.[3,5] Note that for most of the disaster hazards represented in these tables, variation exists only for the relative degree of impact for each public health consequence. Thus, the all-hazard preparedness program focuses not on the specific hazard but on addressing the expected public health and medical consequences. These consequences are managed by projecting an inventory of emergency response capabilities.

CAPABILITY-BASED PLANNING

Using an all-hazard capability-based approach, societies and organizations engage in deliberate **planning** to prepare for and respond to disasters by applying their inherent capabilities to all disaster risks regardless of priority.[6] A capability is the "ability to achieve a desired operational effect under specified standards and conditions through combinations of means and ways to perform a set of tasks."[7]

Table 11-3 lists consequences and public health capabilities commonly addressed during a public health emergency response.[4]

TOPICS FOR DISCUSSION

1. Using Table 11-1, compare the relative public health impacts of tsunamis to that of a flood.
2. Using Table 11-2, describe a thermonuclear detonation in terms of the public health consequences of toxic, thermal, and kinetic hazards.
3. Is it reasonable to conclude that nearly all disasters create the same public health needs? Justify your answer.
4. Is it reasonable to conclude that nearly all disasters require the same public health capabilities? Justify your answer.

Table 11-3. Public Health Consequences and Capabilities Associated With All Disasters

Public Health Consequences	Public Health Capabilities
Common to all consequences	Resource management Mental health services Reproductive health services Social services Occupational health and safety Business continuity
Deaths	Mortuary care Social services Mental health services
Illness and injuries	Health services Injury prevention and control Epidemiology Disease prevention and control
Loss of clean water	Access to safe water
Loss of shelter	Shelter and settlement Social services Security
Loss of personal and household goods	Replacement of personal and household goods
Loss of sanitation and routine hygiene	Sanitation, excreta disposal and hygiene promotion
Disruption of solid waste management	Solid waste management
Public concern for safety	Risk communication Public information Security
Increased pests and vectors	Pest and vector control
Loss or damage of health care system	Health system and infrastructure support
Worsening of chronic illnesses	Health services
Food scarcity	Food safety, security, and nutrition
Standing surface water	Public works and engineering
Toxic exposures	Risk assessment Population protection Health services Hazmat emergency response Occupational health and safety

Source: Keim.[4] Adapted with permission of the publisher.

REFERENCES

1. Slovik P, Peters E. Risk perception and affect. *Curr Dir Psychol Sci.* 2006;15(6):322–325.
2. Keim ME. Building human resilience the role of public health preparedness and response as an adaptation to climate change. *Am J Prev Med.* 2008;35(5):508–516.

3. Federal Emergency Management Agency (FEMA). Guide for all-hazard emergency operations planning. September 1996. Available at: https://www.fema.gov/pdf/plan/slg101.pdf. Accessed January 12, 2023.
4. Keim M. Disaster preparedness. In: Ciottone GR, et al. eds. *Ciottone's Disaster Medicine.* 2nd ed. Philadelphia, PA: Elsevier; 2006.
5. *National Incident Management System.* Washington, DC: Federal Emergency Management Agency; 2008.
6. Murphy C, Gardoni P. Determining public policy and resource allocation priorities for mitigating natural hazards: a capabilities-based approach. *Sci Eng Ethics.* 2007;13:489–504.
7. Henry R. Defense transformation and the 2005 quadrennial defense review. November 1, 2005. Available at: https://press.armywarcollege.edu/parameters/vol35/iss4/4. Accessed January 13, 2023.

12

Global Patterns of Disaster-Related Disease

LEARNING OBJECTIVES

Upon completion, the reader will be able to

1. Define the following terms and phrases:
   - Case fatality rate (i.e., death-to-case ratio)
   - Displacement
   - Incidence
   - Relative frequency
2. Recognize that most disaster-related health statistics are notoriously imprecise.
3. Recognize that the frequency of both natural and technological disasters is increasing.
4. Recognize that during the past 60 years, nearly two-thirds of all disasters were caused by natural hazards.
5. Recognize that natural disasters were the cause of 95% of all deaths, 91% of all injuries, and 99% of all displacement associated with disasters during this period.
6. Recognize that natural disasters were also associated with a much higher mean number of deaths, injuries, and displacements per incident than technological disasters.
7. Recognize that drought, earthquakes, and cyclones were natural disasters associated with the highest total mortality.
8. Recognize that transportation accidents, explosions, and fires were technological disasters associated with the highest total mortality.
9. Recognize that tsunamis and landslides have a very high case fatality rate.
10. Recognize that mining disasters have a very high case fatality rate.
11. Recognize that epidemics and earthquakes were among the natural disasters associated with the highest total morbidity.
12. Recognize that hazardous material releases and transportation accidents were among the technological disasters associated with the highest total morbidity.
13. Recognize that floods were associated with the highest levels of population displacement among natural disasters.
14. Recognize that among technological disasters, fires and explosions were associated with the highest levels of population displacement.

DISASTER-RELATED HEALTH INFORMATION

Descriptions of disaster events are the subject of broad approximations and aggregations. Health information related to these events is often missing or underreported. Disaster-related health data is notoriously imprecise. For example, even simple epidemiological calculations (e.g., mortality, morbidity, and attack rates) are precluded mainly by the consistent lack of denominator (census) data. Estimates of the total number of persons affected and estimated costs of damages are markedly inconsistent and frequently absent. Considering this critical lack of accuracy and validity involving all disaster-related data, the information included in this chapter is offered as a broad description of the general characteristics of the aggregate data. Values for mortality, morbidity, and displacement are presented in terms of global incidence rather than incidence rate.

There are now several global databases, among them EM-DAT and DesInventar.[1,2] Each of these databases possesses inherent challenges influenced by the basic structure of the datasets and the data collection methods. A time bias has been reported among the EM-DAT data acquired before the formal inception of the database in 1973. However, data availability and quality have reportedly increased and improved over time using multiple data sources since then.[3] Notably, 36% of the national datasets in the DesInventar database begin in 1980 or later. The DesInventar dataset has a more significant number of recorded events than the EM-DAT for several disaster types, and the number of considerable disaster hazards is similar for both datasets. However, 3 of the 15 hazards in the DesInventar database relate to soil erosion, sedimentation, and pollution, which are less pertinent to this discussion of disasters. In addition, the Desinventar database includes data for a select 87 countries, compared with 120 countries in the EM-DAT database.[1] This chapter consists of data downloaded from the EM-DAT database, rather than from DesInvestar, primarily because of its wider variety of indicators related to individual hazards and countries. (The intent here is to err on the side of inclusion and sensitivity.) In addition, the study period is limited to the most recent six decades to minimize time bias (and to coordinate with standards for evaluating climate data).

This chapter describes data summaries for 23,503 separate disaster events that occurred among nations worldwide during 1961–2020 from the EM-DAT database.[1] These historical data include all reported disasters caused by natural and technological hazards. Data associated with the COVID-19 pandemic have intentionally been excluded for reasons of scope and comparability. For a disaster to be entered into the EM-DAT database, at least one of the following criteria must be fulfilled: there must be 10 or more people reported killed, or 100 or more people reported affected, or a declaration of a state of emergency, or a call for international assistance.[1]

The World Meteorological Organization describes 30-year "standard reference periods" for use by the international community to maintain consistency in calculating global climate statistics. This chapter intentionally includes the two most recent standard reference periods, ranging from 1961 to 2020, to provide comparability with a reference standard.[4]

THE GLOBAL BURDEN OF DISASTER-RELATED DISEASE

From 1961 to 2020 there were 23,395 disasters reported to have occurred, averaging 390 incidents per year. These events caused a reported 423,920 deaths and 939,389 illnesses and injuries. During this period, an estimated 134 million persons were rendered homeless by disasters. Figure 12-1 depicts the **relative frequency** of disasters among the five continents during that period. Of all the world's disasters, 42% occurred in Asia, which is home to 60% of the global population.

In total, 14,785 (63%) disasters were caused by natural hazards and 8,610 (37%) were caused by technological hazards. Natural disasters caused a reported 4,468,767 deaths and 6,787,941 illnesses and injuries. During this period 132,503,106 persons were rendered homeless by natural disasters. Technological disasters were reported to cause 328,783 deaths and 421,867 illnesses and injuries. During this same time, 502,041 persons were displaced by technological disasters.

The annual **incidence** rate of all disasters is increasing worldwide. As indicated in Figure 12-2, the annual incidences of natural and technological disasters are growing at a remarkably similar rate. This increase has been correlated with the Great Acceleration of human development during the Anthropocene epoch.[5]

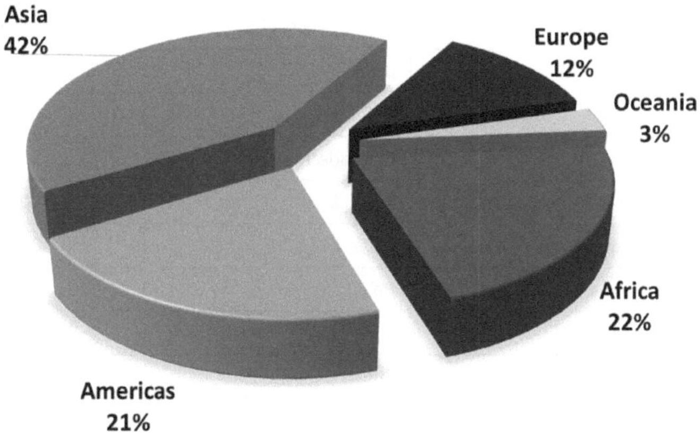

Figure 12-1. Relative Frequency of Disasters According to Continent, 1961–2020

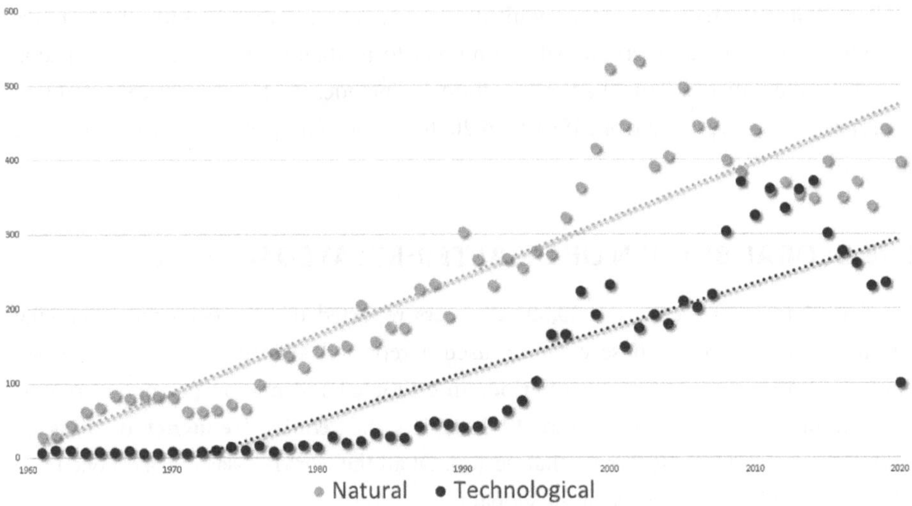

Figure 12-2. Annual Incidence Rate of Natural and Technological Disasters, 1961–2020

Table 12-1 lists the world's 10 deadliest disasters during that period. The deadliest single disaster event occurred in a drought that was responsible for 31% of all global disaster deaths. Drought-prone Ethiopia is listed twice, as is cyclone-prone Bangladesh. All major cyclone disasters occurred in low-lying river deltas. Other significant events involved earthquakes in China, Haiti, and the Indian Ocean, resulting in a tsunami.

Table 12-1. Ten Disasters Associated With the Highest Number of Deaths, 1961–2020

Year	Disaster Subtype	Country	Total Deaths
1965	Drought	India	1,500,000
1995	Famine	DPR Korea	610,000
1970	Tropical cyclone	Bangladesh	300,000
1983	Drought	Ethiopia	300,000
1976	Earthquake	China	242,000
2010	Earthquake	Haiti	222,570
2004	Tsunami	Indonesia	165,708
1983	Drought	Sudan	150,000
1991	Tropical cyclone	Bangladesh	138,866
2008	Tropical cyclone	Myanmar	138,366
1973	Drought	Ethiopia	100,000

COMPARING NATURAL AND TECHNOLOGICAL DISASTERS

Disasters have been traditionally classified according to the causative agent, including natural or technological hazards. However, the World Bank has also coined the description "natural hazards, but unnatural disasters" in recognition that disasters are symptoms of dysfunctional development resulting from human acts of omission and commission.[5,6] In effect, few natural disasters are caused entirely by nature. In addition, the term *natural* is also polysemous and sometimes misconstrued to represent an inevitable event (as opposed to one derived from nature). However, it is helpful to classify disasters that are amenable to comparison.

For comparison, our discussion will use the terms *natural disaster* and *technological disaster* to categorize these events according to their associated hazard group.

Figure 12-3 compares key public health impacts of disasters caused by natural and technological hazards.

Natural disasters were responsible for most disaster-related health impacts during this time. Natural hazards caused 63% of all disasters. However, natural disasters were the cause of 95% of all deaths, 91% of all injuries, and 99% of all displacement associated with disasters during this period. Natural disasters were also associated with a much higher mean number of deaths, injuries, and displacement per incident. Natural disasters were responsible for 6 times more injuries, 12 times more deaths, and 88 times more displacements per incident compared with technological disasters. However, the case fatality rate (depicted in Figure 12-3) was relatively similar for the two groups. Notably, 60% of illnesses and injuries reported during natural disasters resulted in death, compared with a 44% death-to-case ratio for technological disasters.

Figure 12-4 depicts the relative frequency of 12 natural and 13 technological hazards associated with disasters during 1961–2020. The most common natural hazard was flood, responsible for 36% of all-natural disasters (and 22% of all disasters overall). Transportation accidents were the most common technological hazard, causing 66% of all technological disasters (and 24% of all disasters).

Figure 12-5 compares the relative health impacts of natural and individual technological disasters.

DISASTER-RELATED MORTALITY

Among natural hazards, drought was responsible for the highest mortality (2,211,424 deaths), representing 31% of all disaster-related deaths. This was followed by earthquakes (1,093,388 deaths) and tropical cyclones (901,439 deaths). By comparison, transportation accidents were the leading cause of mortality related to technological disasters (228,256), representing 24% of all disaster-related deaths. This top cause was followed by explosions (35,360 deaths) and fire (23,759 deaths).

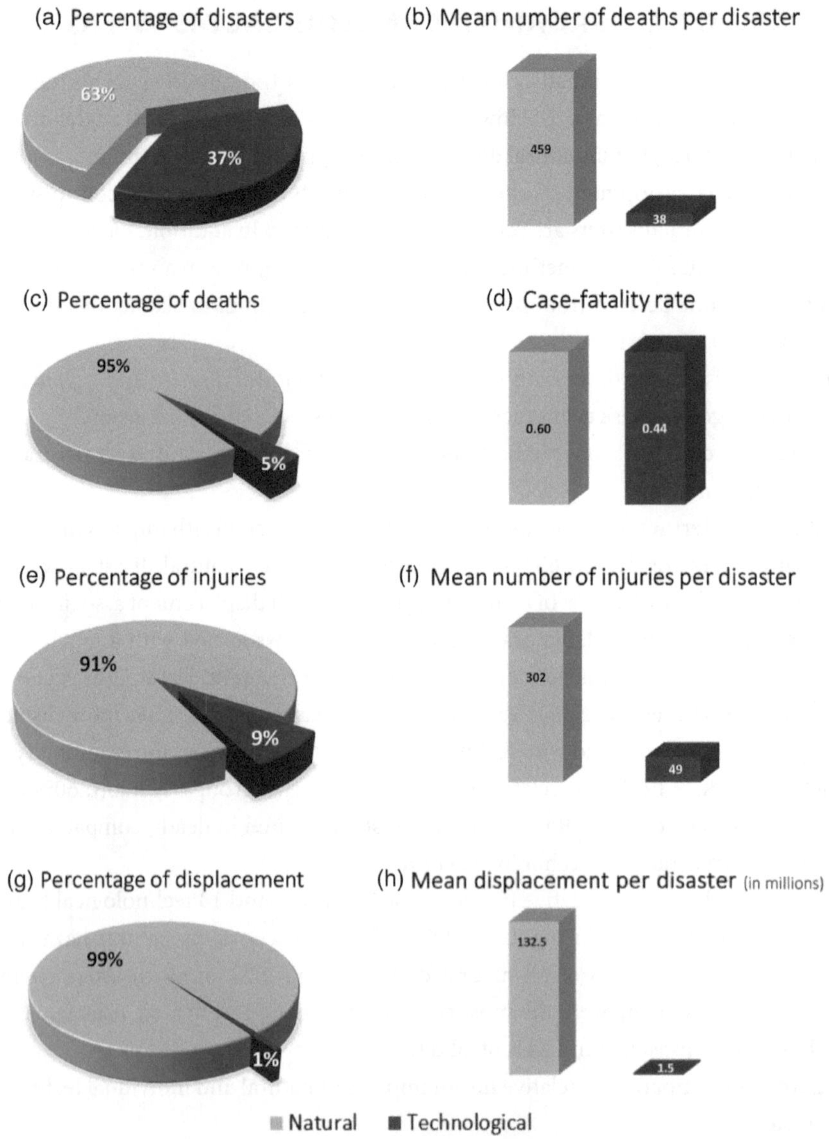

Figure 12-3. Public Health Impacts of Disasters Caused by Natural and Technological Hazards, 1961–2020

Tsunamis were responsible for the highest mean number of deaths per incident (6,105/incident), followed by droughts (3,042 deaths/incident) and earthquakes, with an average of 948 deaths per disaster. Among technological hazards, mass gatherings were associated with the highest mean fatalities per incident (163/incident), followed by structural collapse (45 deaths/incident) and explosions, averaging 38 deaths per incident.

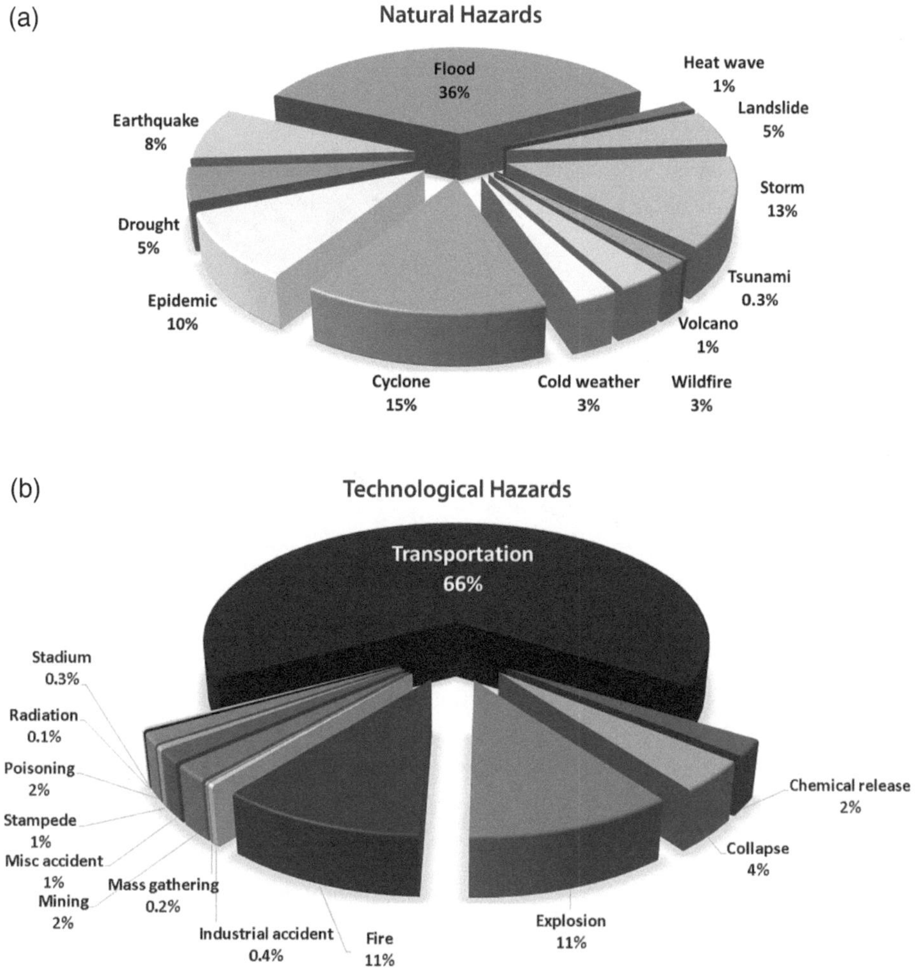

Figure 12-4. Relative Frequency of Disasters Caused by Individual Natural and Technological Hazards, 1961–2020

Case fatality rates for natural disasters identify drought and tsunamis as the most fatal. However, this drought statistic most likely represents an artifact of the data since drought-related morbidity is (presumably erroneously) attributed to only 32 events in the EM-DAT database.[1] Some geological disasters appear particularly deadly. Tsunamis and landslides were associated with a very high case fatality rate, with 80% of all related cases resulting in death. These were followed by volcanic eruptions (54%), heat waves (46%), and tropical cyclones (44%).

Mining disasters were associated with a high case fatality rate reported among technological disasters. Of all cases related to mine disasters, 93% resulted in death. This top cause was followed by transportation accidents (67%) and structural collapse (56%).

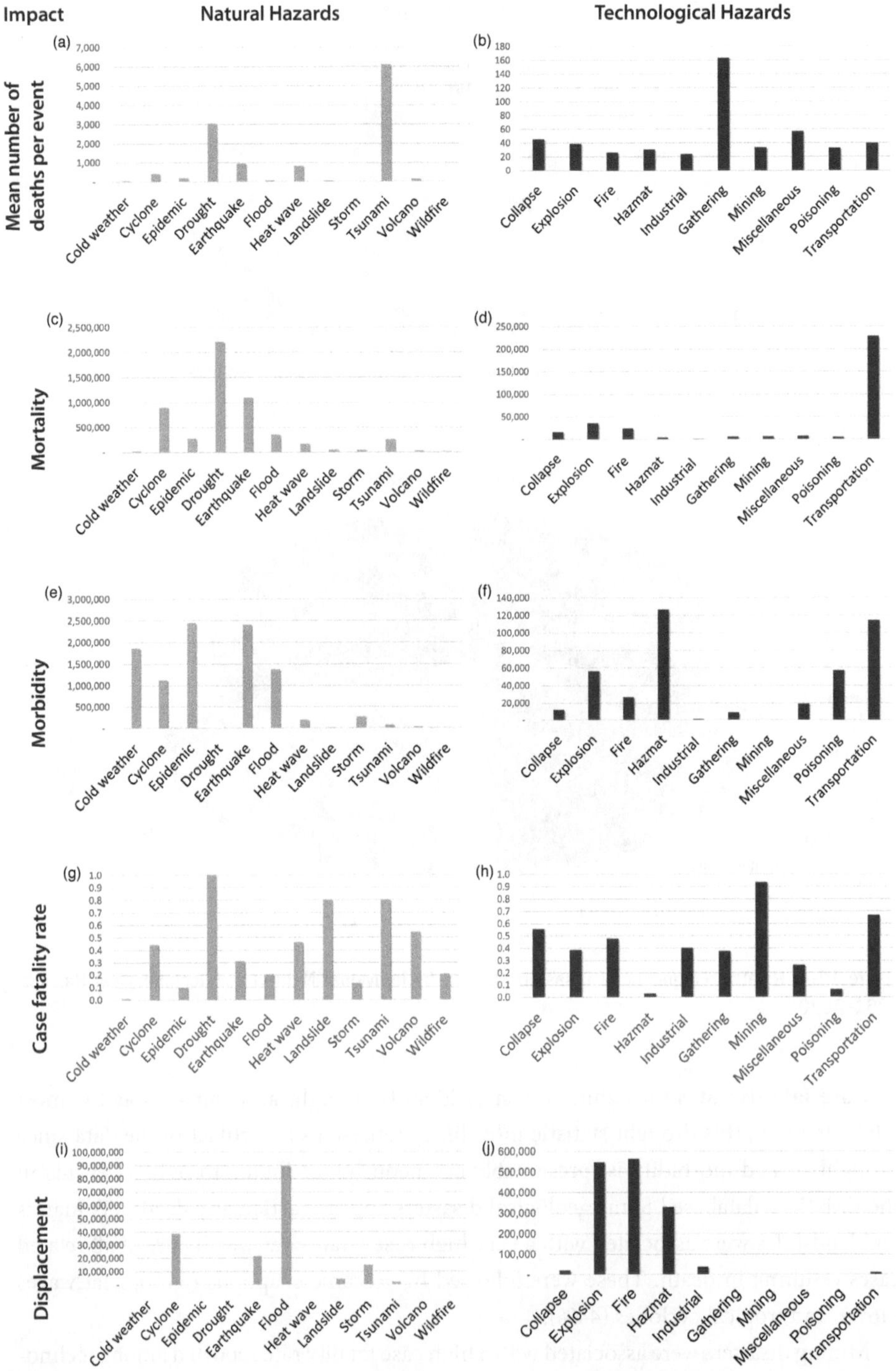

Figure 12-5. Key Public Health Impacts of Disasters Caused by Individual Natural and Technological Hazards, 1961–2020

DISASTER-RELATED MORBIDITY

Among natural hazards, epidemics caused the highest overall morbidity (2,401,757 cases), followed by earthquakes, which were associated with 2,401,757 injuries; cold weather (1,856,682 injuries); floods (1,372,235 injuries); and cyclones (1,126,232 injuries).

By comparison, hazardous material releases and transportation accidents were the leading causes of mortality related to technological disasters (126,431 and 114,210, respectively). This leading cause was followed by 57,070 poisonings and 56,393 injuries resulting from explosions.

DISASTER-RELATED DISPLACEMENT

Floods were responsible for most disaster-related **displacement,** accounting for 68% of that caused by all natural hazards and 67% of all disasters. This was followed by cyclones (38,652,734 persons displaced) and earthquakes (21,488,258 persons displaced). The leading causes of displacement for technological disasters were fire (562,190 persons) and explosions (546,005 persons), followed by hazardous material spills and releases (327,430 persons).

TOPICS FOR DISCUSSION

1. List five characteristics of disasters that affect our ability to collect accurate aggregate health data on a global scale. Justify your answer.
2. Compare the case fatality rates of landslides and earthquakes with that of Ebola and COVID-19 viruses.
3. Why are so many people affected by floods? Justify your answer.

REFERENCES

1. Centre for Research on the Epidemiology of Disasters (CRED). EM-DAT: the international disaster database. 2022. Available at: www.emdat.be. Accessed November 30, 2022.
2. United Nations Office for Disaster Risk Reduction. DesInventar disaster information management system. 2022. Available at: https://www.desinventar.net. Accessed November 30, 2022.
3. Panwar V, Sen S. Disaster damage records of EM-DAT and DesInventar: a systematic comparison. *Econ Disasters Clim Change.* 2020;4:295–317.
4. World Meteorological Organization (WMO). *WMO Guidelines on the Calculation of Climate Normals.* Geneva, Switzerland: United Nations; 2017.
5. Keim ME, Smith TM, Burkle FM. The annual global incidence rate of extreme weather event disasters appears positively correlated with world GDP, 1961–2020. *Prehosp Disaster Med.* 2022;37(4):431–436.
6. World Bank; United Nations. Natural hazards, unnatural disasters: the economics of prevention. 2010. Available at: https://openknowledge.worldbank.org/handle/10986/2512. Accessed November 23, 2022.

V. PRINCIPLES OF EMERGENCY HEALTH

13

Wellness

LEARNING OBJECTIVES

Upon completion, the reader will be able to

1. Define the following terms and phrases:
   - Holistic
   - Indivisible self
2. Recognize three basic tenets of wellness.
3. Compare and contrast four socioecological models for wellness.
4. Describe wellness in terms of creative, coping, social, essential, and physical factors.
5. Describe how the "individual self" uses these five factors of wellness to integrate within larger (i.e., micro, meso, exo, macro, and chrono) contexts of health.
6. Match five wellness factors to their 17 corresponding subfactors.

WHAT IS WELLNESS?

Wellness is "an active process through which people become aware of, and make choices toward, a more successful existence."[1] Compared with health as a state of being (i.e., outcome), wellness is considered an active process (i.e., output).

Wellness is the journey. Health is the destination.

Like health, the concept of wellness was also inspired by the World Health Organization's definition of health as a state of complete well-being. In this sense, wellness seeks to optimize well-being. This is accomplished according to three basic tenets: (1) a conscious, self-directed process, (2) a **holistic** approach, and (3) a positive and affirming perspective.

Hettler described six dimensions of wellness to include emotional, occupational, physical, spiritual, intellectual, and social aspects.[1] This model recognizes a range of dimensions that directly affect our sense of completeness. These dimensions involve our ecosocial environment and intellectual, spiritual, and emotional health. This wellness approach helps remind us of the interconnectedness of each dimension and the influence of these factors as determinants of health for a "state of complete well-being." It offers a comprehensive approach to healthy living that empowers the proactive role of the individual in preventing disease and promoting health.

ECOSOCIAL MODELS FOR WELLNESS

As a holistic approach, the wellness process is intended to influence aspects of well-being. Various models of wellness differ according to which elements are included. Multiple authors have offered slightly different factors according to their perspectives. Table 13-1 summarizes how these factors differ and build upon Hettler's original "dimensions" of wellness.[1-3] Wallerstein's interpretation broadened the focus from the individual to include the community's social sphere and political influences.[2] By comparison, Kuartei described a concept of integrated wellness within the narrative of his life experience involving Western medical training and his native Pacific island beliefs and culture.[3] Kuartei's approach recognized Hettler's and Wallerstein's aspects of wellness while also adding behavioral health (from medicine) along with concepts from the Palauan "nest of life"—a sacred gift of wellness from the land, the sea, the skies, and

Table 13-1. A Comparison of Various Ecosocial Models for Wellness

Aspects of Wellness	Hettler's Dimensions[1] 1976	Wallerstein's Environments[2] 2003	Kuartei's Environments[3] 2005	Stoewen's Dimensions[1] 2017
Behavioral			■	
Community		■		
Cultural			■	
Emotional	■		■	■
Environmental				■
Financial				■
Individual		■		■
Intellectual				■
Mental	■		■	
Natural			■	
Occupational	■			
Physical	■	■	■	■
Political		■	■	
Sacredness			■	
Social	■	■	■	■
Spiritual	■		■	■
Vocational				■

the society.[3] Finally, Stoewen describes wellness measures to include postmodern concepts such as financial, intellectual, and vocational well-being.[1]

The breadth of this table exemplifies the subjective variation of well-being that depends largely on an individual's sense of self and life experience.

WELLNESS AND THE INDIVISIBLE SELF

While we each may be able to offer our personal perceptions of wellness, in 1923 Adler proposed that holism (the indivisibility of self) and purposiveness were central to understanding human behavior and that such understanding required an "emphasis on the whole rather than the elements, the interaction between the whole and parts, and the importance of man's social context."[4,5]

Whitmer and Sweeney performed an extensive review based on Adler's "Individual Psychology." They identified several characteristics that correlated positively with healthy living, quality of life, and longevity. Their findings formed the basis of a counseling theory called the Wheel of Wellness.[6]

Although the relationship between the components of the Wheel of Wellness and the assumed circumplex structure was not supported by empirical analysis, the results of the original analyses were encouraging. Subsequent statistical analysis identified five apparent second-order factors (i.e., creative, coping, physical, social, and essential factors) and one unidimensional higher-order factor called wellness.[6]

These characteristics are organized into a model known as the **indivisible self**. A Venn diagram is often used to depict the relationship between the Indivisible Self and external influences of five second-order factors positioned within five contexts. (See Figure 13-1.)

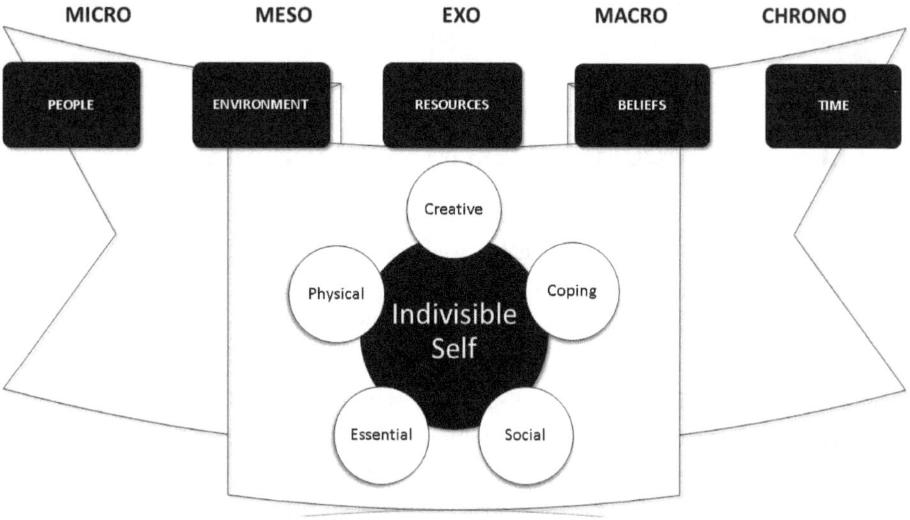

Figure 13-1. Wellness Within the Context of Health

Table 13-2. Wellness Factors and Corresponding Subfactors

The Indivisible Self				
Creative Wellness	**Coping Wellness**	**Social Wellness**	**Essential Wellness**	**Physical Wellness**
Control Emotions Thinking Positive humor Work	Leisure Realistic beliefs Self-worth Stress management	Friendship Love	Spirituality Self-care Gender identity Cultural identity	Exercise Nutrition

This concept emphasizes the indivisible self that functions as a holistic organism (rather than merely a sum of determinants). It illustrates how all these factors come into play within multiple environmental contexts during a person's life span. Figure 13-1 depicts the Adlerian wellness model (the Indivisible Self and its five second-order determinants) within Bronfenbrenner's ecosocial model of health. (i.e., process-person-context-time, PPCT).

Table 13-2 lists five second-order determinants of wellness (DoW) and their corresponding 17 third-order subfactors.

Wellness is determined by five factors: creativity, coping, social, essential, and physical attributes. The creative self is a combination of attributes that each form to make a unique place among others in their social interactions.[5,7] This determinant has five components: thinking, emotions, control, positive humor, and work. There are four components to the coping self: realistic beliefs, stress management, self-worth, and leisure.[5] Social wellness includes two components: friendship and love, which can be conceived as existing on a continuum.

The essential self is a second-order determinant of wellness that includes four components: spirituality, self-care, gender identity, and cultural identity. Adler viewed the basic self as essential to holism and wellness. The physical self includes the factors of exercise and nutrition.

AN ECOSOCIAL MODEL OF WELLNESS DURING DISASTERS

As noted in Chapter 3, health is determined. It must be proactively promoted and potentiated. Like Schultz's production of health, wellness must also be "produced."[8] And one of the three basic tenets of wellness is "a conscious, *self-directed* process."

Wellness and health both contribute to a higher quality of life. Wellness is derived from an indivisible self that also experiences the disaster phenomenon within its full context. This wellness experience is influenced by self-directed essential, physical, creative, coping, and social behaviors. Individuals often utilize multiple subfactors at once and in combination to optimize wellness continuously (compared with within discrete locations or contexts).

Individuals apply these factors to manage health risks and optimize wellness before, during, and after disaster hazards occur. In the case of disasters, creativity is an asset that harnesses the value of intellect, emotions, humor, control, and work. Coping is also a well-recognized disaster skill that must integrate realistic beliefs regarding losses and recovery, challenges to self-worth, stress management, and restrictions on leisure time. Social wellness in a disaster setting often presents as an evident outpouring of unconditional love and friendship. But such events are also frequent settings for intentional harm, exploitation, and manipulation of victims. Ironically, essential wellness (which Adler saw as key to being whole) is not universally addressed within most disaster management systems. While some systems recognize spirituality in the context of religious outreach and recognize self-care as a laudable goal, gender and cultural identity are rarely formally integrated within the recognition of self among disaster victims. Finally, the physical wellness of disaster-affected populations is usually focused on meeting the bare minimums for nutrition and rarely addresses the relationship between disaster-related exertion and rest.

Most activities associated with wellness and disasters are driven by a conscious effort on the part of disaster victims. These self-directed contributors to wellness are supported mainly by disaster-related activities that are otherwise myopic in their focus on managing the disaster-related disease. Few approaches to emergency management seek to identify and prioritize an ecosocial model of wellness and health regarding hazardous exposures.

Let us consider an example of ecosocial wellness during a disaster. In this case, we will consider the scenario of a cyclone that has resulted in widespread damage and population displacement. (See Appendix A: Table A-2.)

Concerning creative wellness, most disaster-affected populations displaced from their home describe an overwhelming loss of control. Even the activities of daily living are now unpredictable as cyclone victims assess the damages and pick up the pieces.

The work of daily living under emergency circumstances is augmented by additional work necessary to recover. Homes and landscapes are destroyed. Infrastructure is affected. The cleanup work is hot and strenuous. Even the essential elements of daily living (e.g., water, meals, toilets, shelter) become complex tasks with stressful attributes.

This increased activity is also associated with a higher pace of intellectual activity and emotional investment. It is in recognizing the value of positive humor that we are taken back to the reality of an indivisible self—one that suffers and, at the same time, laughs and creates. Emotions are on edge as disaster-affected families relate to this new reality and adjust their thinking and actions accordingly. Leisure time largely disappears for displaced families as most efforts are directed toward the emergency. Irrational beliefs and worries often percolate with issues of value and self-worth as breadwinners look to the future as they provide for their families. Family relationships are both tested and reaffirmed. In close alignment with these behaviors are those related to coping that originate with internal beliefs of value and worth that are influenced by coping skills of leisure and stress management. Balanced exercise and nutrition also play a key role in optimizing disaster-affected populations' wellness. Finally, there are factors proximal and intrinsic to the individual that affect wellness directly during disasters, as painful psychological losses are soothed by a selfless outpouring of friendship and love (or become inflamed by a lack thereof).

Finally, disasters often pose core existential questions about our very nature, raising the voices of spirituality, self, and identity in protective actions that remind and reassure us of the meaning, purpose, stability, and continuity of our life experiences. Many disaster survivors turn to their spiritual beliefs as they look for meaning in dramatic and life-altering events. By contrast, self-care is too often replaced with self-sacrifice as people attempt to respond stoically to the damage and loss. Self-identity plays a key role in helping individuals retain some ongoing stability in their lives. Physical wellness is replaced by a functional triage where valuable assets such as physical activity and nutrition are redirected toward reaction and not necessarily the physical wellness of an indivisible self. As a result, it is not uncommon or unexpected for most disaster victims to describe their wellness as lacking in terms of creativity, coping, social, essential, or physical factors.

TOPICS FOR DISCUSSION

Choose one disaster type from Appendix A, and describe how each of the five factors of wellness is influenced by the following contexts:

- Local: the effect of family, friends, and neighbors
- Institutional: the effect of education, religion, government, and business
- Global: the effect of politics, culture, global events, environment, media, and community
- Chronometrical: the effect of time as perpetual, positive, and purposeful

REFERENCES

1. Stoewen D. Health and wellness. *Can Vet J*. 2015;56:983–984.
2. Wallerstein N. Empowerment to reduce health disparities *Scand J Public Health Suppl*. 2002;59:72–77.
3. Kuartei S. Environmental sacredness and health in Palau. *Pacific Health Dialog*. 2005;12(1).
4. Adler A. *Understanding Human Nature*. 6th ed. London, UK: George Allen & Unwin; 1954.
5. Myers JE, Sweeney TJ. The indivisible self: an evidence-based model of wellness. *J Individual Psychol*. 2004;60(3):234–245.
6. Sweeney T, Whitmer J. Beyond social interest: striving toward optimum health and wellness. *Individual Psychol*. 1991;47:527–540.
7. Myers J. The indivisible self: an evidence-based model of wellness. *J Individual Psychol*. 2005;61(3):269–279.
8. Schultz J, Sullivan L, Galea S. *Public Health: An Introduction to the Science and Practice of Population Health*. New York, NY: Springer Publishing; 2021.

14

Health Equity

LEARNING OBJECTIVES

Upon completion, the reader will be able to

1. Define the following terms and phrases:
   - Equity
   - Health equality
   - Justice
   - Susceptibility
2. Compare and contrast health equality and health equity.
3. Recognize obstacles to health that create disparities related to culture, resources, and needs.
4. Recognize that health inequity is more accurately described in terms of the specific determinants of health (DoH) involved rather than less specific terms related to "vulnerable populations."

AN ECOSOCIAL MODEL OF HEALTH EQUITY

In the 1990s, Whitehead offered that health equity "implies that ideally, everyone should have a fair opportunity to attain their full health potential and more pragmatically that no one should be disadvantaged from attaining this potential if it can be avoided."[1] The US Healthy People 2020 program defines health equity as attaining the highest level of health for all people.[2] In this sense, the goal of health equity extends a state of complete well-being to the entire population. Just as wellness seeks to optimize the individual's well-being, health equity aims to develop that sense of well-being in a whole population. Health equity recognizes that in addition to the social determinants that create health, there are also significant ecosocial obstacles to health and well-being. These obstacles create health disparities, "differences in health status that are closely linked with social, economic or environmental disadvantage."[3]

These differences exist between groups of people who systematically experience more significant obstacles to health based on their race, ethnicity, religion, socioeconomic status, gender, age, disability, sexual orientation, gender identity, or geographic location compared with the collective majority. Obstacles to health vary among individuals and groups within the population. Table 14-1 briefly lists some of these significant obstacles to health.

Table 14-1. Character of Health Disparities Related to Needs, People, Environment, Resources, and Culture

Ecosocial Context	Determinant	Character of Disparity	Obstacle to Health
MACRO	Beliefs	Culture and values Policies and practices Laws and governance Role of the state Public trust Graft and corruption Social justice	Bias and discrimination
			Insularity
			Economic system
			Lack of human rights
			Lack of duty to protect
			Lack of duty to treat
			Lack of universal health care
			Unequal resource distribution
			Governance
			Conflict
EXO	Resources	Quality of resources Access to resources Quantity of resources Continuity of resources Security Institutional justice	Agriculture
			Communications
			Economic
			Education
			Environmental
			Financial
			Health care
			Housing
			Human resources
			Industrial
			Infrastructure
			Military
			Political
			Social
			Technological
MESO	Environment	Accessibility Stability Quality Control Safety Sustainability Occupational health Environmental justice	Built environment
			Community
			Health care facilities
			Home
			Prisons
			Markets
			Natural environment
			Neighborhood
			Social structure
			Workplace

(Continued)

Table 14-1. (Continued)

Ecosocial Context	Determinant	Character of Disparity	Obstacle to Health
MICRO	People	Social needs Personal assistance Social identity Guidance and advice Communication Leadership Friendship, love Commerce Safety Interpersonal justice	Advocates
			Care providers
			Coworkers
			Criminality
			Family and friends
			Family composition
			Health care workers
			Language
			Leaders
			Media
			Neighbors
			Patients
			Public safety
			Retailers
			Socioeconomic status
INDIVIDUAL	Person	Survival needs Functional needs Health needs Wellness needs Individual justice	Behavior
			Nutrition, hydration
			Environmental health
			Education
			Language
			Functional ability
			Social capital
			Employment
			Health care
			Housing
			Violence
			Family composition
			Personal safety
			Essential support services

Health equity is not synonymous with health equality. **Health equality** describes fair and equal *outcomes* across an entire population. By comparison, health equity describes a fair and equal *process* for seeking equal outcomes.

> Equity is the journey. Equality is the destination.

While recognizing that life choices and chance may bring unequal outcomes, the goal of health equity is to avoid health disparities—that is, differences in health that are closely linked with social, economic, or environmental disadvantage.[4] Closely related to the subject of health equity is that a person's wealth effectively determines the person's overall health. Simply put, wealth equals health.

And in turn, one's level of health affects one's ability to create wealth. There is overwhelming evidence that economically disadvantaged groups have poor survival chances, a higher mortality rate, a poor quality of life, and overall diminished health and well-being compared with other members of society.[5] In fact, poverty is one of the most critical risk factors for disaster-related morbidity and mortality, regardless of society or nation.[6]

HEALTH INEQUITY AND DISASTER VULNERABILITY

Obstacles to health are sustained and exacerbated by misinformed public opinion and misdirected public policies that tend to overemphasize the biological and physical factors while underemphasizing the social, cultural, economic, environmental, and political determinants of health. Society is too willing to "medicalize" social needs and criminalize social deficiencies.[3]

The resultant system tends to spend a lot to provide reactive medical services instead of making an **investment in health**.[7] In addition to addressing social needs with a patchwork of disaster medical care, society tends to stigmatize those in need. These persons have become popularly referred to as "vulnerable populations." The root of the word *vulnerability* comes from "vulnus," the Latin for *wound*. Using a medical model, this "wound" is treated as damage or losses sustained by the individual. There is an implied sense that these individuals are wounded and somehow less than the whole.

> "The difference between the right word and the almost right word is the difference between lightning and a lightning bug."[8]
>
> –Mark Twain

This model assumes that health differences (like vulnerability) are self-generated and individual rather than a complex mix of ecosocial determinants over time.[9] While this may appear more suitable for the disposition of the crisis, this medical approach does not address the social, cultural, or economic and political determinants of the cause. By comparison, an ecosocial model recognizes that vulnerability is not merely an individual attribute but rather a complex collection of conditions created over time.[9,10]

The terms *vulnerability* and *susceptibility* have been used inconsistently across and within diverse disciplines. When applied to individual health, susceptibility often refers to the chance of disaster-related disease when exposed to a hazard and in particular is biologically based. By contrast, disaster-related vulnerability additionally takes into account the likelihood of exposure (e.g., dose) as well as its potential health impact (e.g., response).[11] Thus, the definition of vulnerability is expanded to include the characteristics of the victim and the nature and likelihood of the hazardous exposure. With these ecosocial determinants of health rolled up under one singular and subjective definition of vulnerability, so-called vulnerable populations are then encouraged to somehow become resilient in a way that will address not only proximate causes of disease under their direct control but also the distal ecosocial causes of disaster-related disease that are created mainly by persons other than the disaster victim.

This difference in terminology is not insignificant. The medical approach does more than narrow the range of opportunity. Populations treated as medically "wounded" are more likely to become patients in a health care system and are more likely to undergo medical interventions (regardless of effectiveness).[12]

Health inequities have been well documented according to race and ethnicity, class and socioeconomic status, sexual orientation and gender identity, immigration and documentation status, or residence. However, labeling some groups as vulnerable may also lead group members to internalize stereotypes and may thus be unintentionally detrimental to health equity.[11]

Perhaps Grumbach's definition of a vulnerable population as "*wounded by social forces* placing them at a disadvantage for their health" is a more accurate representation of this human condition resulting from ecosocial, not merely biological or behavioral, determinants.[13] In this sense, health equity is derived from an ecosocial model of health that recognizes the influences of social, technological, economic, environmental, political, and cultural determinants that either decrease or increase the likelihood of disaster-related disease over time.

According to testimony from the US Congress, disaster survivors experience varying degrees of impact and assistance because of their race, creed, color, ethnicity, physical or mental ability, and socioeconomic standing. There are many examples where varying types of assistance are delayed, denied, or disbursed inequitably to disaster-impacted populations.[14] And while federal agencies providing disaster relief are subject to clear nondiscrimination clauses (e.g., the Stafford Act and the Americans with Disabilities Act), lawmakers have also recognized the need to provide additional assurances intended to eliminate disparities in assistance.[14]

Health outcomes are not created by medical care alone. Health is the result of a complex mix of ecosocial determinants. These determinants are often administered within a natural bias of cultural context. Health equity occurs as an intentional act of social justice, with the distribution of resources directed according to the needs of the individual (as compared with the market or the state).

TOPICS FOR DISCUSSION

Describe how the following components of health equity affect the likelihood of disaster-related disease:

- Social equity
- Technological equity

REFERENCES

1. Bregman P. Health disparities and health equity: concepts and measurement. *Annu Rev Public Health*. 2006;27:167–194.
2. US Dept of Health and Human Services (HHS). Determinants of health. In: *Healthy People 2020*. 2020. Archived. Available at: https://www.healthypeople.gov/2020/about/foundation-health-measures/Determinants-of-Health. Accessed November 23, 2022.
3. Tobin-Tyler E, Teitelbaum J. *Essentials of Health Justice*. Burlington, MA: Jones and Bartlett Learning; 2019.
4. Birkhead G, Morrow C, Pirani S. *Essentials of Public Health*. 4th ed. Burlington, MA: Jones and Bartlett Learning; 2021.
5. Dickman S, Himmelstein D, Woolhandler S. Inequality in the healthcare system in the USA. *Lancet*. 2017;389:1431–1444.
6. Keim M. Disaster preparedness. In: Ciottone G, ed. *Disaster Medicine*. Philadelphia, PA: Mosby-Elsevier; 2006.
7. Kirsch T, Keim M. US governmental spending for disaster-related research, 2011–2016: characterizing the state of science funding across 5 professional disciplines. *Dis Med Public Health Prep*. 2019;13(5-6):912–919.
8. Mark Twain quotes. Available at: https://www.goodreads.com/quotes/4957-the-difference-between-the-almost-right-word-and-the-right. Accessed December 21, 2022.
9. Kushel M, Iezzoni L. Disability in patients with disability. In: King T, Wheeler M, eds. *Medical Management of Vulnerable and Underserved Populations*. New York, NY: McGraw-Hill; 2007:384.
10. Bronfenbrenner U. Ecological systems theory. In: Vasta R, ed. *Six Theories of Child Development: Revised Formulations and Current Issues*. London, UK: Jessica Kingsley Publishers; 1992:187–249.
11. Chae D, Snipes S, Chung K, Martz C, LaVeist T. Vulnerability and resilience: use and misuse of these terms in the public health discourse. *Am J Public Health*. 2021;111(10):1736–1740.
12. Jamoulle M. Quaternary prevention, an answer of family doctors to overmedicalization. *Int J Health Policy Manage*. 2015;4:1–4.
13. Grumbach K, Braveman P, Adler N, Bindman A. In: King T, Wheeler M, Bindman A, eds. *Medical Management of Vulnerable and Underserved Populations: Principles, Practice and Population*. New York, NY: McGraw-Hill; 2007:3.
14. Subcommittee of the House of Representatives Committee on Transportation and Infrastructure. *Experiences of Vulnerable Populations in Disasters*. Report 116-62. Washington, DC: US Government Publishing Office; 2020. Available at: https://www.govinfo.gov/committee/house-transportation?path=/browsecommittee/chamber/house/committee/transportation. Accessed November 23, 2022.

15

Determinants of Emergency Health

LEARNING OBJECTIVES

Upon completion, the reader will be able to

1. Define the following terms and phrases:
   - Determinants of wellness (DoW)
   - Target capability
2. Recognize examples of disaster-related determinants of health (DOH).
3. Recognize examples of the long-term effects of disasters on wellness.
4. Recognize three sets of risk factors for long-term impact on wellness.

DETERMINANTS OF HEALTH

In Chapters 8–10, we discussed the (upstream) causal pathways and (downstream) natural history of disaster-related disease that occurs because of hazardous exposures. We considered pathways that lead to disaster-related exposures and the nature of the disease afterward. In Chapters 13–14, we evaluated an ecosocial model for wellness and health equity. This chapter applies examples of these disaster-related determinants within a holistic ecosocial model for emergency health.

Determinants of health (DoH) are often described as comprising individual risk factors as well as social DoH. But as detailed in the preceding chapters, disaster-related health outcomes are determined by a complex mix of human interactions, the environment, societal resources, and cultural beliefs. Obstacles to health are not singular and discrete social hurdles to overcome. Instead, these obstacles result from many systemic influences that are not under the control of the individual disaster victim. Encouragement to become "resilient" in the face of systemic threats is a poor alternative to interventions that move distal from the proximate cause (i.e., exposure) to address the upstream and downstream factors that either improve or worsen the likelihood of positive health outcomes.

Table 15-1 provides a list of disaster-related health determinants organized according to an ecosocial model. The table also introduces **target capabilities** associated with interventions performed by the individual person and by public health. In this table, DoH are described in terms of risk factors (e.g., obstacles to health). This entry could

Table 15-1. Examples of Disaster-Related Health Determinants and Associated Interventions

DETERMINANT	PERSONAL	MICRO	MESO	EXO	MACRO	PERSONAL	PUBLIC
Obstacles to Health	**Individual Factors**	**Human Interactions**	**Community Environment**	**Societal Resources**	**Cultural Beliefs**	**Individual Capability**	**Public Health Capability**
Impaired mobility	Functional ability	Family and friends	Built environment	Environmental	Accessibility	Rapid evacuation	Population protection measures
Stress-related illness	Behavior	Psychosocial support	Social network	Psychological	Norms	Stress management	Risk communication
Racial prejudice	Race	Neighbors	Neighborhood	Governmental	Equality	Social capital	Environmental justice
Ethnic discrimination	Ethnicity	Community	Local practices and tradition	Human	Human rights		Health equity
Chronic disease	Health status	Health care providers	Health care system	Medical	Wellness	Medical care	Health care quality and access
Child hunger	Age	Teachers	Schools	Nutritional	Food	Livelihood	Food security
Sex and gender	Sex and gender	Social support	Advocacy	Political	Equity	Gender identity	Women's health
Elder abuse	Age	Care providers	Community services	Organizational	Aging	Mobility	Senior outreach programs
Misinformation	Education	Teachers, media	Education system	Informational	Risk	Risk perception	Health marketing
Access to care	Income	Service providers	Socioeconomic status	Financial	Economics	Wealth	Essential services
Crime	Security	Police	Public safety	Legal	Justice	Protection	Health protection
Social isolation	Socialization	Peers	Peer group	Social	Self	Resilience	Health promotion
Loss of health care workers	Occupation	Patients	Austere conditions	Technological	Fairness	Personal protective equipment	Epidemic prevention and control

also just as easily include a protective factor (e.g., contributors to health). Note that for each health determinant listed in the far-left column, there is a range of ecosocial influences related to the individual, personal interactions, the community, the society, and the culture. For example, in the case of impaired mobility, risk factors related to the individual may involve the person's functional ability to ambulate. Human interactions involving family and friends influence this individual's health outcomes, as do accessibility challenges of the built environment and societal resources available to assist. A cultural belief in equal accessibility drives the availability of societal resources.

In addition to specifying the ecosocial influences on health, Table 15-1 shows two categories of interventions that help reduce disaster-related health risks: personal capability and public health capability. Personal capability describes those abilities and attributes that a person may use to lessen disaster-related health risks for the individual. Public health capabilities are those target abilities applied by public health agencies to reduce disaster-related health risks for an entire population. A person with impaired mobility, for example, is likely less capable of performing rapid evacuations that often become necessary during disasters. Public health agencies can participate in population protection measures involving risk communication, evacuation, and mass care (e.g., shelter, food, water). Besides emergency response, looking upstream, public health can help to identify populations with functional needs and coordinate services that will improve mobility beforehand. In addition, public health impact assessments can assess the degree of accessibility in the built environment. Implementing a developmental approach that includes health in all policies helps to ensure future safety (and health) as a default.

DETERMINANTS OF WELLNESS

It is important to keep in mind that health is only one component of the quality of life. Another factor includes our individual perception of wellness. This perception of wellness is influenced by five factors: coping, creating, and having (or lacking) social, essential, and physical wellness. It can be reasonably surmised that populations who experience disaster-related exposures are likely to perceive a loss of wellness, and in many cases they also experience clinical disease. The condition may go undiagnosed. As a result, essential wellness-related factors may be underappreciated and go unnoticed. (See Table 13-2.)

Disasters are frequently highly emotional experiences that often require fast thinking and hard work, all within the context of an overall loss of control. For example, disasters may remarkably affect elements of physical wellness related to exercise and nutrition. Leisure time disappears as personal goals are reevaluated for a more pragmatic set of life objectives. All these events are considered stressful and often call to bear issues of the "indivisible self" related to self-worth, spirituality, identity, humor, and love.

DISASTERS AND WELLNESS

It's not difficult to recognize that people experience more than diseases when disasters occur. Disasters are rare, unpredictable events that have the potential to affect the health of many people . . . forever. People experience multiple losses simultaneously. They lose their homes, health, family members, and community—all at once. The experience itself is often traumatic and highly emotional. Disasters cause not only disease but also illness—that is, the "subjective sense of feeling unwell that often motivates a patient to consult a physician."[1] This sense often continues long after so-called recovery has been considered to have occurred. One longitudinal study found that 15% to 20% of people affected by a natural disaster developed symptoms of post-traumatic stress disorder.[2]

The long-term effects of disasters on wellness are likely even more significant than other health effects. For many people, the emotional trauma continues long after the so-called recovery effort has ceased. Following are three sets of risk factors for long-term impact on wellness:

1. Objective and subjective characteristics of the disaster: these include the proximity of the victim to the disaster site, the duration of the disaster, the degree of physical injury, and the witnessing of death or injury.[3]
2. Characteristics of the post-disaster response and recovery environment: among these are community cohesion, secondary victimization, disruption of social support systems,[4] and lack of homeownership and/or duration of displacement from home.[2]
3. Characteristics of the individual or group: included in this category are the individual's history of psychological problems, the elderly, the unemployed, single parents, and children separated from their families.[3]

In one study of the health effects of flooding in 30 locations in the United Kingdom, psychological effects were much more commonly reported after flooding than physical ones. Women also appeared to report markedly more illness than men at the worst time of flooding.[2]

Heightened psychological stress may also increase morbidity and mortality after a disaster.[3] Bennett studied 316 flood respondents and 454 nonflood controls for morbidity and mortality for one year. He found a higher mortality rate among residents of the flooded sections, especially the elderly.[4] There are also indications that this psychological impact on wellness often continues for many years. Psychiatric examinations of 224 children two years after a flood in West Virginia showed that their experiences had severely emotionally impaired 80% of them.[3] Five years after tropical storm Agnes ravaged Pennsylvania, perceived health problems were reported more commonly by disaster-affected respondents than by nonaffected controls.[4]

Considerable evidence affirms the impacts of anxiety and depression among disaster-affected populations. Studies in Europe and North America have revealed illness among flood-affected populations that meet the criteria for post-traumatic stress disorder.[5] Studies in Poland suggest long-term adverse effects on the well-being of children age 11 to 14 and 11 to 20 years, with increases in post-traumatic stress disorder, depression, and dissatisfaction with life. In the United States similar findings were reported among children age 9 to 12 after Hurricane Floyd.[5]

EMERGENCY HEALTH AND WELLNESS

Emergency health recognizes a range of dimensions that directly affect our sense of completeness (e.g., social, ecological, intellectual, spiritual, and emotional). Given this range of dimensions, emergency health must address more than merely disease. To be complete, emergency health must also address wellness using an ecosocial approach that is (1) conscious and self-directed, (2) holistic, and (3) positive and affirming. Emergency health aims to identify and manage these determinants to ensure the highest quality of life possible before, during, and after disasters.

TOPICS FOR DISCUSSION

Should wellness be a public health goal? Justify your opinion in each case:

- Before disasters
- During disasters
- After disasters

REFERENCES

1. The Association of Facilities of Medicine of Canada (AFMC). AFMC primer on population health: glossary. 2023. Available at: https://phprimer.afmc.ca/en/glossary. Accessed February 15, 2023.
2. Tunstall S, Tapsell S, Green C, Floyd P, George C. The health effects of flooding: social research results from England and Wales. *J Water Health.* 2006;4(3):365380.
3. Gerrity E, Flynn BW. Mental health consequences of disasters. In: Noji E, ed. *Public Health Consequences of Disasters.* New York, NY: Oxford University Press; 1997:101–121.
4. Ohl C, Tapsell S. Flooding and human health: the dangers posed are not always obvious. *BMJ.* 2000;321:1167–1168.
5. Ahern M, Kovats RS, Wilkinson P, et al. Global health impacts of floods: epidemiologic evidence. *Epidemiol Rev.* 2005;27:36–46.

16

Disaster Risk Management

LEARNING OBJECTIVES

Upon completion, the reader will be able to

1. Define the following terms and phrases:
    - BS 11200
    - Crisis management
    - Consequence management
    - Defects
    - Disaster management
    - Disaster risk management
    - Disaster risk reduction (DRR)
    - Emergency management
    - ISO 31000
    - Management
    - Mitigation
    - Plan
    - Performance management
    - Presidential Decision Directive 39 (PDD-39)
    - Prevalence
    - Process control
    - Process management
    - Residual risk
    - Risk
    - Risk acceptance
    - Risk assessment
    - Risk avoidance
    - Risk communication
    - Risk management
    - Risk reduction
    - Risk transfer
    - Risk treatment
    - Terrorism Incident Annex

2. Recognize the following key components of a disaster risk management program:
   - Hazard analysis
   - Impact assessment
   - Capacity assessment
   - Vulnerability assessment
   - Countermeasure determination
   - Cost-effectiveness analysis
   - Risk communication
   - Risk management plan
   - Implementation and monitoring
3. Differentiate crisis management from incident management.

PREVENTIVE CONTROL AND SYSTEMS MANAGEMENT

Public health and medical interventions that effectively manage disaster-related losses are inextricably part of a more extensive system for managing disease. Like other sectors, these health sector systems apply the principles of preventive control to manage outcomes before they occur. (See Figure 10-1.)[1]

Management is "designing and maintaining an environment (or system) in which individuals working together in groups efficiently accomplish selected aims."[2] Simply stated, management is a system used to accomplish the goals of a group. Managers, including public health emergency managers, are responsible for developing, maintaining, and improving this process.

It is essential to recognize that these outcomes lie in the future and therefore remain associated with an inherent degree of uncertainty.

Activities that decrease uncertainty are known to improve the likelihood of accomplishing an outcome. Management is a process used to reduce the uncertainty of outcomes through organization and coordination of the activities intended to achieve defined objectives.[3] The manager's role is to avoid this uncertainty in the outcome by reducing variability during the process. **Process management** is an approach based on systems that measure and control processes to achieve an intended goal or outcome. **Process control** (to best achieve the intended outcome) is considered one of the five key roles of any manager.[2]

Managers are responsible for controlling and improving the performance of a process. **Performance management** is based on the principle of preventive control, which aims to decrease the chance of **defects** before they occur. Preventive control assumes that most negative deviations from the **plan** can be fixed by applying management fundamentals. It seeks to prevent adverse outcomes by intervening (upstream) before the incident occurs.

As managers in various sectors, including public health and health care, have experienced the value of preventive control and continued to look upstream for interventions, so has the practice of disaster management grown to integrate the principles of preventive control, its aim to decrease the chance of disaster-related losses before they occur.

In 1994 the first World Conference on Natural Disaster Reduction was held in Yokohama, Japan. It affirmed that "disaster prevention, **mitigation**, and preparedness are better than disaster response in achieving the goals and objectives of the decade. Disaster response alone is insufficient, as it yields only temporary results at a very high cost."[3] Since then, **disaster risk reduction** has become the mainstay for international development related to disasters.

Unfortunately, despite over three decades of global policy development, the National Academies of Sciences, Engineering, and Medicine recently noted that "while some **disaster management** and public health preparedness programming may be viewed as tangentially related, a multisectoral and interdisciplinary national platform for coordination and policy guidance involving disaster risk reduction in the United States does not exist."[3,4]

RISK MANAGEMENT

In simplest terms, risk is the probability that an outcome will occur. This outcome is uncertain. We therefore measure and express risk in terms of both probability and uncertainty. In this sense, **risk** represents "the effect of uncertainty on outcomes."[5] **Uncertainty** is a state or condition that involves a deficiency of information and leads to inadequate or incomplete knowledge or understanding. (Sound familiar?) Uncertainty exists whenever the knowledge or experience of an event, consequence, or likelihood (e.g., a disaster) is inadequate or incomplete.[5,6] This uncertainty does not allow us to make an evidence-based determination regarding the accuracy and validity of our process. Expressions of risk, therefore, include estimations of uncertainty. This relationship may be represented as $p(\text{risk}) = \int p(\text{outcome}) \pm \text{uncertainty}$. If the outcome of interest does occur, $p(\text{risk}) = 1.0$, the outcome is then referred to as an incident (i.e., an event or a case). (See Figure 16-1.)

The occurrence, rate, or frequency of new outcomes (e.g., cases of disease) is **incidence**. The frequency of this outcome among a population (during a particular period) is called **prevalence**.

Risk is the probability that an outcome will occur as an incident.

Risk management is the activity directed toward assessing, communicating, and treating risks.[3] It is now a multisectoral standard known as ISO 31000, a set of international standards relating to risk management.[5] **ISO 31000** is the systematic approach

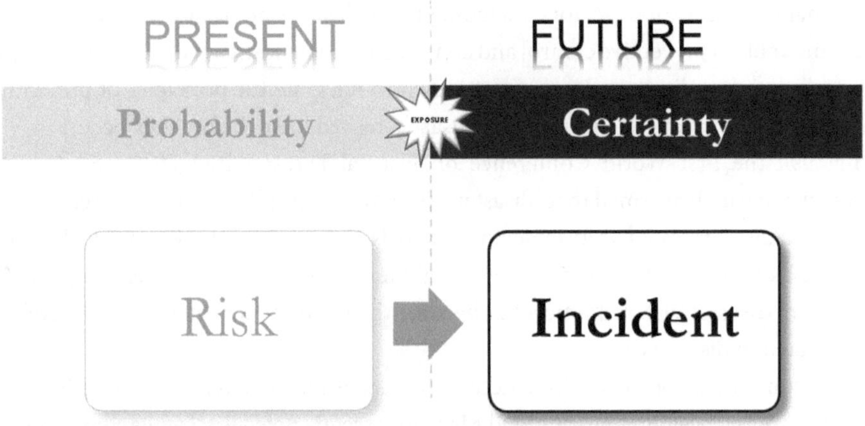

Figure 16-1. Risk as the Current Probability of a Future Outcome

and practice of managing uncertainty to minimize potential harm and loss. This involves evaluating alternative actions, selecting options, and implementing guided risk assessment. The three main phases of risk management involve **risk assessment**, **risk communication**, and **risk treatment**.[7] Risk assessment is the process of the probability of an outcome, usually under a specific set of conditions and for a certain time frame. Risk assessments are intended to express risk in terms of forecasting the statistical probability for a specific, measurable, and time-based outcome.

Risk communication is an interactive process involving the exchange among individuals, groups, and institutions of information and expert opinions about the nature, severity, and acceptability of risks and the decisions taken to combat them.[8] Risk treatment measures are put in place to control risk whenever possible. These, in turn, include the following key components of risk management[8]:

- Risk avoidance: avoiding the risk altogether
- Risk reduction: reducing the negative effect of the risk
- **Risk transfer**: transferring the risk to another party
- Risk acceptance: accepting some or all the consequences of a risk

DISASTER RISK MANAGEMENT

It follows that disaster risk is defined as the probability of this mismatch of needs and resources. Disasters are part of a continuum of effects resulting from this mismatch of needs and ecosocial resources. To summarize, the relationship is as follows:

1. Hazards create losses.
2. Losses create needs.
3. Resources meet needs.[7]

Disaster risk (e.g., disaster-related disease) occurs when hazardous exposures create needs that exceed the resources of the affected population. **Disaster risk management** is the systematic process of using resources to lessen the adverse impacts of hazards and the possibility (i.e., the risk) of disaster.[9]

The risk of disaster-related disease occurs when people are exposed to health hazards within this imbalance. Effective disaster risk management requires not only the management of the immediate problem (e.g., disaster-related disease) but also the imbalance of needs and resources that ultimately correlate with underlying determinants of health.[3,7]

Disaster risk management applies the general principles of risk management to disasters. It is a comprehensive approach that entails developing and implementing interventional strategies for the entire disaster life cycle, before and after hazard impact.[10] Disaster risk management includes pre-impact risk measures involving avoidance, reduction, and transfer and post-impact measures including risk transfer retention. Once risks have been identified and assessed, techniques can be communicated and implemented to manage or "treat" the risk.

Table 16-1 describes disaster risk management's components, including assessment and control.[10]

Table 16-1. Key Components of a Disaster Risk Management Program

Component	Activities
Hazard Analysis • Hazard identification • Hazard probability	• Identifying hazards with the potential to cause loss or damage of an asset. • Determining frequency of past hazard events.
Impact Assessment • Asset assessment • Loss assessment	• Determining critical assets, (e.g., population, medical facilities). • Identifying expected loss or damage of each asset for each hazard. • Prioritizing assets based on consequence of loss.
Capacity Assessment	• Identifying strengths, attributes, and resources available to respond to and recover from a disaster.
Vulnerability Assessment • Susceptibility • Severity	• Estimating degree of vulnerability of each asset for each hazard. • Identifying preexisting countermeasures and their level of effectiveness.
Countermeasure Determination • Avoidance/reduction • Transfer/retention	• Identifying new countermeasures that may be taken to eliminate or lessen hazards and/or vulnerabilities.
Cost-Benefit Analysis	• Identifying countermeasure costs and benefits. • Prioritizing options.
Risk Communication	• Preparing a range of recommendations for decision makers and/or the public.
Risk Management Plan	• Developing a plan for disaster risk treatment for each phase of the emergency cycle.
Implementation and Monitoring	• Implementing and monitoring the risk management program is according to plan.

Source: Keim.[10] Adapted with permission of Wolters Kluwer Health.

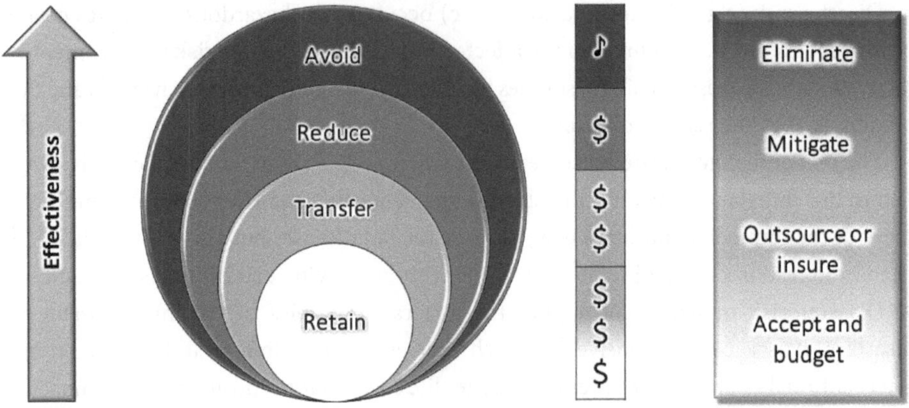

Figure 16-2. Relationship Between Risk Management and Cost Categories and Intervention Effectiveness

Ideally, disaster risk management is based on a prioritization process.[7] Once risks are identified, they are assessed regarding the potential severity of loss and the probability of occurrence.[11] The risks with the most significant loss and the greatest likelihood of occurrence are handled first, and risks with lower loss and lower probability of occurrence are addressed in descending order. In practice, the process can be complicated. Once risks have been identified and prioritized, techniques to manage the risk fall into one or more of these four major categories: avoidance, reduction, transfer, or retention.[7,8]

Figure 16-2 depicts the relationship between the four risk management categories and cost-effectiveness. Hazard avoidance is the least expensive and most effective means for risk management over the long term. (One may also posit that it is the most humane approach as well). Risk retention—that is, risk acceptance—is often the costliest and the least effective means for reducing the risk of an adverse outcome.

Risk Avoidance

Some risks may be avoided altogether. Recall that Chapter 3 examined the epidemiological triad model of disease. In that model, the risk of disease occurs at the center of a notional Venn diagram (see Figure 3-4),[3] when at-risk populations are exposed to hazards. Risk is entirely avoided by (1) avoiding the hazard, (2) avoiding exposure, or (3) avoiding vulnerability. Risk is avoided by separating these three proximate causes. In other words, risk is avoided by preventing the hazard, the exposure, or the vulnerability. For example, flood risk is avoided by floodplain management systems that prevent inundations, fire risk is avoided by construction codes that prevent building fires, and epidemic risk is avoided by immunization measures that prevent vulnerability related to transmission.

Risk Reduction

Disaster risk reduction involves methods that reduce the severity of the loss or the likelihood of the loss from occurring. It aims to detect the hazard early enough to control its advance and reduce the resulting health burden.[12] Risk reduction activities seek to mitigate the health consequences of disasters that cannot be prevented.

While people may not always be able to prevent all hazards from occurring, the health sector can play an important role in reducing public health risk.[10,11,13] The risk of a public health disaster occurs when vulnerable populations are exposed and susceptible to environmental hazards.[12] The role of public health in disaster risk avoidance is primarily risk reduction. This risk reduction involves not only disease prevention but also health protection and health promotion, achieved by identifying risk factors and advocating for healthy people, homes, communities, and commerce free from disaster risk.[12,14]

Risk Transfer

Insurance contracts and risk retention pools are described as mechanisms for risk transfer.[8] By purchasing an insurance contract, people can transfer and share risk across a large population. Risk pools are also used to share risk among a group. This form of risk transfer is different from traditional insurance in that no premium is assessed in advance; instead, losses are assessed to all group members once they occur.[8,11] Risk transfer measures also correspond well to disaster cycle activities involving preparedness.[11,12]

Risk Retention

Risk retention (i.e., risk acceptance) involves accepting disaster loss when it occurs and then attempting to respond and recover, if possible. All **residual risks** that are not avoided or transferred are retained by default.

Residual risks include the actions and cost of emergency/crisis management, response, and recovery. In other words, risk acceptance involves actions taken after the disaster has occurred (i.e., after the incidence). Examples of risk retention activities include providing medical care or temporary shelter to disaster-affected populations. Risk-retention thus corresponds well to the disaster cycle phases of response and recovery.[11,12]

Plans are used for implementing disaster risk management interventions. These interventions involve appropriate controls or countermeasures to manage each risk. An effective risk management plan should include a schedule for control implementation and responsible persons for those actions. Risk communication is a key part of disaster risk management, and thus public awareness of disaster risk and risk treatment options is necessary.

Crisis Management

Crisis management is a form of risk management. Like risk management, crisis management began as a national standard for business.[5] British Standard 11200-2014 (i.e., BS 11200) is now used worldwide by many organizations as guidance for crisis management. **BS 11200** defines a crisis as an "inherently abnormal, unstable and complex situation that represents a threat to the strategic objectives, reputation or existence of an organization."[15] According to BS 11200, crises are not synonymous with incidents and present unique challenges that require different approaches.

Figure 16-3 depicts an augmented version of Figure 16-1, including the crisis phenomenon.

The terms *crisis management* and *consequence management* initially entered the US national security lexicon by the promulgation of **Presidential Decision Directive 39 (PDD-39)** in 1995.[16] According to PDD-39, crises represented a credible or imminent threat that had *not* yet occurred.[17] Accordingly, crisis management refers to measures that manage resources needed to anticipate, prevent, or resolve a credible or imminent threat. Thus, crisis describes the relative probability of an adverse event. In other words, crisis describes risk, not incidence.

Like other forms of risk management, the goal of crisis management is to prevent an adverse outcome from ever occurring (i.e., to avoid its incidence). Once an incident has occurred, efforts are redirected to manage the consequences. Initially, PDD-39 separated the pre- and post-event responsibilities for crisis management and consequence management between two federal agencies. Later, the Terrorism Incident Annex of the

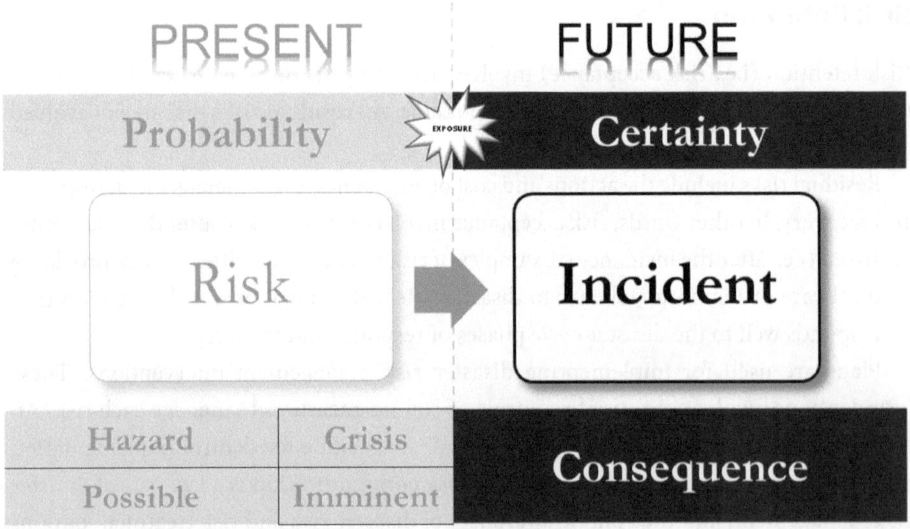

Figure 16-3. A Comparison of Risk, Crises, and Consequences

Federal Response Plan converged both crisis and consequence management into one system of pre- and post-event **emergency management** and assigned the responsibility to one federal agency, the Federal Emergency Management Agency, commonly known as FEMA.[18]

TOPICS FOR DISCUSSION

1. Discuss the importance of preventive control involving systems that operate under a high degree of uncertainty.
2. Explain how risk management is intended to lower the incidence of an adverse outcome.
3. What is the role of alert and warning in differentiating crises from hazards?

REFERENCES

1. Keim, M. *Disaster Planning: A Practical Guide for Effective Health Outcomes.* Cambridge UK: Cambridge University Press; 2021.
2. Koontz H, Weihrich H. *Essentials of Management.* 5th ed. New York, NY: McGraw-Hill; 1990.
3. Keim M. Managing disaster-related health risk: a process for prevention. *Prehosp Disaster Med.* 2018;33(3):326–334.
4. National Academies of Science, Engineering, and Medicine. *Exploring Disaster Risk Reduction Through Community-Level Approaches to Promote Healthy Outcomes: Proceedings of a Workshop—in Brief.* Washington. DC: National Academies Press; 2016.
5. Standards Australia Committee OB-007. *Risk Management.* AS/NZS 4360:2004. Sydney, Australia, and Wellington, New Zealand: Standards Australia International; 2004.
6. ISO. International Standards Organization. ISO 31000: Principles and guidelines. 2009. Available at: https://www.iso.org/standard/43170.html. Accessed November 30, 2022.
7. Keim M. Defining disaster-related health risk: a primer for prevention. *Prehosp Disaster Med.* 2018;33(3):308–316.
8. Dorfman MS. *Introduction to Risk Management and Insurance.* 9th ed. Englewood Cliffs, NJ: Prentice Hall; 2007.
9. United Nations Office of Disaster Reduction (UNDRR). Building risk knowledge: terminology. 2022. Available at: http://www.unisdr.org/eng/library/UNISDR-terminology-2009-eng.pdf. Accessed November 30, 2022.
10. Keim ME. Disaster risk management for health. In: David S, ed. *Textbook of Emergency Medicine.* Chicago, IL: Wolters Kluwer Health (Lippincott); 2010.
11. Keim ME. Disaster risk management. In: Briggs S, ed. *Advanced Disaster Medical Response for Providers.* 2nd ed. Woodbury, CT: Cine-Med Publishing; 2014.
12. Keim ME. Building human resilience the role of public health preparedness and response as an adaptation to climate change. *Am J Prev Med.* 2008;35(5):508–516.
13. Keim ME. Environmental disaster. In: Frumkin H, ed. *Environmental Health: From Global to Local.* San Francisco, CA: Wiley & Sons; 2010:843–875.

14. Srinivasan S. Creating healthy communities, healthy homes, healthy people: initiating a research agenda on the built environment and public health. *Am J Public Health.* 2003;93(9):1446–1450.
15. Hamidovic H. An introduction to crisis management. *ISACA J.* 2012;5:1–4.
16. Seiple C. Consequence management: domestic response to weapons of mass destruction. *Parameters.* 1997;27(3).
17. White House. Presidential Decision Directive / NSC-39. Washington, DC: White House; 1995.
18. Federal Emergency Management Agency (FEMA). Terrorism Incident Annex to the Federal Response Plan. Washington, DC: Federal Emergency Management Agency; 1997.

17

Risk Assessment

LEARNING OBJECTIVES

Upon completion, the reader will be able to

1. Define the following terms and phrases:
   - Accuracy
   - Analytical risk assessment
   - Decision tree
   - Disaster-related health risk
   - Disaster risk
   - Hazard analysis
   - Hazard identification
   - Hazard-impact matrix
   - Health risk
   - Impact analysis
   - Index
   - Measures of outcome
   - Measures of process
   - Predictability
   - Ratio scale
   - Reliability
   - Resource allocation
   - Risk characterization
   - Risk equation
   - Risk index
   - Utility
2. Describe the use of risk assessment in public health.
3. List three main components of a risk assessment.
4. Recognize the interrelationship between the components of disaster risk.
5. Differentiate health risk from disaster-related health risk.
6. Recognize the limited utility of health-related disaster risk assessments as a result of uncertainty.
7. Differentiate a risk scale from a risk index.

8. Describe a method for disaster-related health risk assessment based on traditional public health measures (e.g., annual disease incidence rates).
9. Using a hazard-impact matrix, compare the relative probability and impact of multiple disasters.

RISK ASSESSMENT

Risk assessment is estimating the probability of an outcome under a specific set of conditions and for a certain time frame (in this case, the annual impact of a hazardous agent on a particular population). Thus, health risk assessments express risk regarding the probability of a specific health outcome. They should also include an estimation of the degree of uncertainty related to this assessment.[1]

Risk assessment is a key component of public health. Health risk assessments are widely used to guide public health programming and multidisciplinary studies of environmental impact and developmental decision-making.[2] **Analytical risk assessment** is a well-validated tool routinely used among specific subsets of public health, including those for chemical, radiological, and microbiological risk assessment. However, this is not the case for risk assessments involving disasters in general or, more specifically, for public health emergencies involving environmental hazards, such as those encountered in technological, hydrometeorological, and seismic events.[2]

While there are now multiple examples of qualitative and semi-quantitative assessments being used to predict disaster-related health risks, few models express health risk in terms of the actual probability of health outcomes and the uncertainty of evidence.[2] This ambiguity has limited the utility of most public health disaster risk assessments. Historical data regarding disaster-related hazard incidence are typically much more readily available than disease incidence. Denominator data are notoriously absent or unreliable. This information void complicates our ability to prioritize and allocate health resources effectively before, during, and after the disaster. This results in an acceptably accurate hazard identification and prioritization, but inaccurate and nonreproducible estimations of health-related impact.

COMPONENTS OF RISK ASSESSMENT

Risk assessments consist of the following three main components: (1) **hazard analysis**, (2) **impact analysis**, and (3) **risk characterization**.

Hazard analyses typically include two stages: hazard identification and hazard characterization. **Hazard identification** involves the recognition of those hazards that are likely to occur within a given location. **Hazard characterization** consists in identifying the frequency of those hazards and then describing the adverse health effects that may result from exposure to them.[3,4]

Impact analysis seeks to quantify the degree of damage or losses (e.g., disease) that may be expected when a population is exposed to a hazard. For health, these potential losses include disaster-related morbidity and mortality. Impact analysis therefore consists of an assessment of those risk factors (besides the hazard) that are known to influence disaster-related health outcomes (i.e., exposures and health determinants).[2]

Risk characterizations combine the various factors affecting the disaster-related disease—namely, hazards, exposure, vulnerability, and capacity—into one measure of joint probability. This characterization allows for a standardized comparison among various disaster risks, including morbidity and mortality.[2]

Ideally, disaster risk management is based on a prioritization process.[5] In addition to enabling prioritization, risk assessment offers a process for ongoing research involving the interaction of health determinants, risk, and protective factors that may contribute to future adverse health outcomes. Finally, risk assessment provides a framework for monitoring and evaluating the performance of interventions intended to reduce adverse health outcomes.[1]

DISASTER RISK

To summarize, recall that (1) hazards create losses, (2) losses create needs, and (3) resources meet needs.[5] **Disaster risk** is the probability that a hazard will occur, resulting in needs exceeding resources. Disaster impact is the net loss that results when needs exceed resources. (See Figure 17-1.)[4,6–8]

Referring to Figure 17-1, note that disaster risk has two primary components: disaster hazards and their corresponding impacts. In this relationship, disaster risk increases

<table>
<tr><td rowspan="6">HAZARD</td><td colspan="10">IMPACT</td></tr>
<tr><td colspan="4">Needs</td><td colspan="6">Resources</td></tr>
<tr><td colspan="2">Exposure</td><td colspan="2">Vulnerability</td><td colspan="6">Capacity for Resilience</td></tr>
<tr><td rowspan="2">Concentration, Magnitude, or Potency</td><td rowspan="2">Time</td><td rowspan="2">Susceptibility</td><td rowspan="2">Severity</td><td rowspan="2">Avoidance</td><td rowspan="2">Reduction</td><td rowspan="2">Transfer</td><td colspan="3">Retention</td></tr>
<tr><td>Absorption</td><td>Adaptation</td><td>Transformation</td></tr>
<tr><td colspan="2">Dose</td><td colspan="2">Response</td><td colspan="6">Treatment</td></tr>
<tr><td>Increases risk</td><td colspan="2">Increases risk</td><td colspan="2">Increases risk</td><td colspan="6">Decreases risk</td></tr>
</table>

Source: Based on Keim[4,6,7] and Winderl.[8]

Figure 17-1. Relationship Between Components of Disaster Risk

as the likelihood of the hazard or its impact is increased. The impact of a disaster is primarily determined by a pathognomonic mismatch of needs and resources. Exposures increase the needs at a given corresponding vulnerability. Resources tend to increase along with the capacity of the affected population. This capacity helps to treat and therefore decrease risk. Further help comes from assessments of hazardous exposures (measuring dose) and estimates of vulnerability (measuring response) to that dose. Assessments of capacity include **measures of the process**. At the same time, assessments of overall risk involve **measures of outcome**).

DIFFERENTIATING DISASTER RISK FROM DISASTER-RELATED HEALTH RISK

Health risk differs from disaster risk in that by definition disaster risk is a measure of not only the probability of adverse health outcomes (e.g., health risk) but also the ability of the target population to avoid a mismatch of needs (caused by losses) and resources (e.g., the capacity needed to prevent disease).

Health risk is customarily reported as the proportion of initially disease-free individuals who develop disease over a defined period. This proportion is calculated as the annual case incidence rate (e.g., mortality rate, morbidity rate) and described as the percentage of individuals within a given population who develop disease over a defined time. In other words, health risk equals the likelihood of disease during a given time frame.

Note that the disaster **risk equation** differs from Wharton's general risk equation in that disaster risk also includes the effect of post-event capacity in its determination of impact. By comparison, Wharton's risk equation (and health risk assessments, generally) deal only with pre-event probability.[9] (See Figure 16-1.) Calculations of disease incidence do not include various elements of post-event risk treatment that may be applied (e.g., transfer and acceptance).

It is, therefore, important to recognize that disaster risk is not synonymous with disaster-related health risk. When applied to public health, health risk, $p(R_H)$, is the probability that in a specific time frame, an adverse health outcome will occur among a population that is exposed to a hazardous agent.[5]

When applied to disasters, **disaster-related health risk**, $p(D_H)$ can be described as the probability of disease, given that a disaster $p(D)$ has occurred (i.e., $p(D_H) = p(R_H) \mid p(D) = 1$).[1] Thus, disaster-related health risk, $p(D_H)$, is often expressed as the annual disaster-related case incidence rate and described as the proportion of individuals within a given population (and over a defined time) who experience morbidity and mortality, first, as a result of direct hazard exposure and, second, as a consequence of a mismatch between community needs and resources caused by the disaster hazard. (See Figure 5-1.)

THE "TWILIGHT ZONE" OF DISASTER RISK ASSESSMENT

Things often appear less evident in the twilight. And into that darkness, uncertainty settles. It is reasonable to compare our current disaster risk assessment with this "twilight zone." The utility of disaster risk assessment is often complicated by first- and second-order uncertainty. There is an overall lack of predictability and a high degree of ambiguity.[2] To date, none have been validated as predictive of quantifiable health risk related to disasters.[2]

These challenges have also limited our general scientific understanding of risk assessment. For the past decade most disaster-related health studies have repeatedly investigated nearly the same set of risk factors (now broadly referred to as vulnerability and resilience). By contrast, very few epidemiological studies have included measures of capacity and exposure. "Imagine, if you will," a world where environmental health assessments routinely omit exposure science! As Rod Serling (host of the 1960s TV series with the same name) would say, "Welcome to the "*Twilight Zone.*"

Epidemiological assessments of disaster-related health risk routinely underreport risk factors related to the environment and agent (exposure and hazard) while focusing almost entirely on the characteristics of the individual victim (e.g., vulnerability).[2] Thus, these risk assessments rarely describe the role of society in the problem. Instead, the focus is directed on an inherently "wounded" individual. Most epidemiological investigations involving disasters focus on the demographics and emergent needs of the population. These studies are insufficient to collect the full range of data necessary for an accurate and valid prediction of disaster-related health risk. "Imagine, if you will," a world where public health does not measure health risk. Welcome to the "disaster zone."

The **utility** of existing health-related disaster risk assessment models is obviously limited by challenges involving first- and second-order uncertainty. This uncertainty is often due to a lack of **predictability** (reflected in the standard deviation) and **accuracy** (reflected in the standard error) of these assessments. This uncertainty has limited the predictive value of most public health disaster risk assessments. This phenomenon has resulted in the development of acceptably accurate hazard identification and prioritization but unacceptably inaccurate and non-reproducible estimations of health-related impact.

APPROACHES FOR ASSESSMENT OF DISASTER-RELATED HEALTH RISK

Multiple approaches have been used for performing a disaster risk assessment. These approaches include using ordinal measures such as scales and indices and a nominal method designed to overcome uncertainty. Ideally, a health risk may also be calculated from historical data and expressed as a scale in terms of mean annual incidence and standard deviation.

Typically, both scales and indices employ multiple observations or items of measurement. However, disaster-related indices are often not based on empirical measures but somewhat subjective estimates that are more prone to first- and second-order uncertainty. Disaster-related risk indices typically consist of unproven assumptions regarding the pathways of causation.[2,10–13] Thus, most indices used to assess disaster-related disease lack predictive value that would guide accurate cost accounting necessary to justify large-scale **resource allocation** or investment.

Compared with a **risk index**, **risk ratio** scales have also been used to describe the risk of disaster-related disease. These scales describe one measurable outcome (e.g., the probability of disaster-related health outcome). This outcome is then expressed as a specific and quantifiable public health indicator (e.g., morbidity and mortality rates). And while the uncertainty of these values may remain relatively high because of a lack of predictability (reflected in the standard deviation), accuracy (reflected in the standard error) is improved using this scale compared with an ordinal index of subjective estimates. This accuracy results in enhanced **reliability** (and transparency) of the assessment. A numerical scale also allows for statistical calculations and statements that describe the relative degree of uncertainty. This test is not possible using ordinal indices.[1]

Finally, when disaster data are entirely unavailable (or unreliable), disaster planners often apply a capability-based approach to planning that helps to compensate for the relatively high degree of uncertainty. This unpredictability is best met by planning to accomplish those objectives within our ability to achieve—that is, our capability—rather than the scenario's constraints. In emergency response, capability-based planning allows for the flexibility necessary to address a wide range of unpredictable scenarios.[1]

An Evidence-Based Approach for Assessing Disaster-Related Health Risk

Figure 17-2 depicts an algorithm for assessing disaster-related health risk based on traditional public health measures (e.g., annual disease incidence rates). This approach includes four traditional components of risk assessment: context, hazard analysis, impact analysis, and risk characterization. The risk assessment is based on the availability of historical data (e.g., hazard and disease incidence rates). These data are then evaluated for certainty. To summarize the entire risk assessment process:

1. Context: select the population at risk (P) and the disaster-related health outcome (D_H).
2. Hazard analysis: calculate or estimate the mean annual hazard incidence rate, $p(H)$, for population, P.

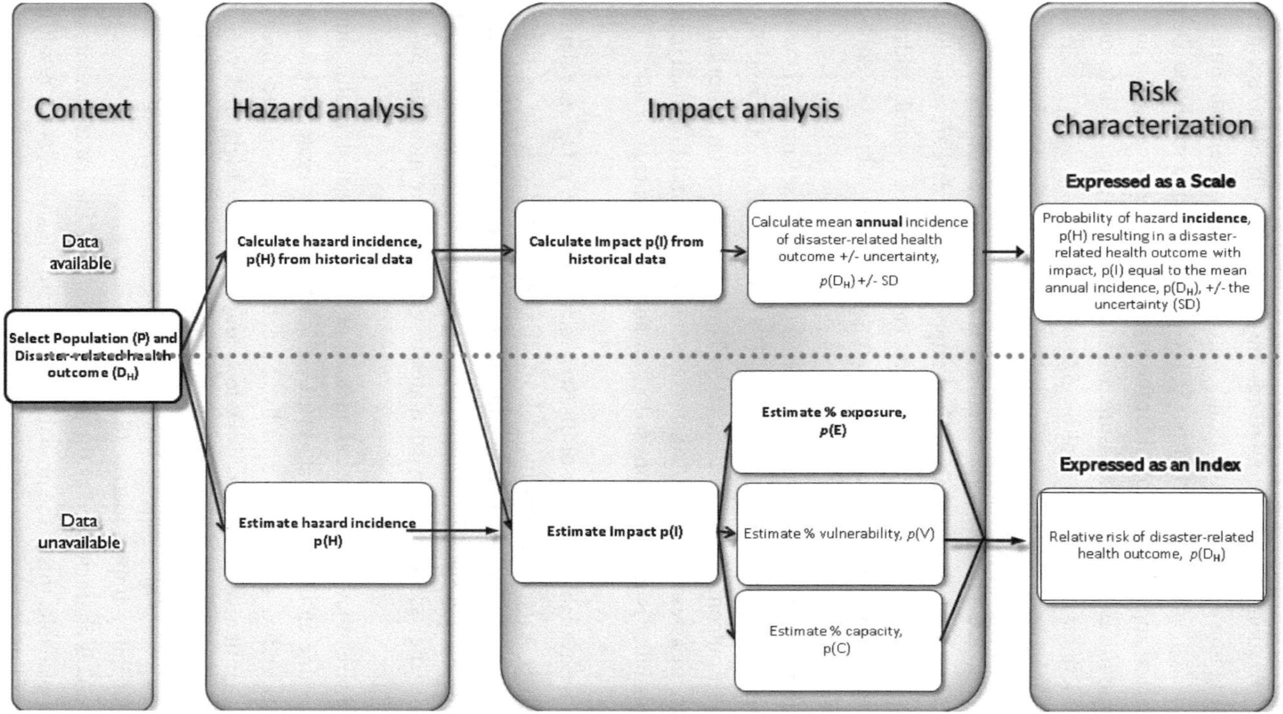

Source: Keim et al.[1] Reprinted with permission of Cambridge University Press. © Cambridge University Press 2021.

Figure 17-2. Decision Tree for Assessment of Disaster-Related Health Risk

3. Impact analysis: calculate or estimate the mean annual incidence rate of disaster-related health outcome, $p(D_H)$ +/– the standard deviation (*SD*).
4. Risk characterization: express overall risk as the joint probability of hazard incidence, $p(H)$, resulting in a disaster-related health outcome equal to the mean annual incidence rate, $p(D_H)$ +/– the uncertainty (*SD*). Consider using a modified Delphi or similar empirical approach to control for the variability of expert input. In absence of data, combine the estimates of exposure, vulnerability, and capacity into one index of relative risk of disaster-related health outcome, $p(DH)$.

This **decision tree** includes two main pathways. The top expresses risk as a scale and the bottom as an index. The appropriate pathway is selected based on the availability of health data related to each disaster hazard. In the upper pathway, data are available. In the lower pathway, data are unavailable. In all cases, calculations of central tendency and variance (i.e., means and standard deviation) are preferable to subjective estimates of relative degrees of impact.[1]

This algorithm begins by deciding the context for the assessment. This context includes selecting the specific target population (*P*) to be served and the specific disaster-related health outcome being studied (D_H). Then, depending on historical hazard data availability, the assessor either calculates or estimates the hazard's annual incidence, $p(H)$. This probability is usually expressed as an annual percentage or as a "100-year event."

When data are available, this risk of disaster-related disease, $p(D_H)$, is calculated as a ratio scale. This scale expresses the risk of disaster-related disease as the annual percent-probability of a hazard that would result in a health impact of average size (i.e., mean value) for that specific hazard. Then depending on the availability of historical impact data, the assessor either calculates or estimates the mean annual disease incidence, $p(D_H)$.

Where data are unavailable, causal factors of disaster-related health outcomes (i.e., exposure, vulnerability, and capacity) are estimated and aggregated to be expressed as a relative risk index. This index broadly characterizes disaster-related disease risk along a semi-quantitative scale (e.g., very low, low, moderate, high, and very high). Indices describe the risk applied to the hazard incidence and its associated impact (e.g., low probability to high impact). The risk may then be compared for different hazards using a probability-impact matrix. (See Figure 17-3.)

Finally, the risk is characterized as the joint probability of the hazard and its impact. When data are available, this is the probability of hazard incidence, $p(H)$, resulting in a disaster-related health outcome with impact, $p(I)$, equal to the mean annual incidence of disaster-related disease, $p(D_H)$. When historical data are unavailable, estimates of exposure, vulnerability, and capacity are combined into one index of relative risk of disaster-related health outcomes, $p(D_H)$.

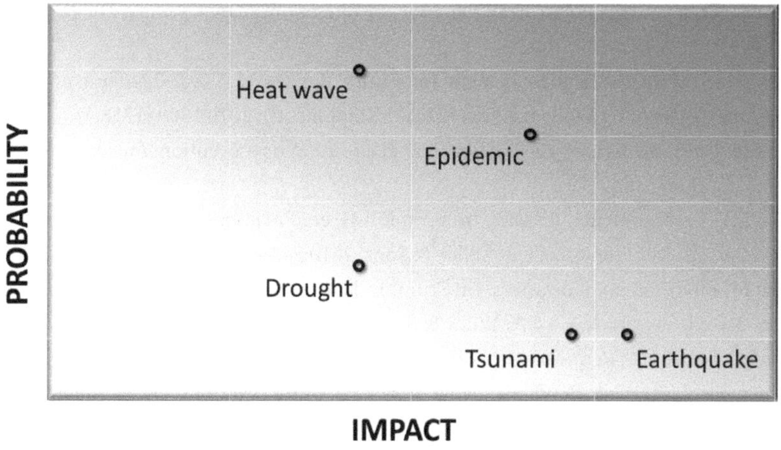

Figure 17-3. Example of a Hazard-Impact Matrix for Five Natural Disasters

Figure 17-3 provides an example of a simple hazard probability-impact matrix. High-probability/high-impact events (noted in the upper right corner) are prioritized highest. By contrast, low-probability/low-impact events (depicted in the bottom left corner) are given the least priority. This prioritization is often described in a **hazard-impact matrix** with probability represented on the *y*-axis and impact represented on the *x*-axis.

TOPICS FOR DISCUSSION

1. Discuss the relative risk of floods using the following information:
   - The incidence of a "100-year flood"
   - Percentage of the population that is "exposed"
   - Percentage of the population that is "vulnerable" to floodwater
   - Percentage of the population with the "capacity" to avoid an adverse health outcome
2. Describe the relative certainty of your estimates in terms of
   - Predictability
   - Accuracy

REFERENCES

1. Keim M. *Disaster Planning: A Practical Guide to Effective Health Outcomes*. Cambridge, UK: Cambridge University Press; 2021.
2. Keim M. Assessing disaster-related health risk: appraisal for prevention. *Prehosp Disaster Med*. 2017 33(3):317–325.

3. Keim M. Developing a public health emergency operations plan: a primer. *Pac Health Dialog.* 2002;9(1):124–129.
4. Keim ME. Disaster risk management for health. In: David S, ed. *Textbook of Emergency Medicine.* Chicago, IL: Wolters Kluwer Health (Lippincott); 2010:1309–1318.
5. Keim M. Defining disaster-related health risk: a primer for prevention. *Prehosp Disaster Med.* 2018;33(3):308–316.
6. Keim ME. Environmental disaster. In: Frumkin H, ed. *Environmental Health: From Global to Local.* 2nd ed. San Francisco, CA: Wiley & Sons; 2010:843–875.
7. Keim M. Environmental disasters. In: Frumkin H, ed. *Environmental Health: From Global to Local.* 3rd ed. San Francisco CA: Wiley & Sons; 2016:667–692.
8. Winderl T. *Disaster Resilience Measurements: Stock Taking of Ongoing Efforts in Developing Systems for Measuring Resilience.* New York NY: United Nations Development Program; 2014.
9. Wharton F. Risk management basic concepts in general principles. In: Ansell J, Wharton F, eds. *Risk Analysis Assessment and Management.* Chichester, UK: Wiley & Sons; 1992:100.
10. Keim M, Lee V, Cruz M, et al. The CDC/ATSDR public health vulnerability mapping system. 2007. Available at: https://ininet.org/the-cdcatsdr-public-health-vulnerability-mapping-system-using.html. Accessed December 20, 2022.
11. Geospatial Research Analysis and Services Program. The Social Vulnerability Index. 2017. Available at: https://svi.cdc.gov. Accessed November 30, 2022.
12. Badia A, Pallares-Barbera M, Valldeperas N, Gisbert M. Wildfires in the wildland-urban interface in Catalonia: vulnerability analysis based on land use and land cover change. *Sci Total Environt.* 2019;673:184–196.
13. Keim M, Lovallo A. Validity of the National Health Security Preparedness Index as a predictor of excess COVID-19 mortality. *Prehop Dis Med.* 2021;36(2):141–144.

18

Risk Communication

LEARNING OBJECTIVES

Upon completion, the reader will be able to

1. Define the following terms and phrases:
   - Monitoring and evaluation
   - Risk communication
2. Differentiate risk communication from crisis communication.
3. Differentiate risk communication from risk messaging.
4. Recognize four theories of risk communication.
5. Recognize eight qualitative factors that affect risk perception and public concern.
6. Recall seven cardinal rules of risk communication.
7. Recognize the role of risk communication in terms of an ecosocial model of health.
8. Recognize risk communication as a continuous discussion of wellness and illness.

DEFINING RISK COMMUNICATION

Once disaster-related health risk has been identified and assessed, these results must be communicated to decision makers and at-risk populations. However, communicating risk in practical and unmisleading ways is often challenging. "Communicating information about environmental risk to the people most affected by it is one of the major challenges faced by risk managers and community decision-makers."[1,2] Risk assessment is a complex process, let alone one not communicated well to the lay public.

From the risk management perspective, risk communication aims to help populations understand risk and participate in "decisions about how the risk should be managed."[1] A basic understanding of risk is therefore necessary to understand risk communication.

The World Health Organization has described risk communication as "the exchange of information, advice, and opinions between experts, community leaders, officials, and the people at risk." Risk communication has also been described as a "science-based approach for communicating effectively in situations of high stress, high concern or controversy."[3] Simply put, risk communication is the public discussion of an uncertain future outcome.

Risk communication should be differentiated from crisis communications intended to serve an organization's needs "during any unexpected incident potentially upsetting an organization's employees, customers, operations, reputation, finances, or community."[4] In simple terms, risk communication is intended for populations, whereas crisis communication is designed for organizations.

In addition, it is also essential to recognize the difference between risk communication and risk messaging. Risk messaging is the systematic process for planning, creating, and distributing information in a one-way flow, such as in broadcasting. By contrast, risk communication is an interactive process of exchanging information and opinion among individuals, groups, and institutions at multiple levels.[1] Risk communication should therefore be considered cyclical rather than linear. This iteration allows the population at risk to address a wide range of issues that are often of significant concern. The following are categories of concern that are commonly related to risk: health, safety, environment, family, community, economics, trust, benefits, control, fairness, respect, and accountability. Each of these elements adds another level of complexity to communicating effectively, even during a nonemergency.

Risk communication is a conversation, not a broadcast.

FOUR THEORIES OF RISK COMMUNICATION

Risk theorists have proposed four theories of risk communication.[1] Each of these theories is based on people's observed behavior when they "are upset, angry, fearful, outraged, under high stress, involved in conflict, or feel great concern."[1] People in these situations often (1) have difficulty processing information, (2) experience distrust, (3) give greater weight to negative information, and (4) perceive risk in both an objective and a subjective manner.[1] It appears that our perceptions regarding safety and risk are highly subjective, just as our perceptions of wellness and illness are. Very interesting! Human values deeply influence both. Following is a list of eight qualitative factors that affect risk perception and public concern:

1. Are measures voluntary or mandatory?.
2. Is the incident within or outside someone's control?
3. Is the risk familiar or unfamiliar?
4. Is the risk well distributed or unevenly distributed among the population?
5. Is the risk periodic or catastrophic?
6. Is the risk natural or human-made?
7. Is the risk generated by a trusted versus an untrustworthy source?
8. Does the risk affect adults only or does it also affect children?

According to these qualitative factors, public perception of a lower subjective risk therefore involves risk that is voluntary, natural, familiar, moral, and fair.[1]

SEVEN CARDINAL RULES OF RISK COMMUNICATION

Covello was the first to propose seven cardinal rules of risk communication intended to help address this level of complexity.[5] Covello's seven cardinal rules of risk communication are listed as follows:

1. Accept and involve the public as a legitimate partner in the decision-making process.
2. Listen to your audience.
3. Be truthful, honest, frank, and open.
4. Coordinate, collaborate, and partner with other credible sources.
5. Meet the needs of the media.
6. Speak clearly and with compassion.
7. Prepare, plan, and evaluate the performance of your communication.

These rules by Covello are directed toward three main goals: (1) placing the risk within a familiar context, (2) advising about risk reduction behavior, and (3) encouraging a dialog.[1] Compared with the ad hoc element of emergency response, the most effective interventions result from an ongoing program or campaign. Risk communication programs should begin by developing an outreach plan. Outreach plans typically identify the goals, target audience, message content, message medium, mechanisms for follow-up, and **monitoring and evaluation** activities.

It is important to establish realistic goals for risk communication. There is no single overriding approach for making risk communication easy. Risk messages seek to compress what is often technical information, which can lead to misunderstanding, confusion, and distrust. For this reason it is mistaken to expect improved risk communication to reduce conflict and smooth risk management. The National Research Council identified two significant problems of risk communication: problems deriving from institutional and political systems and issues among risk communicators and recipients.[3] Institutional and political systems are known to limit the possible responses to the risk in question or require that specific actions be taken in given circumstances, often regardless of effectiveness. Problems related to risk communicators and recipients commonly involve credibility, understandability, attention span, and access to information.[3]

RISK COMMUNICATION FOR AN ECOSOCIAL MODEL OF HEALTH

The role of risk communication has expanded over the years beyond that of a system used in times of emergency. Public health risk communication has expanded to include various ecosocial determinants related to the individual, people, environment, resources, and population beliefs. (See Figures 9-1 and 10-3.)[6]

Risk communication is a continuous discussion of wellness and illness. Our goal of "producing health" requires not only management of the immediate problem (downstream) but also proactive management of the person's (upstream) determinants of health and proximate causes, or etiology. (See Figure 8-1.) Wellness is our pathway to that destination of health. In that case, risk communication is our tour guide, preventing us from becoming lost, preparing us for the steep climbs, protecting and promoting our progress. Burkle described these actions within the context of Carr's disaster cycle as the more inclusive role of a "health crisis manager."[7] The time for risk communication is not only after the disaster. In most examples, proactive alerts and warnings are much more cost-effective than survival advice offered after the fact.

An ecosocial approach to risk communication aligns the process with a person's context and life stage to address any potential mismatch between objective and subjective risk.[1] Risk communication can be designed that specifically address the determinants of health associated with the individual person within that person's own familiar contexts of family, community, environment, society, and belief system. (See Figure 3-3.) Public dialogs are created that include individual, micro, meso, exo, macro, and chrono contexts. This exchange of information and opinion occurs among individuals, groups, and institutions, often coinciding and at multiple levels.[3] During this exchange, each and every stakeholders can learn more about each other's perceptions of risk, wellness, and illness and reference their own experiences with those of the community and society.

TOPICS FOR DISCUSSION

Describe examples of how each of the eight qualitative factors that affect risk perception occurred during the COVID-19 pandemic.

REFERENCES

1. Environmental Protection Agency (EPA). *Risk Communication in Action.* Cincinnati, OH: National Risk Management Research Laboratory; 2007.
2. Reckelhoff-Dangel C, Petersen D. *Risk Communication as a Risk Mamangement Tool.* Washington, DC: Environmental Protection Agency; 2005.
3. National Research Council. *Improving Risk Communication.* Washington, DC: National Academies Press; 1989.
4. Fernandez L, Merzer M. *Crisis Communication Handbook.* Coulsdon, UK: Jane's Information Group; 2003.
5. Covello V. *Seven Cardinal Rules of Risk Communication.* Harrisburg, PA: Pennsylvania Dept of Environmental Resources; 1988.
6. Frieden T. A framework for public health action: the health impact pyramid. *Am J Public Health.* 2010;100(4):590–595.
7. Burkle F. Challenges of global public health emergencies: development of a health crisis management framework. *J Exp Med.* 2019;249:33–41.

VI. THE PRACTICE OF EMERGENCY HEALTH

19

Tenets of Emergency Health

LEARNING OBJECTIVES

Upon completion, the reader will be able to

1. Define the following terms and phrases:
   - Community-based
   - Disability
   - Environmental justice
   - Evidence-based decision-making
   - Health in all policies (HiAP)
   - Measures of effectiveness
   - Outcome
   - Outputs
   - Population health
2. Recall the seven principles of emergency health depicted as the acronym $HOPE^4$.
3. Identify four stages of prevention, in terms of upstream and downstream location on the disease pathway.
4. Describe two phases of disaster risk management in terms of upstream and downstream locations on the disease pathway.
5. Compare six prevention goals with the four pillars of emergency health.

SEVEN TENETS OF EMERGENCY HEALTH

Emergency health is intended to be a return to public health basics. The aim is to reinforce the tried-and-true governing principles of public health that have shown to be effective means for addressing public health threats. Chapter 3 introduced the four pillars of emergency health: prevention, promotion, protection, and provision. This chapter delves deeper to discuss the underlying public health principles that guide the practice of emergency health.

Following is a list of the seven tenets of emergency health that may be recalled according to the mnemonic $HOPE^4$. (See Table 19-1.)

1. Health in all policies
2. Outcome oriented

3. Population health
4. Evidence-based decision-making
5. Equity
6. Environmental justice
7. Ecosocial perspective

Health in All Policies

The first tenet of emergency health is the notion of health in all policies (HiAP). HiAP recognizes that a multitude of factors beyond healthcare create health. In many cases, health is created (or destroyed) by other sectors beyond the scope of traditional public health activities.[1] HiAP is an approach for addressing the ecosocial determinants of health (DoH) that are the key drivers of health outcomes and health inequities. It promotes collaboration between public health practitioners and nontraditional partners. Public health 3.0 describes the role of local public health agencies to serve as they convener and the catalyst for **community-based** interventions and population health. The HiAP approach includes five key elements: (1) promoting health and equity, (2) engaging in intersectoral collaboration, (3) encouraging co-benefits for multiple partners, (4) engaging stakeholders, and (5) creating change. In essence, to be healthy, communities must meet the needs of the population, needs that are not entirely dependent on the health care sector. To thrive, communities must meet the basic needs of all. They must also ensure a safe and sustainable environment that supports adequate economic and social development levels. Social relationships and responsibilities must ensure health and social equity in supportive and respectful ways.[1]

HiAP is a critical principle of emergency health. Emergency health recognizes that disaster-related mortality is not merely dependent on the actions of health care or public health entities. It is a complex problem with multiple contributing factors drawn from across all sectors of society. To address only health policy would ignore many of the most effective means for controlling disease. HiAP allows for an all-sector approach and all-sector benefit.

Outcome-Oriented Methods

Outcome-oriented methods encourage public health practitioners to be clear on the protection outcomes we are trying to achieve, to have a theory about how to achieve those outcomes, and to plot a course of action toward them. These methods derive from results-based protection, commonly referred to as RBP. RBP is a problem-solving approach to address the complex and ever-changing environment surrounding protection issues in humanitarian action.[2] It emphasizes starting from the perspective of the affected community while encouraging learning and adapting, investing in relationships,

Table 19-1. The Relationship Between Emergency Health, Prevention, Exposures, and Risk

Location on Disease Pathway	Upstream				Downstream	
Impact on Disease	Lowers incidence				Lowers prevalence	
Phase of Risk Management	Risk reduction				Risk acceptance	
Health Status	Wellness		At risk		Illness	
Stage of Prevention	Primordial prevention		Primary prevention		Secondary prevention	Tertiary prevention
Prevention Goal	Reduce adverse health determinants	Increase protective factors	Reduce risk factors	Reduce hazardous exposures	Reduce disease, given exposure	Reduce progression, given disease
Dose-Response Effect	Decreases *y*-intercept	Decreases slope	Decreases slope	Decreases *x*-max	Increases LD^{50}	Decreases *y*-max
Relationship to the Individual	Extrinsic	Intrinsic	Intrinsic	Extrinsic	Intrinsic	Intrinsic
Emergency Health Pillar	Prevention	Promotion	Protection		Provision	

and strategic collaboration to achieve protection outcomes. In RBP, protection outcomes are defined as "reduction in risk."[2]

In contrast to this outcome-oriented method, task-based approaches fail to recognize that goals are also a tangible product of personal values. Individuals' attitudes, beliefs, and cultural backgrounds inform their goals. And while a group of individuals may begin at the same time working toward the future on the same issue, the outcome can become highly variable without some metric for completion.[3] The mental construct of what that future outcome may look like is influenced by multiple individuals' attitudes, beliefs, and cultural backgrounds. The more complex the plan becomes (as it adds more stages and individual perspectives), the higher the risk of uncertainty regarding the planned outcome. Outcome-oriented methods identify clear outcomes and plot a course of action toward them. This approach is well suited for the complex and ever-changing environment surrounding humanitarian action protection issues.[2] It also helps to focus our interventions on the measurable reduction of morbidity and mortality as the primary intended outcome.

Chapter 1 described many of the problems associated with managing public health emergencies, which tend to be focused on the number of people treated rather than the number of lives saved or mortality prevented. Public health emergencies represent one of the few public health burdens where effectiveness and outcome measures are not the primary drivers of merit for practice and research. Most emergency operations studies utilize anecdotal and experiential recall rather than hard data to evaluate system performance. And emergency funding is rarely tied to **measures of effectiveness.**

Measurable outcomes are the foundation of emergency health, with its primary mission to lower disaster-related morbidity and mortality. All system activities are intended to contribute directly to this primary focus. Interventions must be evaluated for **measures of efficiency** and effectiveness in this fundamental public health goal. All public health emergency response activities should be subject to **measures of success.** All general allocations and programming related to disasters should be evaluated regarding cost-effectiveness for reducing disaster-related mortality.

Population Health

Population health has been described as "the health outcomes of a group of individuals, including the distribution of such outcomes within the group, and includes "health outcomes, patterns of DoHs [determinants of health], and policies and interventions that link these two."[4] These populations are often delineated by geographic region, but they can also be other groups, such as employees, ethnic groups, disabled persons, or racial minorities. In addition, many DoH impact individuals in part at a population level.

Population health researchers tend to use a set of methods and approaches that have the following essential characteristics: (1) an examination of systematic differences in outcomes across populations, (2) the "complexity of interactions among determinants, biological pathways linking determinants to population health outcomes, and (3) the influence of different determinants over time and throughout the life cycle."[5]

Evidence-Based Decision-Making

Eddy's 1990 article in the *Journal of the American Medical Association* first identified the principles of evidence-based guidelines and population-level policies. An evidence-based approach to medicine and public policy was considered as "explicitly describing the available evidence that pertains to a policy and tying the policy to evidence instead of standard-of-care practices or the beliefs of experts."[6] The pertinent evidence must be identified, described, and analyzed. The policymakers must determine whether the evidence justifies the policy.

This convergence of clinical practice and public policy has evolved to suggest that a broader systems-based approach is needed to inform health system design and improvement. The Agency for Healthcare Research and Quality defines evidence-based medicine as "an interdisciplinary approach which uses techniques from science, engineering, biostatistics and epidemiology, such as meta-analysis, decision analysis, risk-benefit analysis, and randomized controlled trials to deliver 'the right care at the right time to the right patient.'"[7]

Performance improvement uses measurable evidence to correct problems before they manifest deficiencies. This is based on the principle of process control, which assumes that most negative deviations can be fixed by applying management fundamentals. Performance is typically measured and managed during the short term through monitoring and during the long term through evaluation.[3]

Empirical data are the evidence that drives process analysis. Without proof of performance (e.g., efficiency, effectiveness, **utility**), public health officials are left to operate systems without their knowing the reliability and validity of costly population-based interventions. Often this uncertainty does not offer up adequate evidence for decision makers that will justify the significant public investment necessary to address the need. Without process control, the management of disaster-related disease predictably results in a high degree of variability, with random cause variation in full play. Within this void, interventions are based on the process (e.g., number of patients treated), not measurable outcomes (e.g., number of deaths prevented). In other words, disaster-related disease is left to continue unabated by a system that is not driven by health outcomes data or consistent with the evidence.

Equity

In the 1990s Margaret Whitehead offered that health equity "implies that ideally, *everyone* should have a fair opportunity to attain their full health potential and more pragmatically that no one should be disadvantaged from attaining this potential if it can be avoided."[8]

The US Department of Health and Human Services Healthy People 2020 program defines health equity as the "attainment of the highest level of health for *all* people."[9] In this sense, health equity extends the goal of complete well-being to the entire population. Just as wellness seeks to optimize the individual's well-being, health equity aims to raise that optimum for everyone fairly and impartially. Health equity recognizes that there are also significant ecosocial obstacles to health in addition to the ecosocial determinants that create health. These obstacles create health disparities that are "differences in health status that are closely linked with social economic or environmental disadvantage."[10]

These differences exist between groups of people who, compared with the majority, have systematically experienced more significant obstacles to health on the basis of their race, ethnicity, religion, socioeconomic status, gender, age, **disability**, sexual orientation or gender identity, or geographic location.

For many years disaster researchers have recognized a disparity among specific population demographics related to the burden of disaster-related disease (e.g., poverty). The goal of health equity is to avoid health disparities—that is, to avoid those differences in health that are closely linked with social, technological, economic, environmental, political, or cultural disadvantages.[11] As such, health equity is not synonymous with health equality. Health equality describes fair and equal outcomes across an entire population. By comparison, health equity describes a fair and equal process for seeking equal outcomes.

Measurable outcomes are the foundation of emergency health. And as such, measures of equal outcomes across a population represent a core metric for health equity (or lack thereof). While random cause variation may also cause some unequal outcomes, the goal of health equity is to avoid health disparities by addressing those special cause variations associated with ecosocial DoH.

Environmental Justice

Along with health equity, public health is also characteristically founded on social justice.[11] In this case, social justice describes a process for seeking equal health outcomes. This concept of social justice recognizes that significant factors outside of individuals' control can impede the fair distribution of outcomes.

Environmental justice seeks to codify a system for ensuring health equity. The US Department of Energy describes environmental justice as "the fair treatment and meaningful involvement of all people regardless of race, color or national origin or income risk concerning the development implementation and enforcement of environmental laws regulations and policies."[12]

Environmental justice also provides an established frame of reference work for comparing other related DoH that contribute to the balance of impartial justice across the entire population.

Environmental factors often play an enormous role in determining individual health outcomes among populations affected by disasters. It then follows as a reasonable assumption that environmental justice should also play a key role in developing, implementing, and enforcing disaster-related interventions.

Ecosocial Perspective

The ecosocial model of health recognizes an individual's biological and psychological development as a core makeup that is affected and modified by the immediate physical and social environment and subsequent interactions with more distal environments and contexts. It is based on principles of human development that characterize the individual person within a context of progressively broader ecosocial determinants.

An ecosocial model of health considers personal characteristics, environmental context, and life stage.[13] This perspective emphasizes the multiple determinants (e.g., environments and personal characteristics), the multiple social levels (e.g., individuals, groups, societies), and the complexity of human situations (e.g., culture, attitudes, beliefs). Also important is that an ecosocial model for health incorporates the role of life stage and aging as a key DoH.

Furthermore, epidemiological patterns of disaster-related disease reflect proximal as well as distal factors at play. For emergency health, an ecosocial model recognizes the role of personal characteristics, environmental context, and life stage as determinants of disaster-related disease. The ecosocial perspective also provides a more detailed framework for identifying, assessing, monitoring, and managing disaster-related causes and risk factors.

RELATIONSHIP BETWEEN EMERGENCY HEALTH, WELLNESS, PREVENTION, AND RISK

Table 19-1 depicts the overall relationship between emergency health, wellness, disease prevention, and risk management, as described in this book. The top line divides Table 19-1 into events that occur either upstream (before exposure) or downstream (after exposure). (See Chapter 3.) Upstream DoH tend to lower disease incidence, while downstream determinants reduce the prevalence. (See Chapters 9 and 10.) Upstream and downstream factors may also be considered within the context of disaster risk management, which broadly divides upstream factors into those dedicated to risk reduction and downstream factors into those activities dedicated to risk acceptance. (See Chapters 23–24.) These factors are also implemented at various stages of health status, beginning with the stage of wellness and then extending to illness. (See Chapter 3.) Following exposure, downstream populations may experience changes in health status related to clinical disease. (See Chapter 2.) Activities intended to address these various risk and protective factors may be considered within the context of disease prevention that occurs in stages. (See Chapter 20) Prevention goals associated with primordial prevention involve reducing adverse DoH and increasing individual protective factors. Goals related to primary prevention seek to reduce individual risk factors and hazardous exposures.

Secondary prevention goals involve the reduction of disease, given exposure; and finally, tertiary prevention includes the goal of reducing progression, given disease. (See Chapter 18.) Each disease stage may also be a key factor within a hazard dose-response curve. The *y*-intercept of the curve represents those DoH that establish a baseline of risk existing at the time of exposure. The dose-response curve's slope reflects the protective and risk factors of the individual that affect the degree of physiological response per dose of hazard. The maximum point on the *x*-axis constitutes the maximum dose of hazard delivered during exposure, and the maximum point on the *y*-axis represents the maximum response to the hazardous exposure, which in this case is mortality. The LD_{50} (i.e., lethal dose for 50% of those exposed) is identified as the intersection between the mean dose and mean response. (See Chapter 5.)

Each of the four pillars of emergency health for the individual at risk involves a different order of relationship to the individual. In the case of disease prevention, interventions are proved effective for a full range of primordial, primary, secondary, and tertiary prevention activities. Health promotion activities focus on increasing protective factors and reducing the individual's risk factors. Populations are then protected from hazardous exposures; in cases where this is not possible, clinical interventions become necessary.

TOPICS FOR DISCUSSION

Choose one type of natural or technological disaster and then describe ways the seven tenets of emergency health (i.e., HOPE[4]) may apply to this disaster.

REFERENCES

1. Rudolph L, Caplan J, Ben-Moshe K, Dillon L. *Health in All Policies: A Guide for State and Local Governments.* Washington, DC, and Oakland, CA: American Public Health Association and Public Health Institute; 2013.
2. What is RBP? Interaction. 2022. Available at: https://protection.interaction.org/what-is-rbp. Accessed December 1, 2022.
3. Keim M. *Disaster Planning: A Practical Guide to Effective Health Outcomes.* Cambridge, UK: Cambridge University Press; 2021.
4. Kindig D, Stoddart G. What is population health? *Am J Public Health.* 2003;93(3):380–383.
5. Adler N, Marmot M, McEwan B, Stewart J. Socioeconomic status and health in industrial nations: social, psychological, and biological pathways. *Ann NY Acad Sci.* 1999:896.
6. Eddy D. Practice policies: guidelines for methods. *JAMA.* 1990;263(13):1839–1841.
7. Mondoux S, Shojania K. Evidence-based medicine: a cornerstone for clinical care but not for quality improvement. *J Eval Clin Pract.* 2019;25(3):363–368.
8. Bregman P. Health disparities and equity: concepts and measurement *Annu Rev Public Health.* 2006;27:167–194.
9. US Department of Health and Human Services (DHH). Determinants of health: Healthy People 2020. 2020. Archived. Available at: https://www.healthypeople.gov/2020/about/foundation-health-measures/Determinants-of-Health. Accessed November 30, 2022.
10. Tobin-Tyler E, Teitelbaum J. *Essentials of Health Justice.* Burlington, MA: Jones and Bartlett Learning; 2019.
11. Birkhead G, Morrow C, Pirani S. *Essentials of Public Health.* 4th ed. Burlington, MA: Jones and Bartlett Learning; 2021.
12. US Departmentt of Energy. *What Is Environmental Justice?* Washington, DC: Office of Legacy Management; 2022.
13. Bronfenbrenner U. Ecological systems theory. In: Vasta R, ed. *Six Theories of Child Development: Revised Formulations and Current Issues.* London, UK: Jessica Kingsley Publishers; 1992:187–249.

20

Disease Prevention

LEARNING OBJECTIVES

Upon completion, the reader will be able to

1. Define the following terms and phrases:
   - Distal health determinants
   - Determinants of clinical outcome (DoO)
   - Determinants of disparity (DoD)
   - Determinants of exposure (DoEx)
   - Determinants of health, wellness, and equity (DoHWE)
   - Determinants of wellness (DoW)
   - Modeling
   - Shelter in place
2. Recognize prevention to include five stages: primordial, primary, secondary, tertiary, and quaternary.
3. Recognize the goals, focus, and target groups for each prevention stage.
4. Recognize that disease prevention may be applied according to an ecosocial model of health and equity.
5. Recognize that the five stages of prevention are intended to optimize disaster-related health determinants, exposure, disease, clinical outcome, wellness, and disparity.

FIVE STAGES OF DISEASE PREVENTION

Disease prevention includes a wide range of activities aimed at reducing health risks, improving outcomes, and ensuring equity. Prevention occurs in five main stages: primordial, primary, secondary, tertiary, and quaternary.[1–3] The four pillars of emergency health are based on activities performed during the five stages of prevention. This chapter discusses disease prevention as a comprehensive framework for "producing" emergency health—that is, taking actions that avert or mitigate public health emergencies and disasters. Subsequent chapters describe the individual stages of prevention according to the four pillars of emergency health; thus they discuss primordial and quaternary prevention (i.e., health promotion), primary prevention (i.e., health protection), and secondary and tertiary prevention (i.e., provision of care).

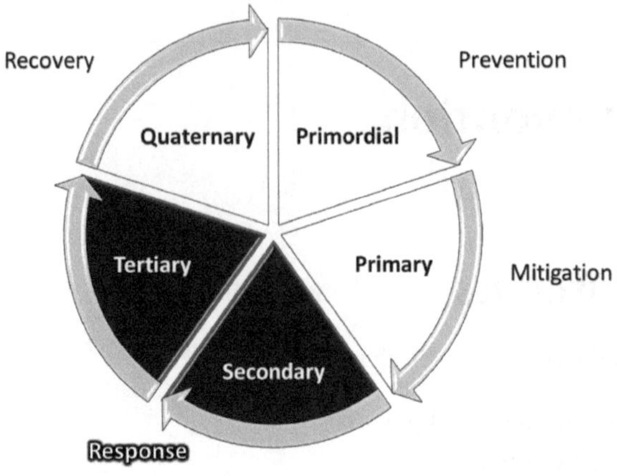

Figure 20-1. The Prevention Wheel

The cyclical process of comprehensive disease prevention can be considered as a wheel. (See Figure 20-1.) The health impact is cumulative for each stage of prevention as the focus shifts from health determinants to hazardous exposures, disease, clinical outcomes, wellness, and health equity. The prevention wheel's overall goal is to optimize health and wellness through preventive control of modifiable risk and protective factors. This goal is accomplished as a continuous iterative cycle. With each rotation of the prevention wheel, the goal is to create a system that averts or mitigates public health emergencies by default, thereby lessening the need for emergency response (i.e., secondary and tertiary prevention).

Primordial prevention involves optimization of health determinants by modifying risk factors and promoting protective factors that are the "distal determinants" (i.e., causes of the cause) of health.[4] Some sectors tend to lump all activities related to prevention into this stage. By comparison, many in public health consider prevention in terms of disease, including five distinct stages.

Primordial prevention optimizes the distal health determinants. Primary prevention involves preventing hazardous exposures. This is accomplished either by preventing the hazard or by preventing exposure if the hazard has already occurred. Secondary prevention involves preventing disease, given that exposure has occurred. Tertiary prevention then involves preventing further progression (e.g., prolonged impairment, permanent disability, or death) given that disease (including injury) has occurred.[2] Quaternary prevention involves preventing the "overmedicalization" of disaster-affected individuals (and the iatrogenic impairment of affected populations) who experience illness without an identifiable disease.[3] Quaternary prevention involves "producing" wellness and preventing health inequity after a disaster. Table 20-1 represents the goals, focus, and target groups for each corresponding stage of prevention.

Table 20-1. Stages of Prevention According to Focus, Target Population, and Emergency Management Goal

<table>
<tr><th>Timing</th><th>Stage of Prevention</th><th>Prevention Goal</th><th>Identifiable Disease</th><th>Focus</th><th>Target</th><th colspan="2">Emergency Management Goal</th></tr>
<tr><td rowspan="2">Up-stream</td><td>Primordial</td><td>Optimize health determinants</td><td>No</td><td>Determinants of health (DoH)</td><td>Population</td><td>Prevention</td><td rowspan="5">Preparedness</td></tr>
<tr><td>Primary</td><td>Prevent hazardous exposures</td><td>No</td><td>Determinants of exposure (DoEx)</td><td>Population</td><td>Mitigation</td></tr>
<tr><td rowspan="4">Down-stream</td><td>Secondary</td><td>Prevent disease, given exposure</td><td>No</td><td>Determinants of disease (DoD)</td><td rowspan="2">Person</td><td rowspan="2">Response</td></tr>
<tr><td>Tertiary</td><td>Prevent progression, given disease</td><td>Yes</td><td>Determinants of clinical outcome (DoO)</td></tr>
<tr><td rowspan="2">Quaternary</td><td>Prevent illness, given no disease</td><td>No</td><td>Determinants of wellness (DoW)</td><td>Person</td><td rowspan="2">Recovery</td></tr>
<tr><td>Prevent health inequity</td><td>No</td><td>Determinants of disparity (DoD)</td><td>Population</td><td></td></tr>
</table>

All the determinants just mentioned are collectively referred to as **determinants of health, wellness, and equity (DoHWE)**. Considering Table 20-1, prevention activities can be applied before, during, and after a hazardous exposure occurs. Upstream stages of prevention (occurring before exposure) include primordial and primary prevention. Downstream stages include secondary, tertiary, and quaternary prevention, which are applied after exposure. Only tertiary prevention involves the presence of clinically identifiable disease. The focus of prevention activities varies according to the stage of prevention, ranging from health determinants to health hazards, to disease, to outcomes, and then to wellness and health equity. Primordial and quaternary prevention targets the distal DoHWE, while primary, secondary, and tertiary prevention deals mainly with the proximate cause of disease. Secondary and tertiary interventions are targeted to involve affected persons (e.g., disaster patients or victims), while primordial, primary, and quaternary interventions extend to include the entire population at risk. And again, each stage of prevention roughly corresponds to a matching emergency management goal, an approach based on Carr's original "disaster cycle."

Primordial Prevention

Primordial prevention involves "producing" the **distal health determinants**. This type of prevention is accomplished using an ecosocial approach that recognizes the ecology of the individual within that individual's social network, community, society, belief system, and life stage. Primordial prevention implies that all persons have the right to a fair opportunity to attain their full health potential. Just as wellness is intended to optimize the individual's well-being, so primordial prevention is intended to maximize the population's well-being. Primordial prevention recognizes that, in addition to the ecosocial determinants that create health, there are also significant obstacles to health that create disparities. These disadvantages are magnified during times of disaster and often result in health inequity. Primordial prevention describes a fair and equal process for seeking optimal outcomes. It is intended to prevent the "causes of the cause" of disease that occur at all ecosocial levels, whether personal, micro, meso, exo, macro, or chrono.

For example, let us consider flood disasters. The literature describes the risk of flood-related mortality as strongly associated with multiple health determinants, like age, race, socioeconomic status, and national level of economic development. Simply put, flood deaths are more likely to occur among poor, elderly members of racial minorities, especially in low-resource nations. Primordial prevention seeks to identify those at-risk populations and to address the full range of modifiable health determinants, including all ecosocial levels (i.e., the individual as well as the individual's people, environment, resources, beliefs, and life stage). It has been said that "disasters seek out the poor and bind them in their poverty." Primordial prevention is designed to counter the selectivity of this "search."

Primary Prevention

Primary prevention involves preventing hazardous exposures that are the proximate cause of disease. Chapter 3 examined the epidemiological triad—the interaction between the individual, the hazardous agent, and the individual's environment—as the proximate cause of disease. Recall that disease occurs when an individual is exposed to an environment containing agents that are hazardous to health. The goal of primary prevention is to prevent population exposure to health hazards. Ideally, this is accomplished by preventing the hazard altogether (e.g., preventing the flood). When hazard avoidance is not possible, primary prevention is instead focused on preventing exposures to the hazard. This often requires an interdisciplinary approach for identifying, characterizing, monitoring, and avoiding exposure to human health hazards. It includes investigational aspects (like monitoring, forecasting, **modeling**, and dose reconstruction) as well as structural (e.g., engineering controls, construction methods, and architectural design) and nonstructural (e.g., public policy, education, and population protection measures) means for reducing hazards and exposures.[5]

Primary prevention seeks to identify those at-risk populations and to address their **determinants of exposure (DoEx)** according to ecosocial factors at all levels (i.e., the individual as well as the individual's people, environment, resources, beliefs, and life stage).

Again, consider the example of flood disasters. Floodplain management is a system for optimizing upstream water sources, wetlands, weirs, and dams to prevent flood hazards. In cases where floods cannot be prevented, primary prevention involves measures to avoid human exposures (e.g., early warning and population evacuation). Other flood-related examples of primary prevention measures are these:

- Risk communication (e.g., forecasting, alert, warning)
- Epidemiology (e.g., notifiable disease surveillance, injury surveillance)
- Community mitigation (e.g., social distancing and quarantine)
- Population protective measures (e.g., evacuation or **shelter in place**)
- Environmental safety (e.g., hazard monitoring, land use regulation)
- Personal protective measures (e.g., respiratory protection)
- Health care (e.g., screening, testing, prophylaxis, counseling)

Secondary Prevention

Secondary prevention aims to prevent disease, given that exposure has already occurred.[6] These activities typically occur during the subclinical phase in the natural history of disease. (See Figure 3-4.)[7] Secondary prevention also focuses on the proximate cause of disease—namely, hazardous exposures. Secondary prevention includes immediately necessary actions to (1) remove the affected population from ongoing exposure or risk of harm and (2) avert disease onset once exposure has already occurred. For example, patient decontamination is one intervention intended to remove hazardous chemicals from the body, thus preventing ongoing exposure. In another example, prophylactic medications can be given early after exposure to some biological hazards to prevent disease. In yet another example, normalizing a person's body temperature can prevent disease if performed early enough after exposure to cold hazards.

Secondary prevention often involves rapidly deployed emergency response capabilities like search and rescue, mass casualty management, active surveillance, mass care, or hazardous material response. Such actions enable early detection and preventive control of an exposure event. This emergency response is predominantly focused on immediate and short-term needs. Here are some flood-related examples of secondary prevention measures:

- Risk communication (e.g., forecasting, alert, warning)
- Epidemiology (e.g., active surveillance, case investigation)
- Search and rescue (e.g., swift water rescue)
- Population protection measures (e.g., evacuation or shelter in place)
- Environmental safety (e.g., decontamination, infection control measures)
- Community mitigation (e.g., case isolation)
- Mass care for displaced persons (e.g., shelter, food, water, sanitation, hygiene)
- Health care (e.g., screening, testing, prophylaxis, counseling)

Tertiary Prevention

Tertiary prevention seeks to prevent additional risk once the adverse health event has occurred. The goal of tertiary prevention is to prevent the progression of impairment, disability, and death, given that disease has occurred.[6] This prevention stage aims to reduce morbidity, avoid complications, and restore function.[5] Simply put, tertiary prevention involves the treatment of disease.

However, this simple statement defines a complex network of curative and rehabilitative health, economics, technology, and social services—all intended to prevent additional or ongoing impairment, disability, and death after the disease occurs. Like secondary prevention, tertiary prevention involves measures taken during the response phase of emergency management. Tertiary prevention focuses on the **determinants of clinical outcome (DoO).** Following is a list of examples of activities that accomplish tertiary prevention:

- Risk communication (e.g., treatment guidelines, public messaging)
- Epidemiology (e.g., active surveillance, outbreak investigation)
- Community mitigation (e.g., personal protective equipment, social distancing, isolation)
- Mass care for displaced persons (e.g., shelter, food, water, sanitation, hygiene)
- Health care (e.g., triage, first aid, diagnosis, therapeutics, hospitalization)

Quaternary Prevention

Quaternary prevention is an action taken to identify a patient at risk of overmedicalization, protect the patient from new "medical invasion, and suggest ethically acceptable interventions."[3] Jamoulle initially proposed the concept of quaternary prevention for patients who experience illness in the absence of identifiable disease.

Quaternary prevention activities were initially designed to mitigate or avoid the consequences of unnecessary or excessive intervention in the health system.[3] However, as was widely reported during the COVID-19 pandemic, adverse health consequences may also occur as the result of unnecessary or excessive intervention from other systems during a disaster (e.g., a political system or an incident management system).

This chapter focuses on the use of quaternary prevention to resolve or reduce the experience of illness among disaster-affected populations. In other words, quaternary prevention can be applied to promote wellness and prevent health inequity after a disaster event.

Disasters can be life-altering events. Many people experiencing a disaster perceive a significant degree of illness even without any identifiable disease. This sense of illness is a complex mix of uncertainty, change, mismatches of needs and resources, and many other ecosocial factors. Such an individual is also at pronounced risk for medicalizing these complex ecosocial problems. For example, physical symptoms of chronic fatigue syndrome were attributed to 25 patients in just one county affected by Hurricane Andrew.[8] This study reported an increased "illness burden" noted during "physician-related relapses." All interventions remained exclusively medical despite direct patient perceptions of illness. There appeared to be complementary upstream interventions available that could also address the **determinants of wellness (DoW)**. (See Table 13-1.)

While quaternary prevention is expected to occur during the recovery phase of emergency management, a lack of clinical cases during this time is all too often misinterpreted as recovery of the public health. This oversight is not insignificant, since most recovery phase activities characteristically require long-term commitments of resources. It is often just as easy to deny significant ecosocial dysfunction when wellness is narrowly defined as the absence of clinical disease.

In addition to addressing determinants of wellness, quaternary prevention can also be applied to the **determinants of disparity (DoD)** that result in health inequalities after a disaster. The approach to quaternary prevention can be used to overcome obstacles to health. For example, students who experienced flood-related job loss or disruption had a higher proportion of psychological symptoms than those who did not experience job loss or disruption, controlling for individual loss such as injury, home loss, or evacuation.[9] Depending on the institutional bias of the implementing system, the solution to this problem could vary from clinical approaches (e.g., psychiatry) to occupational ones (e.g., business continuity). Quaternary approaches could be used to avoid or mitigate job disruption that would prevent psychological symptoms rather than merely treating them.

To summarize, disease prevention is a comprehensive framework for "producing" emergency health. This approach applies an ecosocial model of health intended to avoid or mitigate adverse health determinants, exposures, disease, clinical outcomes, wellness, and disparity. The focus varies according to the individual stage of prevention. (See Figure 2-1.) Primordial and quaternary prevention focus on the distal health determinants and equity. By comparison, primary, secondary, and tertiary prevention concentrate on the proximate causes of disease.

TOPICS FOR DISCUSSION

Discuss how each of the five stages of prevention (i.e., primordial, primary, secondary, tertiary, quaternary) can be applied to the following disaster hazards:

- Lead poisoning in a municipal water system
- A tropical cyclone in an urbanized river delta
- An oil spill in coastal wetlands
- A respiratory virus in a high-resource nation

REFERENCES

1. Association of Faculties of Medicine of Canada. AFMC primer on population health. 2017. Available at: http://phprimer.afmc.ca/Glossary. Accessed December 1, 2022.
2. Kisling L, Das J. *Prevention Strategies*. Treasure Island, FL: StatPearls Publishing; 2022. Available at: https://www.ncbi.nlm.nih.gov/books/NBK537222. Accessed December 1, 2022.
3. Jamoulle M. Quaternary prevention, an answer of family doctors to overmedicalization. *Internatl J Health Policy and Manage*. 2015;4:1–4.
4. Strasser T. Reflections on cardiovascular diseases. *Interdisciplinary Sci Rev*. 1978;3:225–230.
5. Keim M. Environmental disasters In: Frumkin H, ed. *Environmental Health: From Global to Local*. 3rd ed. San Francisco, CA: Wiley & Sons; 2016:667–692.
6. Keim M, Abrahams J, Castilla-Echenique J. How do people die in disasters and what can be done? 2016. Available at: http://disasterdoc.org/how-do-people-die-in-disasters. Accessed December 1, 2022.
7. Keim M. Managing disaster-related health risk: a process for prevention. *Prehosp Disaster Med*. 2018;33(3):326–334.
8. Lutgendorf SK, Antoni MH, Ironson G, et al. Physical symptoms of chronic fatigue syndrome are exacerbated by the stress of Hurricane Andrew. *Psychosom Med*. 1995;57(4):310–323.
9. Peek-Asa C, Ramirez M, Young T, Cao Y. Flood-related work disruption and poor health outcomes among university students. *Prehosp Disaster Med*. 2012;27(6):503–508.

21

Health Promotion

LEARNING OBJECTIVES

Upon completion, the reader will be able to

1. Define the following terms and phrases:
   - Anthropocene epoch
   - Good governance
   - Great Acceleration
   - Health impact assessment
   - Health literacy
   - Health promotion
   - Healthy settings
   - Investment in health
   - Multisectoral
   - Ottawa Charter
   - Planetary health
   - Primary health care
   - Shanghai Declaration
   - Supportive environments for health
   - Sustainable development
   - Sustainable development goals (SDGs)
   - Well-being
2. Recall the primary focus for the five stages of prevention.
3. Recognize the association between the four pillars of emergency health and the five stages of prevention.
4. Recognize the nine prerequisites of health named by the Ottawa Charter.
5. Recognize 10 core elements of health promotion.
6. Recognize eight characteristics of good governance.
7. Recognize the association between sustainable development, prevention, and disaster risk management.

DEFINITION OF HEALTH PROMOTION

The 1986 **Ottawa Charter** recognized that to reach the World Health Organization's definition of health as "a state of complete physical, mental and social well-being," people must be able to identify and realize their aspirations, satisfy their needs, and change or cope with their environment.[1,2] In other words, the Ottawa Charter recognized that health is a human right and an essential resource for everyday living. It called for public health to "advocate (to boost the factors which encourage health), enable (allowing all people to achieve health equity), and mediate (through collaboration across all sectors)."[1]

The Ottawa Charter also identified five priority action areas as follows: (1) building healthy public policy, (2) creating supportive environments for health, (3) strengthening community action, (4) developing personal skills, and (5) reorienting health care services toward the prevention of illness and promotion of health.[1]

In 1998 the World Health Organization defined **health promotion** as "enabling people to increase control over, and to improve their health."[3] Simply stated, health promotion addresses the "distal determinants" (i.e., causes of the cause) of health. This definition implies that activities of human development govern the determinants of health. Our social goals should therefore consider the implications for our collective health and well-being. In 2016 the **Shanghai Declaration** recognized health and well-being as essential to sustainable development. It also recognized health as a political issue. The Shanghai Declaration reaffirmed health as "a universal right, an essential resource for everyday living, a shared social goal, and a political priority for all countries."[4]

ACTIVITIES OF HEALTH PROMOTION

Prevention

Regarding prevention, health promotion activities are designed to affect the distal determinants of health, wellness, and equity (DoHWE) that correspond with the primordial and quaternary stages of prevention. (See Figure 21-1.)

In these terms, health promotion focuses on optimizing the ecosocial DoHWE that relate to the individual person and that person's social network, community, environment, and culture. Actions related to primordial prevention are intended to "produce" the distal determinants of health. And quaternary prevention activities involve "producing" the distal determinants of wellness and equity. Primordial prevention acknowledges that in addition to the ecosocial determinants that create health, there are also significant ecosocial obstacles that create disease and disparity before the disaster occurs. Quaternary prevention recognizes that significant ecosocial obstacles create illness and inequity after the disaster occurs) Both stages of prevention promote the distal DoHWE. And both stages involve a process of enabling people, individually and collectively, to promote the DoHWE for everyone in the population.

Timing	Upstream		Downstream		
Prevention	Primordial	Primary	Secondary	Tertiary	Quaternary
Focus	Determinants of health	Determinants of exposure	Determinants of disease	Determinants of clinical outcome	Determinants of wellness and equity
Emergency health	Promotion	Protection	Provision of care	Provision of care	Promotion
Proximity	Distal	Proximal	Proximal	Proximal	Distal

Figure 21-1. Pillars of Emergency Health According to Stage of Prevention

The Ottawa Charter recognized nine prerequisites for health. These fundamental conditions and resources form a foundation upon which health can be "produced." These prerequisites for health include peace, shelter, education, food, income, a stable ecosystem, sustainable resources, social justice, and equity.[1]

Health promotion activities have been described to include 10 core elements: health in all policies, **healthy settings**; good governance; health literacy, investment for health, planetary health, primary health care, sustainable development, well-being, and health equity.[3–6] These health promotion activities are also important determinants of disaster-related health.

Health in All Policies

Health in all policies (HiAP) is "an approach to public policy development across sectors, which systematically takes into account the health implications of decisions, seeks synergies and avoids harmful health impacts to improve population health and health equity."[3] "The goal of HiAP is to ensure that decision-makers are informed about the health, equity, and sustainability consequences of various policy options during the policy development process."[6]

HiAP acknowledges that many DoHWE are governed by sectors other than public health and health care. Health agencies rarely have the mandate, authority, or organizational capacity to make systemic changes that can promote healthy living through healthy environments.[6] That responsibility falls mainly to other sectors. Sometimes, health is included in decision-making via **health impact assessment**. These methods and procedures offer insight by which a policy, program, product, or service may be judged concerning its effects on the health of the population in question.[3]

HiAP is intended to improve accountability, legitimacy, transparency, access to information, participation, sustainability, and collaboration across all sectors. HiAP can also promote efficiency as well as improve performance and outcomes.[6] In one example, the California Health in All Policies Task Force developed a framework for health promotion based on five key characteristics. Accordingly, a healthy community (1) meets the basic needs of all, (2) sustains environmental quality, (3) ensures economic and social development, (4) promotes health and social equity, and (5) offers social relationships that are supportive and respectful.[6]

Healthy Settings

The concept of healthy settings offers another approach to public policy development regarding the "meso" determinants of health related to the physical environment. (See Figures 9-1 and 10-3.) These healthy settings are "where people actively use and shape the environment and thus create or solve problems relating to health."[3] Comparable to the Healthy People programs, these settings include healthy homes, workplaces, cities, and islands.[7,8] These settings create **supportive environments for health** that provide protection from hazards and enable people to expand their capabilities to address health determinants. For example, a healthy city is defined as "one that is continually creating, expanding, and improving those physical and social environments and community resources that enable people to mutually support each other in performing all the functions of life and in developing to their maximum potential."[3] Cities should "produce health" by creating a health-supportive environment, offering a good quality of life, providing basic sanitation and hygiene, and ensuring access to health care.

Good Governance

Health promotion also includes actions that promote **good governance**.[3,5,9] Good governance involves effective decision-making and the process by which decisions are implemented. Like HiAP, the concept of good governance is predicated on the fact health is determined by multiple factors outside the control of the health sector. Good governance allows societies to make collective, evidence-based decisions that affect the health of individuals and shape patterns of disease distribution and mortality.[5]

The United Nations describes eight major characteristics of good governance. Good governance is (1) participatory, (2) consensus-oriented, (3) accountable, (4) transparent, (5) responsive, (6) effective and efficient, (7) equitable and inclusive, and (8) follows the rule of law.[10]

Good governance is a key factor affecting disaster-related health outcomes. For example, many of the risks related to the COVID-19 pandemic were reportedly associated with lack of good governance.[5,11] Major donors and international financial institutions, like the International Monetary Fund or the World Bank, base their fiancial assistance on the condition that the recipient ensures good governance.[10]

Health Literacy

Health literacy encompasses the "personal knowledge and competencies that accumulate through daily activities, social interactions, and across generations."[3] Health literacy enables people to understand and use information in ways that promote health and well-being. Health literacy benefits not only the individual but also the individual's social network. (i.e., ecosocial micro environment). According to the 2016 Shanghai Declaration, health literacy is critical for informed decision-making and "empowers people and communities."[3,4] Health literacy is more than being able to access information. It includes the ability to critically judge health information and resources and interact with others to express personal and societal needs for promoting health. In this sense, health literacy is accomplished by hearing, understanding, and communicating it to others. Health literacy is intended to be transformative for health and society in many ways. Actions that enhance health literacy are intended to transform knowledge and data, thinking and acting, as well as technology and science.[4]

Investment in Health

The 2016 Shanghai Declaration emphasized the wide-ranging benefits of investing in health. "**Investments in health** can lead to societal transformation." Investments in health contribute to (1) sustainable development, (2) interconnectedness, (3) inclusivity, (4) productivity, and (5) gender and social relations.[4]

The **Anthropocene epoch** is the designation for the newest planetary geological age, an age during which human activity has dominated the earth. During this time human development has achieved remarkable gains involving life expectancy, poverty, and child mortality.[12] The global gains in health over the past century have indeed been impressive. Life expectancy in the healthiest countries has increased steadily. At the same time, differences in life expectancy between those countries and much of the rest of the world have narrowed.[13]

Focused attention by health systems can lead to dramatic improvements in health at a modest cost.[13] Health promotion has delivered a remarkable return on investment. Healthy people are productive people.[4] However, this development also includes maladaptive elements such as the overuse of natural resources, pollution, biodiversity loss, and the negative impacts of energy sources.

Key challenges remain for health policy, among them high levels of inequality in health conditions across and within countries. Global trends of increasing gross domestic product are correlated with an increased risk of disaster-related mortality, not a decrease.[12] There remains a need for societal investments to include health and health equity.

Planetary Health

Within the Anthropocene age, humanity's impact on Earth's geology and ecosystems has been designated the Great Acceleration. This characterization represents the simultaneous increase in an extensive range of human activity, first recorded in the mid-20th century.[14] **Planetary health** is a new multidisciplinary field focused on addressing the impacts of human disruptions to the earth's natural systems on human health and all life on Earth. Planetary health is based on recognizing the earth's natural systems that define the safe environmental limits within which humanity can flourish.[3] It is based on the understanding that human health depends on flourishing natural systems. The underlying goal of planetary health is a world where everyone thrives by protecting and regenerating the earth's natural systems.[15] The concept of planetary health is directly aligned with **sustainable development goals (SDGs).** The SDGs provide a framework for addressing the goals by bringing together various disciplines, including health, environment, and economics, to tackle global issues holistically.

Sustainable Development

The 1987 Brundtland Report defined sustainable development as "development that meets the needs of the present without compromising the ability of future generations to meet their own needs."[16] It is an organizing principle that is, like planetary health, intended to advance human development while sustaining the ability of natural systems to provide the resources and services on which society depends.

> "Healthy life is an outcome of sustainable development, as well as a powerful and undervalued means of achieving it. We need to see health both as a precious asset and as a means of stimulating economic growth and reducing poverty."[16]
>
> - Dr. Gro Harlem Brundtland, WHO Director-General Emeritus

The 2002 World Summit on Sustainable Development concluded that "an integrated multi-hazard, inclusive approach to address vulnerability, risk assessment, and disaster management, including prevention, mitigation, preparedness, response, and recovery, is an essential part of a safer world in the twenty-first century."[17] The 2016 Shanghai Declaration further reinforced the link between health and sustainable development.[4]

The United Nations has provided 17 SDGs as a roadmap for human development.[18] These SDGs address the root causes of dysfunctional development and maladaptation that are also, not coincidentally, the root causes of disasters.[12]

Primary Health Care

Primary health care is an overall approach to the organization of health systems that encompasses the three aspects: (1) establishing a **multisectoral** policy and taking action to address the broader determinants of health; (2) empowering individuals, families, and communities; and (3) meeting people's essential health needs throughout their lives.[3] Primary care is a subset of primary health care. It involves essential first-contact care provided in a community setting. Primary health care is a holistic approach that includes health promotion, disease prevention, treatment, management, rehabilitation, and palliative care.[3]

Well-being

Well-being is a positive state experienced by individuals and societies. Well-being is often used synonymously with the concept of wellness, "an active process through which people become aware of, and make choices toward, a more successful existence."[19] The concept of well-being helps to remind us of the interconnectedness of a "state of complete well-being."[2] It offers a comprehensive approach to healthy living that empowers the proactive role of the individual. Well-being encompasses quality of life and the ability of people and societies to contribute to the world in accordance with a sense of meaning and purpose.[3] And, similar to health, it is a resource for daily life determined by various personal, social, environmental, societal, and institutional factors.[20]

Health Equity

Health equity is the absence of unfair, avoidable, or remediable differences in health status among population groups defined socially, economically, demographically, or geographically.[3] Like health, health inequity is also determined by a full range of personal and ecosocial factors.[20] Simply put, health equity is attaining the highest level of health for all people.

Recall that health equity differs from health equality. Health equality describes fair and equal outcomes. Health promotion is a comprehensive approach to balance the unfair distribution of opportunity in societies. Health equity addresses those distal determinants of health that drive this maldistribution. By comparison, health equity describes a fair and equal process for seeking equal outcomes.

TOPICS FOR DISCUSSION

Describe how each of the 10 core elements of health promotion could be applied to lower disaster-related morbidity and mortality for the following disaster hazards:

- Tropical cyclones (i.e., hurricanes)
- Mass gatherings
- Hazardous materials release

REFERENCES

1. World Health Organization (WHO). Ottawa Charter for health promotion. 1987. Available at: https://www.who.int/publications/i/item/ottawa-charter-for-health-promotion. Accessed December 1, 2022.
2. World Health Organization (WHO). Preamble to the Constitution of the World Health Organization. 1946. Available at: https://www.who.int/about/governance/constitution. Accessed December 1, 2022.
3. World Health Organization (WHO). *Health Promotion Glossary*. Geneva, Switzerland: World Health Organization; 1998.
4. World Health Organization (WHO). Promoting health in the SDGs: report on the 9th Global Conference for Health Promotion, Shanghai, China. November 21–24, 2017. Available at: https://www.who.int/publications/i/item/promoting-health-in-the-sdgs. Accessed December 1, 2022.
5. World Health Organization (WHO). Health promotion. 2022. Available at: https://www.who.int/health-topics/health-promotion. Accessed December 1, 2022.
6. Rudolph L, Caplan J, Mitchell C, Ben-Moshe K, Dillon L. Health in all policies: improving health through intersectoral collaboration. *NAM Perspect.* 2013.
7. US Department of Health and Human Services (DHH). Determinants of health. In: *Healthy People 2020*. 2020. Archived. Available at: https://www.healthypeople.gov/2020/about/foundation-health-measures/Determinants-of-Health. Accessed December 1, 2022.
8. Srinivasan S. Creating healthy communities, healthy homes, healthy people: initiating a research agenda on the built environment and public health. *Am J Public Health.* 2003;93(9):1446-1450.
9. Landman T, Splendore L. Pandemic democracy: elections and COVID-19. *J Risk Res.* 2020;23(7–8):1060-1066.
10. United Nations Economic and Social Commission for Asia and the Pacific (UNESCAP). What is good governance? 2009. Available at: https://www.unescap.org/resources/what-good-governance. Accessed December 1, 2022.
11. Mansoor M. Citizens' trust in government as a function of good governance and government agency's provision of quality information on social media during COVID-19. *Gov Inf Q.* 2021;38(4):101597.
12. Keim M, Smith T, Burkle F. The annual global incidence rate of extreme weather event disasters appears positively correlated with world GDP, 1961–2020 *Prehosp Disaster Med.* 2022;37(4):431–436.
13. Jamison D. Investing in health. In: Jamison D, Breman J, Measham A, eds. *Disease Control Priorities in Developing Countries*. 2nd ed. Washington, DC: World Bank; 2006.
14. Steffen W, Broadgate W, Deutsch LM, Gaffney O, Ludwig C. The trajectory of the Anthropocene: the Great Acceleration. *Anthropocene Rev.* 2015;2(1)1–18.
15. Whitmee S, Haines A, Beyrer C, et al. Safeguarding human health in the Anthropocene epoch: report of the Rockefeller Foundation—Lancet Commission on Planetary Health. *Lancet.* 2015;386(10007):1973–2028.

16. Brundtland G. *Report of the World Commission on Environment and Development: Our Common Future.* London, UK: United Nations; 1987.
17. United Nations International Strategy for Disaster Risk Reduction (UNISDR). World Summit on Sustainable Development, Heinrich Boll Foundation. International Strategy for Disaster Reduction, 2002. August 26–September 4, 2002. Available at: https://sdgs.un.org/statements/un-international-strategy-disaster-reduction-unisdr-8377. Accessed December 20, 2022.
18. United Nations. *Plan of Implementation of the World Summit on Sustainable Development.* New York, NY: United Nations; 2002.
19. Stoewen D. Health and wellness. *Can Vet J.* 2015;56:983–984.
20. Bronfenbrenner U. Ecological systems theory. In: Vasta R, ed. *Six Theories of Child Development: Revised Formulations and Current Issues.* London, UK: Jessica Kingsley Publishers; 1992:187–249.

22

Health Protection

LEARNING OBJECTIVES

Upon completion, the reader will be able to

1. Define the following terms and phrases:
   - Health protection
   - Normative safety
   - Perceived safety
   - Safety
   - Safety standards
   - Security
   - Social safety
   - Socio-politicization of risk
   - Substantive safety
2. Compare and contrast the terms *safety* and *security* concerning health.
3. Describe the role of health protection in ensuring environmental justice.

DEFINITION OF HEALTH PROTECTION

Health protection is a form of primary prevention and a core field of public health. It can be defined as "the protection of individuals, groups and populations through expert advice and effective collaboration to prevent and mitigate the impact of infectious disease, environmental, chemical and radiological threats."[1] Health protection is often managed by the public sector. However, many, if not most, of the drivers of health protection are governed by the private sector. And the timing of health protection is decidedly upstream—indeed, at the top of "Malins' cliff."

Health protection is a form of primary prevention for emergency health.

HEALTH PROTECTION INTERVENTIONS

Health protection interventions are designed to prevent hazardous exposures. (See Table 19-1.) This is accomplished by avoiding the hazard altogether and by avoiding exposure to the hazard.

Health protection is intended to serve the entire population and mitigate health hazards' impact (including those associated with disasters). In this sense, health protection has an active role in ensuring equal protection and equitable health outcomes.

Health protection focuses on determinants of exposure (DoEx) as the proximate cause of disease. Protective actions most often require an interdisciplinary approach. Multiple sectors are needed to identify, characterize, monitor, and avoid exposure to health hazards. Thus health protection includes investigational aspects (like monitoring, forecasting, exposure modeling, dose reconstruction, surveillance, and epidemiological investigation) as well as structural means (e.g., engineering controls, construction methods, and architectural design) and nonstructural means (e.g., public policy, education, and population protection measures) for reducing hazards and exposures.[2] Put simply, actions involving health protection are intended to offer safety for everyone in the population. In simplest terms, separating the hazard and associated environmental exposures from people accomplishes this objective. (See Figure 3-4.)[3]

THE IMPORTANT DIFFERENCE BETWEEN SAFETY OR SECURITY

There are subtle yet important issues related to our choice of words regarding health protection. Such choices often relate to the origin of the term *health protection* and are influenced by our personal life experiences and the context of our environment. The Latin origin of the word *protection* roughly translates in English as "to cover in front."[1] During the US-Soviet Cold War, the term *civil defense* was initially used to describe nonmilitary activities intended to protect noncombatants. Later some nations, among them Germany, replaced this term at the national level with *civil protection*, or "protection of the people."[4] Similarly, the Latin origin of the word **safety** translates as "freedom from harm."[1] By contrast, the Latin origin of the word **security** means "freedom from anxiety."[1] Unlike safety's focus on protecting the population, "the study of security lies at the heart of international relations."[5]

Safety protects the people. Security protects the state.

Security

ISO 22300 defines *security hazard* as "a source of potential harm."[6] The source of this harm can include a broad range of social, technological, economic, environmental, and political factors. The World Health Organization more narrowly defines potential sources of harm as health hazards rather than security hazards. That is, the source of harm is "a process, phenomenon or human activity that may cause loss of life, injury or other health impacts."[7]

The term *security* is often used within multiple contexts, such as (1) protection from hostile forces, (2) absence of harm, (3) resilience against damage, (3) secrecy, and (4) a state of mind.

During the 1990s and 2000s, the definition of *global health security* evolved as an extension of US national health security. *Homeland security* originated as a national security term for "the national effort to ensure a homeland that is safe, secure, and resilient against terrorism and other hazards where American interests, aspirations, and ways of life can thrive."[8] However, the marriage of health and security is also the subject of debate. There are concerns regarding the "securitization" and "militarization" of public health.[9,10] Davies described this as a debate between "statist" and "globalist" perspectives, where a state-centric and disease-focused approach clashes with one more concerned with individuals' health challenges.[9] The dynamic could also be described in terms of differences in individual human rights versus the rights of the collective society or state.

Table 22-1 describes the origins and history of the term *global health security* in the United States. Note how the policy emphasis has evolved from what was initially unilaterally directed detection and surveillance systems (implemented downstream) as compared with those that describe a multilateral and cooperative approach to decrease the impact and danger (implemented both upstream and downstream).[11–15]

Safety

Safety is defined as "all measures and practices taken to preserve the life, health, and bodily integrity of individuals."[16] Safe environments effectively prevent hazardous exposures by default. Because the environment is vital in determining health, safety is a core element of disaster-related health protection.

Safety Standards

There is an important distinction between environments that meet **safety standards**, those that are safe, and those that merely feel safe. **Normative safety** is based on applicable norms and standards regardless of the actual safety history. **Substantive safety** occurs when the actual safety history is substantial or acceptable irrespective of whether standards are met. **Perceived safety** is in the eye of the beholder; it is subjective, without consideration of standards or safety history. Finally, there is **social safety**, which entails public safety or security. Social safety addresses the risk of intentional harm (e.g., crime, terrorism, conflict, and warfare). Because of the moral issues involved, social safety (e.g., law enforcement) is often considered more important to some than substantive safety. For example, a death attributable to murder is considered worse than a death in a car crash, even though in many countries traffic deaths are more common than homicides.

Table 22-1. Historical Events Related to Global Health Security

1995	Congress passes the Weapons of Mass Destruction Act.
1996	Dept of Defense established Global Emerging Infections Surveillance System in response to a Presidential Decision Directive regarding emerging infectious diseases.
1998	Anthrax spores are delivered through US mail system.
2000	WHO establishes an international Global Outbreak and Response Network (GOARN) in partnership with 67 international partners (currently >200).
2002	Congress enacts the 2002 Homeland Security Act after the September 11 attacks.
2004	Congress creates the CDC Global Disease Detection (GDD) program to "*gather resources* so countries could prepare for potential infectious disease threats."[11]
2005	WHO revises International Health Regulations (IHR) "to *prevent, protect against, control, and provide* a public health response to the international spread of disease."[12]
2005	Hurricane Katrina devastates New Orleans and kills over 1,800 people.
2006	Congress passes the Pandemic and All-Hazards Preparedness Act, intended to improve capabilities for emergencies, whether deliberate, *accidental, or natural*.
2007	CDC creates the GDD Operations Center for "*detecting* and monitoring global public health events of international importance."[13]
2008	CDC reports GDD accomplishments to include disease *surveillance* for less than eight million persons worldwide.
2014	The Global Health Security Agenda (GHSA) is implemented to *strengthen* public health systems needed to protect global health security.[14]
2018	CDC discontinues 80% of GDD program activities.
2019	COVID-19 pandemic begins.
2020	The 6th GHSA Ministerial Meeting is held in Thailand under the theme "Bridging Cooperative Action for Global Health Security."
2020	WHO defines global health security as "activities required, both *proactive and reactive*, to *minimize the danger and impact* of acute public health events that endanger people's health across geographical regions and international boundaries."[15]

Source: Based on CDC[11,13,14] and WHO.[12,15]

Note: All italics added.

Again, as is the case for human-made disasters, the public tends to judge intentional incidents more harshly.[17]

Emergency health is intended to preserve individuals' life, health, and bodily integrity. As such, the primary objective of emergency health is to produce health for the individual, not to ensure a state's security. Safety, then, is the outcome to be achieved. Security is but one path to achieving safety.

There are good reasons for setting safety priorities independent of security measures in order not to be directed toward specific solutions too soon. For example, until 2005 none of the counterterrorism policies listed in Table 22-1 were intended to develop a comprehensive framework for avoiding all hazards. The capacity to manage disasters caused by natural hazards (e.g., extreme weather as a consequence of climate change) and technological hazards (e.g., hazardous material releases) has mainly remained unimproved by health security programs that focus on hazards that are most effectively weaponized: chemical, biological, radiological, and nuclear weapons, though primarily biological hazards. For this reason, the US Congress passed the 2006 Pandemic and All-Hazards Preparedness Act following the death of nearly 2,000 people during Hurricane Katrina.

A second reason for separating priorities between safety and security is to enable comparison between priorities of values and priorities of measures.[3] Measures for health differ from measures of security, as do their measures of success and failure.

ENVIRONMENTAL JUSTICE

The US Environmental Protection Agency defines **environmental justice** as "the fair treatment and meaningful involvement of all people regardless of race, color, national origin, or income, with respect to the development, implementation, and enforcement of environmental laws, regulations, and policies."[18] Environmental justice implies that everyone has the "same degree of protection from environmental and health hazards, and equal access to the decision-making process to have a healthy environment."[18]

Environmental justice describes a state of fairness concerning the environmental determinants of health (i.e., the ecosocial meso context). Environmental justice focuses on eliminating disparities regarding the DoEx. Simply put, the goal of environmental justice is to protect everyone in the population at risk. And while it may not always be possible to predict and prevent all environmental DoEx accurately, it certainly is possible to predict and prevent disparities of exposure that so often occur as the result of social determinants. Investigating the ecosocial factors that sustain or diminish health has become a growing area of public health research.[19] One early example of a growing environmental justice movement occurred in 1982 when civil rights activists organized to stop the state of North Carolina from dumping hazardous chemicals in the county with the highest proportion of African Americans.[19] Soon afterward, an interdisciplinary body of literature was developed that documented the unequal impacts of environmental pollution on different social classes and racial/ethnic groups. A substantial body of literature has since emerged documenting the existence of environmental risk and health inequalities.[20] In 1996, Firpo et al. described this phenomenon as the "**socio-politicization of risk**" concerning the incidence of chemical disasters in rapidly industrialized countries. In these nations, less elaborate measures for protecting the environment, human health, and safety are important in economic negotiations and often lead to the unfair international division of risks.[21] There are indications that the costs of major chemical accidents, particularly its human costs, are not as expensive in industrializing countries.[21] Some have likened this to an incentive for industrialized countries to "export risk" overseas or to less advantaged populations within the same nation.[21,22]

TOPICS FOR DISCUSSION

1. Why is it important to differentiate between security and safety?
2. How does environmental justice relate to the determinants of disparity?

REFERENCES

1. Harper D, ed. Online etymology dictionary. 2022. Available at: https://www.etymonline.com. Accessed November 23, 2022.
2. Keim M. Environmental disaster. In: Frumkin H, ed. *Environmental Health: From Global to Local.* San Francisco, CA: Wiley & Sons; 2010:843–875.
3. Keim M. Managing disaster-related health risk: a process for prevention. *Prehosp Disaster Med.* 2018;33(3):326–334.
4. Fekete A. Safety and security target levels: opportunities and challenges for risk management and risk communication. *Int J Disaster Risk Reduction.* 2012;2:67–76.
5. Degaut M. What is security? Article in Portuguese. *Revista Brasileira de inteligência.* 2015;9:9–28.
6. International Organization for Standardization. ISO 22300:2018: Security and resilience—vocabulary. 2018. Revised by ISO 22300:2021. Available at: https://www.iso.org/standard/77008.html. Accessed November 23, 2022.
7. World Health Organization and Food and Agriculture Organization of the United Nations (WHO/FAO). Hazard characterization for pathogens in food and water: guidelines. 2003. Available at: https://apps.who.int/iris/bitstream/handle/10665/42693/9241562374.pdf. Accessed November 23, 2022.
8. Reese S. Defining homeland security: analysis and congressional considerations. Congressional Research Service Reports R42462. 2013. Available at: https://digital.library.unt.edu/ark:/67531/metadc86623. Accessed November 23, 2022.
9. Davies SE, Kirk J. Global health security. *Oxford Bibliographies.* 2021. Available at: https://www.oxfordbibliographies.com/view/document/obo-9780199756797/obo-9780199756797-0204.xml. Accessed November 23, 2022.
10. Cohen H, Gould R, Sidell V. Bioterrorism initiatives: public health in reverse? *Am J Public Health.* 1999;89(11):1629–1631.
11. Centers for Disease Control and Prevention (CDC). Global disease detection program history & accomplishments. December 17, 2021. Available at: https://www.cdc.gov/globalhealth/healthprotection/gdd/gdd-accomplishments.html. Accessed February 2, 2023.
12. World Health Organization (WHO). International Health Regulations (2005). Available at: https://www.who.int/publications/i/item/9789241580410. Accessed February 2, 2023.

13. Centers for Disease Control and Prevention (CDC). Event-based surveillance. December 17, 2021. Available at: https://www.cdc.gov/globalhealth/healthprotection/gddopscenter/how.html. Accessed February 2, 2023.
14. Centers for Disease Control and Prevention (CDC). About global health security. December 17, 2021. Available at: https://www.cdc.gov/globalhealth/healthprotection/ghs/about.html. Accessed February 2, 2023.
15. World Health Organization (WHO). Health security. Available at: https://www.who.int/health-topics/health-security#tab=tab_1. Accessed February 2, 2023.
16. Safety. 2018. Available at: https://www.safeopedia.com/definition/1104/safety-occupational-health-and-safety. Accessed December 1, 2022.
17. Slovik P, Peters E. Risk perception and affect. *Curr Dir Psychol Sci.* 2006;15(6):322–325.
18. Environmental Protection Agency (EPA). Environmental justice. 2022. Available at: https://www.epa.gov/environmentaljustice. Accessed December 1, 2022.
19. Mohai P, Pellow DN, Roberts JT. Environmental justice. *Annu Rev Environ Resources.* 2009;34(1):405–430.
20. Brulle RJ, Pellow DN. Environmental justice: human health and environmental inequalities. *Annu Rev Public Health.* 2006;27(1):103–124.
21. Firpo M, Machado C. Major chemical accidents in industrializing countries: the socio-political amplification of risk. *Risk Analysis.* 1996;16(1):19–29.
22. Keim ME. Industrial chemical disasters. In: Ciottone G, Darling R, Anderson P, et al., eds. *Disaster Medicine.* 3rd ed. Philadelphia, PA: Mosby-Elsevier; 2006:556–568.

23

Provision of Care

LEARNING OBJECTIVES

Upon completion, the reader will be able to

1. Define the following terms and phrases:
    - Case
    - Event
    - Event-based surveillance (EBS)
    - Indicator-based surveillance (IBS)
    - Humanitarian Charter
    - Performance indicator
2. Describe the provision of care in terms of medical care and mass care.
3. Recognize the role of the health sector in detecting disaster-related cases and events.
4. Compare and contrast indicator-based and event-based surveillance systems.
5. Recall five core capabilities of the health sector for detecting disaster-related cases and events.
6. Recognize the role of the health sector in managing disaster-related cases and events.
7. Recall four special capabilities of the health sector for managing disaster-related cases and events.
8. Recognize that most disaster medical care is provided by family, bystanders, and local caregivers.
9. Recognize the evolving definition (and practice) of disaster medicine.
10. Recognize 16 emergency response functional areas included in the US National Response Framework (ESF8) Public Health and Medical Annex.
11. Recognize four emergency response functional areas included in the US National Response Framework (ESF6): Mass care, Emergency assistance, Temporary housing, and Human Services Annex.
12. Recognize components of the Sphere Humanitarian Charter and Minimum Standards in Humanitarian Response.

DEFINING THE PROVISION OF CARE

After a disaster the emergency response phase characteristically involves a rapid **provision of care** intended to terminate or cease and prevent exposures and to treat existing disease. Figure 5-1 depicts these care categories as associated with two key clusters of disaster-related consequences that affect health outcomes. As per Figure 5-1, health consequences occur because of either direct exposure to health hazards or the loss of basic physical needs and protections such as food, water, shelter, sanitation, and temperature. It is therefore important to recognize that many survivors of the initial direct effects of a disaster hazard remain at high risk for the indirect risks associated with displacement and ecosocial disruption.

Of course, providing care after a disaster is not limited to health care. Disaster-affected populations require care and assistance beyond medical needs.[1] As shown in Tables 11-1 and 11-2, the health impact of disasters includes loss of water, sanitation, shelter, and many other basic needs in addition to exposure to disaster-related disease[2]. Some emergency health needs are fulfilled by a person's social network or community. Within the health sector, some of these needs are also addressed by nongovernmental organizations and the private sector. This chapter focuses on the roles of public health and health care as critical components of the health sector for addressing the health-related impacts of disasters.

Detecting Disaster-Related Cases and Events

Public health and health care providers assist not only in the management of disaster consequences but also in the detection of the disaster itself. Detection and management are critical functions that public health and health care providers serve during a disaster.

Disasters characteristically result in health-related consequences that must be rapidly detected, diagnosed, and managed. These consequences include clinical **cases** often associated with specific high-risk **events** of concern. Table 23-1 depicts the role of the public health and health care systems in detecting and managing disaster-related disease.

Table 23-1 summarizes the role of public health and health care providers in detecting and managing both cases and events related to disasters. Cases are detected using an **indicator-based surveillance (IBS)** system, and events are detected using **event-based surveillance (EBS)**. IBS is well structured and used for the detection of individual cases of disease. These cases are traditionally identified by syndrome, clinical diagnosis, or

Table 23-1. Relationship Between Disaster-Related Consequences and the Primary Role of Public Health and Health Care

Consequences	Detection	Management	Role	Surveillance System
Cases	Case detection	Case management	Health care	Indicator-based (IBS)
Event	Event detection	Incident management	Public health	Event-based (EBS)

laboratory confirmation. By comparison, EBS is typically less structured and used for detecting a broad range of events and hazards. For example, public health agencies routinely use EBS to track hazardous material release events. Other sources of event-based surveillance data may include threat- and hazard-monitoring systems, meteorological forecasting, and environmental modeling. Both traditional and nontraditional sources of media may also be included in an EBS system.

The Role of Health Care Providers in Case Detection

Health care providers are vital in detecting cases and events associated with all disaster hazards. In many examples health care providers are the first to detect cases of the disaster-related disease. The signs of disease are detected by clinical diagnosis and managed as clinical cases. They are then reported to public health agencies, most often through an active surveillance system.

The Role of Public Health in Event Detection

In addition to using IBS, public health uses EBS to detect adverse events that could become health hazards. Compared with a reportable case of disease, an "adverse event" is a specific situation of public health concern (i.e., an incident). Accordingly, incident management is defined as those options required to prevent, treat, or control the adverse consequences of an adverse event. Therefore, public health agencies maintain EBS systems to rapidly identify incidents associated with hazardous exposures or disaster-related disease.

The role of the health sector in detecting cases and events can easily be summarized within five core capabilities as follows: (1) intelligence, (2) surveillance, (3) identification, (4) confirmation, and (5) reporting. Table 23-2 describes how these five public health and health care capabilities detect disaster-related consequences.

Table 23-2. Public Health and Health Care Capabilities for Detection

Core Capability	Case Detection	Event Detection
Intelligence	Pre-incident intelligence Medical education	Pre-incident intelligence Hazard awareness and recognition
Surveillance	Health information systems Passive and active surveillance	Environmental monitoring Hazardous substance emergency event surveillance system
Identification	Point of care assays Clinical laboratory tests	Hazard characterization Boundary demarcation Exposure assessment Laboratory reporting
Confirmation	Clinical examination Laboratory evaluation	Epidemiological assessment Scene assessment
Reporting	Hospital Public health	Law enforcement, public safety Emergency management

Managing Disaster-Related Cases and Events

The health sector's role in managing disaster-related cases is more specific than case and event detection according to the individual hazard involved. Case and event management requires a broad range of capabilities, from routine health care to mass vaccination and distribution of pharmaceuticals.

Considering this range, four special capabilities for the management of disaster-related consequences include (1) decontamination/infection control, (2) interventions, (3) specialty services, and (4) evidence management (in criminal cases). Table 23-3 describes these four special capabilities for managing health emergencies.

The Role of Health Care in Case Management

Measures that avoid or terminate hazardous exposures are a common component of emergency response for multiple health hazards. For example, decontamination is used to terminate patient exposures during hazmat disasters. In the case of an epidemic, infection control measures serve a similar purpose of separating individual hosts from the causative agent. (See Figure 2-2.) External decontamination of the patient is a critical first step in treating patients exposed to chemical, radiological, or nuclear hazards. Corollary to this capability is the ability to protect staff while performing decontamination after such events. Cases involving epidemics similarly apply infection control measures that prevent cross-contamination and secondary disease transmission.

Table 23-3. Public Health and Health Care Special Capabilities for Management

Capability	Case Management	Event Management
Decontamination	Personal protective equipment Patient and staff decontamination Infection/contamination control	Incident command systems Hazmat site control Mutual aid
Interventions	Treatment protocols Therapeutics Prophylaxis & vaccines Occupational health and safety Behavioral health	Warning and risk communication Population protection measures Site decontamination & control Crowd control Mass shelter
Specialty Services	Toxicology Traumatology Resuscitology Pulmonology Critical care	Infrastructure assessment Environmental health interventions Cybersecurity Population health assessment
Evidence Management	Intelligence Chain-of-evidence preservation Forensic pathology	Intelligence Crime scene preservation Civilian-military coordination

For all four of these hazards, the appropriate level and adequate training in using personal protective equipment is also essential knowledge for health care providers. For interventions, providers often utilize emergency health care services and standard operating procedures for occupational health and safety. Care providers may also require additional support concerning psychological services, including critical incident stress debriefing. Multispecialty care is also often required after disaster-related injury. Besides routinely involving emergency services, these special events may require additional high-level support from specialty care, including toxicology, traumatology, surgical subspecialties, and critical care. Finally, in some cases involving criminal activity or terrorism, health care providers may also have a role involving evidence management. Clinicians may need to take additional measures to preserve the evidence chain, facilitate accurate forensic testing, and offer other intelligence. In summary, the detection and management of disaster-related disease require the clinician's knowledge and ability to perform as part of an extensive, multisectoral system.

The Role of Public Health in Event Management

Public health agencies use an incident command system to manage adverse events and control access to sites that may be hazardous. They may also call on other agencies (e.g., fire, mass casualty management) for assistance through mutual aid agreements or memorandums of understanding,

Public health interventions related to the event may involve risk communication, population protection measures, site decontamination, crowd control, mass care, and shelter arrangements. Specialized services can include assessment of damaged infrastructure, environmental health interventions, cyber security support, or population-based health assessments performed by epidemiologists. Finally, disaster-related events may be expected to generate intelligence and evidence that must be secured, managed, and coordinated with multiple sectors.

In summary, the detection and management of disaster events require public health actors to have both knowledge and the ability to perform as part of an extensive, multisectoral system.

COMPONENTS OF CARE

As shown in Figure 5-1, the health-related consequences of disasters include disease and displacement. Besides directly causing disease, disaster-related damage and losses can create the potential for additional indirect health risk. As a result, public health emergency response actions frequently include actions intended to meet the immediate needs of food, water, sanitation, shelter, and health care.

MEDICAL CARE

Despite the highly visible nature of national and international response capability, most disaster-related medical care is provided by local health care providers within the first hours after an incident. Just as "all disasters start local," so does all disaster medical care. As a result, most case management of the disaster-related disease is provided by family, bystanders, and local caregivers, not by specialized units. And since most trauma deaths occur within hours, not days after disaster impact, most disaster medical care occurs nearly immediately. Simply put, nearly "all disaster medicine is local." As a result, almost all disaster-related mortality (i.e., traumatic injury) has already occurred when external medical teams arrive and establish operations several days after the incident. At that time, most cases are of low-to-moderate acuity and characteristically involve cleanup injuries, medication refills, primary care, and exacerbations of chronic disease. Regardless of the challenges, prehospital and hospital-based emergency care provision remains an essential component of any disaster response, irrespective of the hazard.

Providing Care for Disaster Victims

Shortly after Haddon's original 1963 work on accident theory (and coinciding with US lessons learned from trauma care in Vietnam), studies of disaster-related disease began to appear in the United States and worldwide.[3-5]

In 1974 the US Congress passed the Disaster Relief Act, which furthered the provision of care for disaster victims. And in 1978 the International Conference on Disaster Medicine held in Cape Town, South Africa, represented one of the field's first formal gatherings. During that same time, disaster epidemiologists from around the world also began to characterize trends in disaster-related disease.[6,7]

In 1983 the Centers for Disease Control (CDC) was asked to create a concept paper entitled "Potential Public Health Threats Following Major Catastrophes." On the basis of their findings, in 1989 (notably one year after the passage of the Stafford Disaster Relief and Emergency Assistance Act, commonly referred to as the Stafford Act), Gregg and French published the CDC monograph entitled "The Public Health Consequences of Disasters."[8,9] During that same year, Auf der Heide published the benchmark operational guide "Disaster Response: Principles of Preparation and Coordination."[10]

During the 1990s, the field began to coalesce worldwide, as demonstrated by Gunn's multilingual dictionary of disaster medicine published in the Netherlands.[11] Gunn's definition reflected the ambitious nature of an evolving discipline, with disaster medicine described as "the study and collaborative application of various health disciplines (e.g., pediatrics, epidemiology, communicable diseases, nutrition, public health, emergency medicine, social mending, community care, and international health) to the prevention, immediate response and rehabilitation of the health problems arising from disaster, in cooperation with other disciplines."[11]

In 1994 a group of authors, including disaster medicine pioneer Frederick (Skip) Burkle and Joseph Waeckerle, then editor of the *Annals of Emergency Medicine*, published the first editorial review of disaster medicine as a subspecialty of emergency medicine.[1] And in 1997, Noji reconvened one-third of the original authors of the 1989 CDC monograph to create an updated edition published by Oxford University under the same title.[12]

Gunn's definition of disaster medicine envisioned a broad scope of medical and public health capabilities to perform "prevention, immediate response, and rehabilitation." However, with some exceptions most self-identified disaster medicine practitioners are involved in training, preparing for, and implementing Gunn's "immediate response."[13]

As discussed in Chapter 1, disaster medicine is populated mainly by part-time volunteers or serves as an extension of full-time academic or clinical duties in medicine, nursing, and emergency medical services. The worldwide number of formally trained subspecialists remains very limited. Professional societies typically have less than 1,000 members worldwide. Public health practices—epidemiology, prevention, environmental health, and public policy, for example—are not a primary focus of most training in disaster medicine. Most disaster-related health publications describe activities directed toward the response phase of disasters. Some 25 years later Burkle repeated his visionary 1994 call to action that "the art and science of disaster medicine include much more than clinical medical issues and require significant contributions from many disciplines." In 2019 he continued to advocate for a "multi-disciplinary framework" to be applied throughout Carr's entire "disaster cycle."[1,14,15]

Considering disaster medicine's observable scope of practice and that most practitioners are local health care providers, perhaps the most valid and accurate definition of disaster medicine is simply that of "health care provided after a disaster." As such, we should ensure that all health care providers are competent in the basic knowledge, skills, and abilities necessary to perform effectively during disasters. Some special aspects can be unique to disasters (e.g., triage, decontamination, prophylaxis, scarce resources, and austere environments). (See Table 23-3.) However, the clinical principles remain largely the same for most health care providers regardless of disaster. For example, given equal resource availability a patient with a second-degree burn caused by an urban fire disaster is likely to be treated similarly to a patient burned by a faulty cookstove during a hurricane disaster. While the logistics, communications, and availability of disaster resources may vary remarkably, our clinical approach does not change significantly from hazard to hazard. Simply put, a broken arm is still broken, regardless of whether it's caused by a fall from "Malins' cliff" or a bus crash at the bottom. Since disasters are often low-probability, high-impact events, it is prudent to maintain a modest but adequate level of emergency medical capability in all communities and pool resources during times of high risk.

In the United States, essential support function 8 of the Public Health and Medical Annex of the National Response Framework (ESF 8) provides supplemental assistance to state, tribal, and local governments in the following core functional areas:

1. Assessment of public health/medical needs
2. Health surveillance
3. Medical care personnel
4. Health, medical, and veterinary equipment and supplies
5. Patient evacuation
6. Patient care
7. Safety and security of drugs, biologics, and medical devices
8. Blood and blood products
9. Food safety and security
10. Agriculture safety and security
11. All-hazard public health and medical consultation, technical assistance, and support
12. Behavioral health care
13. Public health and medical information
14. Vector control
15. Potable water and wastewater and solid waste disposal
16. Mass fatality management, victim identification, and decontaminating of remains
17. Veterinary medical support

MASS CARE

Humanitarian assistance involves providing goods and services to fulfill the essential needs of disaster victims. In the United States, this process is referred to as mass care. The Federal Emergency Management Administration, commonly known as FEMA, defines mass care as "congregate sheltering, feeding, distribution of emergency supplies, and reunification of children with their parent(s)/legal guardians and adults with their families."[16]

Agencies and organizations at the local, state, tribal, territorial, insular area, and federal levels collaborate to assist disaster survivors. In the United States, the four primary functional areas for humanitarian assistance involve essential support functions (ESF 6): (1) mass care, (2) emergency assistance, (3) temporary housing, and (4) human services.[16] The US National Response Framework is a plan that convenes governmental and nongovernmental support agencies and provides a standardized system for coordinating a complex, multisectoral response and recovery.

Internationally, national-level response agencies usually coordinate disaster responses with international resources (e.g., United Nations, nongovernmental agencies, and donors)

Table 23-4. Organization of the Sphere Project Humanitarian Charter and Minimum Standards in Humanitarian Response

Principles and **Foundation**	Humanitarian Charter
	Protection principles
	Core humanitarian standard
Standards	Water supply, sanitation, and hygiene promotion
	Food security and nutrition
	Shelter and settlement
	Health

within a framework of humanitarian assistance. This assistance is often delivered according to a globally recognized set of minimum standards for humanitarian response. These standards are known as the Sphere Project.[17]

The Sphere Project

The Sphere Project (i.e., "Sphere") was initiated in 1997 by a group of humanitarian nongovernmental agencies and the International Red Cross and the Red Crescent movement. These standards were intended to improve the quality of disaster response and have as their basis two core beliefs—namely, that those affected by disaster have the right to assistance and that all possible steps should be taken to alleviate human suffering.[17] Since then, these standards have been published as a handbook that is widely known and internationally recognized. Table 23-4 depicts the organization of the Sphere handbook.

The **Humanitarian Charter** is the foundation of the Sphere handbook. It is a statement of shared principles, rights, and duties of disaster responders and disaster victims. The charter also explains why assistance and protection are critical pillars of any humanitarian action. The handbook specifies a set of population protection principles and lays out a core set of minimum standards. These core standards are supplemented by a group of minimum standards explained in four technical chapters: (1) water supply, sanitation, and hygiene promotion; (2) food security and nutrition; (3) shelter, settlement, and nonfood items; and (4) health action for each of these standards.[17] The charter also identifies corresponding minimum objectives, key actions, and **performance indicators** and provides guidance notes.[17]

The Sphere handbook is designed for use as a guide during the humanitarian response in various disaster situations. Focusing on the period of response, the Sphere minimum standards prioritize activities that meet the urgent needs of disaster-affected populations.[17] As such, provision of care can last from a few days or weeks to many months or even years, particularly in the context of protracted insecurity and displacement.

TOPICS FOR DISCUSSION

Disasters are said to "seek out the poor and bind them in their poverty." Considering this notion, describe the following:

- How ecosocial factors can influence the access to and quality of disaster-related medical care
- How ecosocial factors can influence access to and quality of disaster-related mass care
- The role of the Sphere Humanitarian Charter and minimum standards in addressing disparities related to access and quality of care

REFERENCES

1. Waeckerle J, Lillibridge S, Burkle F, Noji N. Disaster medicine: challenges for today. *Ann Emerg Med.* 1994;23:715–718.
2. Keim M. Disaster preparedness. In: Ciottone GR, et al. eds. *Ciottone's Disaster Medicine.* 2nd ed. Philadelphia, PA: Elsevier; 2006.
3. Haddon W. A note concerning accident theory and research with special reference to motor vehicle accidents. *Ann NY Acad Sci.* 1963;107:635–646.
4. Mason J, Cavalie P. Malaria epidemic in Haiti following a hurricane. *Am J Trop Med Hyg.* 1965;14:533–539.
5. de Ville de Goyet C, Lechat M. Health aspects in natural disasters. *Trop Doctor.* 1976;6: 152–157.
6. Bertazzi PA. Industrial disasters and epidemiology: a review of recent experiences. *Scand J Work Environ Health.* 1989;15(2):85–100.
7. Guha-Sapir D, Lechat M. Reducing the impact of natural disasters: why aren't we better prepared? *Health Policy Plann.* 1986;1:118–126.
8. Centers for Disease Control and Prevention (CDC). *Public Health Consequences of Disasters.* Atlanta, GA: Centers for Disease Control and Prevention; 1989.
9. Centers for Disease Control and Prevention (CDC). Outbreak of diarrheal illness associated with a natural disaster—Utah. *MMWR.* 1983;32(50):662–664.
10. Auf der Heide E. *Disaster Response: Principles of Preparation and Coordination.* St Louis, MO: Mosby; 1989.
11. Gunn SWA. *Multilingual Dictionary of Disaster Medicine and International Relief.* Dordrecht, Netherlands: Kluwer Academic Publishers; 1990.
12. Noji E. The Nature of disaster: general characteristics and public health effects. In: Noji E, ed. *The Public Health Consequences of Disasters.* New York, NY: Oxford University Press; 1997:3–20.
13. Khan F, Amatya B, Gosney J, Rathore FA, Burkle FM, Jr. Medical rehabilitation in natural disasters: a review. *Arch Phys Med Rehabil.* 2015;96(9):1709–1727.
14. Burkle F. Challenges of global public health emergencies: development of a health crisis management framework. *J Exper Med.* 2019;249:33–41.

15. Clack ZA, Keim ME, Macintyre AG, Yeskey K. Emergency health and risk management in sub-Saharan Africa: a lesson from the embassy bombings in Tanzania and Kenya. *Prehosp Disaster Med.* 2002;17(2):59–66.
16. US Department of Homeland Security. ESF6 Annex: Mass Care, Emergency Assistance, Temporary Housing and Human Services Annex. Washington, DC: Dept of Homeland Security; 2016.
17. The Sphere Project. *The Sphere Handbook.* 4th ed. Geneva, Switzerland: Practical Action Publishing; 2018.

24

Target Capabilities of Emergency Health

LEARNING OBJECTIVES

Upon completion, the reader will be able to

1. Define the following terms and phrases:
   - Capability
   - Capability-based planning
   - Target capability
2. Recognize that most US target capabilities for emergency management focus on response.
3. Categorize a list of emergency health target capabilities according to ecosocial factors.

CAPABILITY-BASED PLANNING

Capability-based planning is the cornerstone of most modern approaches to disaster planning.[1] Simply stated, a **capability** is the ability to achieve a given outcome. **Target capabilities** are used to meet predetermined (i.e., targeted) objectives. The Target Capabilities List (TCL) in the United States is a national-level, generic model of emergency management capabilities.[2] No single jurisdiction is capable of accomplishing all TCL capabilities. These are intended as both individual aspirational and collective operational targets.

Like the four pillars of health, these target capabilities are divided into a small group of "mission areas": common capabilities, prevention, protection, response, and recovery. (See Table 24-1.) However, current TCL capabilities actually focus primarily on downstream interventions. For example, the mission area of response contains 60% of the current TCL version. (See Table 24-2.) While providing an organizational framework for many domestic response activities, the 2007 version of US Department of Homeland Security TCL includes few capabilities known to determine health and wellness. In general, the 2007 TCL version focuses on national security related to CBRNE hazards (i.e., chemical, biological, radiation, narcotics, and explosives hazards). Target capabilities in the prevention mission area do not include health outcomes. The protection mission area does not address hazardous exposures other than foodborne. The recovery mission does not include recovery of the individual victim's health, wellness, or functional ability.

Table 24-1. Target Capabilities List for 19 Common Capabilities as Well as Those Involving Prevention, Protection, and Recovery

Common	Prevention	Protection	Recovery
Planning Communications Community preparedness and participation Risk management Intelligence, information-sharing, and dissemination	Information-gathering Recognition of indicators Warning Intelligence analysis and production Counterterror investigation and law enforcement CBRNE detection	Critical infrastructure Food and agriculture safety and defense Epidemiological surveillance and investigation Laboratory testing	Structural damage Assessment Restoration of lifelines Economic and community recovery

Note: CBRNE = Chemical, biological, radiation, narcotics, and explosives detection.

Table 24-1 lists 19 target capabilities, including common capabilities and others involving prevention, protection, and recovery. By contrast, Table 24-2 lists 16 target capabilities for response alone.

This chapter supplements the current Universal Task List (UTL) with additional factors known to influence population health and wellness. Here, reported determinants of health, wellness, and equity (DoHWE) have been summarized from Tables 3-2, 13-1, 13-2, 14-1, and 15-1 into one UTL for emergency health, shown in Table 24-3.

This UTL of candidate factors is discussed within an ecosocial context (i.e., personal to macro). The intent is to derive target capabilities for prevention, promotion, protection, and care provision based on known DoHWE and to offer TCL mission area capabilities that align with the ecosocial determinants of health. Like most DoHWE, an exo-level lack of resources significantly affects health outcomes during all Federal Emergency Management Administration mission areas. However, as illustrated by Figures 9-1 and 10-3, the upstream and downstream health determinants are often the same.[3] For example, the macro-level beliefs of a society can be a major determinant in accessing preventive capabilities as well as for making a response. Thus, target capabilities for health are presented according to five ecosocial contexts (from the victim's perspective instead of the responder's).

Table 24-2. Target Capabilities List for 16 Capabilities Involving Response

Animal disease Critical resource Emergency operations center Public information and warning	Environmental health Evacuation and shelter in place Explosive response Fire response	Incident management Isolation and quarantine Logistics and distribution Public safety and security	Responder safety and health Search and rescue Volunteer management and donations Weapons of mass destruction (WMD) and hazardous materials

Table 24-3 summarizes examples of the ecosocial DoHWE drawn from this textbook. This list is not intended to be all-inclusive or definitive but rather to be representative of the DoHWE likely to be associated with the disaster-related disease. These determinants (and related goals) are intended exemplify a range of risk and protective factors that affect disaster-related disease within an ecosocial context. And it should be realistically recognized that some of these stated outcomes are easier to achieve than others (e.g., health equality versus health equity).

The first column of Table 24-3 (i.e., personal) lists the intrinsic and acquired risk and protective factors inherent to the individual person. The second column (i.e., micro) lists the people that compose a person's social network. The third column ((i.e., meso) relates environmental factors associated with health and wellness. The fourth column (i.e., exo)

Table 24-3. Ecosocial Determinants of Health, Wellness, and Equity

Personal (Individual)	Micro (People)	Meso (Environment)	Exo (Resources)	Macro (Beliefs)
Demographic	Advocates	Built environment	Accessibility	Bias
Age	Antagonists	Clinics	Commerce	Conflict
Ethnicity	Care providers	Ecosystem	Communication	Culture
Gender	Community	Home	Economics	Discrimination
Race	Coworkers	Hospitals	Education	Equality
Sex	Criminals	Infrastructure	Employment	Equity
Psychological	Educators	Institutions	Energy	Governance
Behavior	Family and friends	Markets	Finance	Human rights
Control	Health care workers	Natural environment	Goods	Humanitarianism
Emotion	Institutionalized persons	Neighborhood	Government	Identity
Friendship	Leaders	School	Healthcare	Insularity
Humor	Media	Shelter	Hospitals	Justice
Intellect	Neighbors	Workplace	Housing	Norms
Leisure	Patients		Income	Peace
Love	Public safety		Information	Realistic beliefs
Motivation	Retailers		Legal system	Religion
Self-care	Service providers		Logistics	Risk
Self-worth			Organization	Sacredness
Stress management			Sanitation	Spirituality
Work			Security	Violence
Physiological			Safety	
Exercise			Social capital	
Food			Socioeconomic status	
Functional ability			Technology	
Genetics				
Health				
Health status				
Hygiene				
Nutrition				
Water				

lists resources influencing outcomes. And the fifth column lists belief systems (i.e., macro) that also affect health, wellness, and equity.

Tables 24-4 to 24-8 list target capabilities based on five ecosocial determinants: personal, social, and environmental determinants, resources, and beliefs. Emergency

Table 24-4. Target Capabilities List and Outcome Statement for Individual (Personal) Determinants of Health and Wellness

Target Capability	Outcome Statement for Personal DoH/W
Age	All people have full functional ability regardless of age.
Behavior	All people behave in ways that optimize their health and wellness.
Control	All people control their own health and wellness.
Emotion	All people recognize and express emotion in healthy ways.
Ethnicity	All people have equitable health outcomes regardless of ethnicity.
Exercise	All people exercise daily.
Food	All people have equitable access to nutritional food.
Friendship	All people have friends.
Functional ability	All people have optimal functional ability.
Gender	All people have equitable health outcomes regardless of gender.
Genetics	All people have optimal genetic health.
Health	The health of all people is actively produced and protected from harm.
Health status	All people have optimum health status.
Human	All people have human rights.
Humor	All people have positive humor.
Hygiene	All people have adequate hygiene.
Intellect	All people can understand health risk and messaging.
Leisure	All people have leisure.
Livelihood	All people have a safe and healthy occupation, vocation, or livelihood.
Love	All people feel loved.
Motivation	All people are motivated to prevent and manage disease.
Nutrition	All people are well nourished.
Race	All people have equitable health outcomes regardless of race.
Self-care	All people practice self-care.
Self-worth	All people have self-worth.
Sex	All people have equitable health outcomes regardless of sexual identity.
Stress management	All people manage their stress in productive ways.
Water	All people have safe and equitable access to a sufficient quantity of water.

Note: DoH/W = Determinants of health and wellness.

Table 24-5. Target Capability List and Outcome Statement for Social (Micro) Determinants of Health and Wellness

Target Capability	Outcome Statement for Social DoH/W
Advocates	All persons have advocates for their health and wellness.
Care providers	All persons have providers that are available to assist in their care.
Community	All persons are part of a social community.
Coworkers	All coworkers maintain good interpersonal relationships.
Criminals	Crime is prevented so that everyone's health and safety are protected.
Educators	All persons have access to quality educators.
Family and friends	All persons have a network of family and/or friends.
Health care workers	All persons have timely access to well-trained health care workers.
Institutionalized persons	All institutionalized persons have equitable health and wellness.
Leaders	All persons have access to high-quality leadership.
Media	All persons have access to quality media.
Neighbors	All persons have access to neighbors who will assist them.
Patients	All patients are treated with equitable quality care.
Public safety	Communities are safe from crime.
Retailers	All persons have equitable access to retail markets.
Service providers	All persons have equitable access to commercial services.

Note: DoH/W = Determinants of health and wellness.

Table 24-6. Target Capabilities List and Outcome Statement for Environmental (Meso) Determinants of Health and Wellness

Target Capability	Outcome Statement for Environmental DoH/W
Built environment	The built environment is safe for all people.
Clinics	All people have equitable access to quality health care clinics.
Ecosystem	All people live in a stable ecosystem that is healthy and safe.
Home	All people's homes are healthy and safe.
Hospitals	All people have equitable access to safe and quality hospital facilities.
Infrastructure	All people have equitable access to quality infrastructure.
Institutions	Institutional living is safe and healthy for all people.
Markets	All people have equitable access to quality markets.
Natural environment	The natural environment is safe for all people.
Neighborhood	All people live in safe and healthy neighborhoods.
School	School environments are safe.
Shelter	All people have shelter.
Violence	All people are safe from violence.
Workplace	All workplaces are safe environments.

Note: DoH/W = Determinants of health and wellness.

Table 24-7. Target Capabilities List and Outcome Statement for Resource-Related (Exo) Determinants of Health and Wellness

Target Capability	Outcome Statement for Resource-Related DoH/W
Accessibility	All persons have equal accessibility to the built and natural environment.
Commerce	All persons have fair and equal access to commercial transactions.
Communication	All people can communicate with others.
Economics	All people have the economic stability to be healthy and well.
Education	All people have adequate training and education to be healthy and well.
Employment	All people have livelihoods that adequately supports their health and safety.
Energy	All people use energy for their daily needs.
Finance	All persons have income that adequately supports their health and wellness.
Goods	All people have the goods necessary to be healthy and well.
Government	Good governance is applied to ensure that all people are healthy and well.
Healthcare	All people have access to quality health care.
Housing	Safe and healthy housing is accessible to all persons.
Income	All people have income sufficient to be healthy and well.
Information	All people have equitable access to pertinent information.
Legal system	All persons have access to a civil and criminal legal system.
Logistics	All people have logistical resources to assist their health and wellness.
Organization	All people have organizational resources to assist their health and wellness.
Safety	All people live and work in safe places.
Sanitation	All people have adequate sanitation and hygiene.
Security	All people live secure from intentional harm.
Social capital	All people have social capital.
Socioeconomic status	All people have an adequate socioeconomic status that supports their health and wellness.
Technology	All people have access to technology that supports their health and wellness.

Note: DoH/W = Determinants of health and wellness.

health interventions are intended to influence all five categories of ecosocial determinants during each of the four mission areas (i.e., prevention, promotion, protection, and provision).

These TCLs represent a UTL for addressing a broad range of DoHWE related to disasters. They also provide a roadmap of strategic goals or measures of success for ensuring emergency health in the future. These TCLs and outcome statements describe an objective framework for the health sector to produce and protect health before, during, and after emergencies.

Table 24-8. Target Capabilities List and Outcome Statement for Beliefs (Macro) Related to Determinants of Health and Wellness

Target Capability	Outcome Statement for Beliefs Related to DoH/W
Bias	All people live without unfair bias.
Conflict	All persons live free from conflict.
Culture	All people practice their culture.
Discrimination	All people live without unfair discrimination.
Equality	All people have equal access to the determinants of health and wellness.
Equity	All people have equitable outcomes for health and wellness.
Governance	All people have good governance.
Human rights	All people have the human right to health and wellness.
Humanitarianism	All people have equitable access to humanitarian assistance.
Identity	All people can express their personal identity.
Insularity	All people have access to a diversity of people, beliefs, and views.
Justice	All people have justice.
Norms	All people live within healthy and safe social norms.
Peace	All people live in peace.
Realistic beliefs	All people have realistic beliefs.
Religion	All people can practice religion.
Risk	All persons have fair and equitable risk for disaster-related disease.
Sacredness	All people have sacredness.
Sexual bias	All people are free from bias or discrimination due to their sex.
Spirituality	All people have spirituality.

Note: DoH/W = Determinants of health and wellness.

TOPICS FOR DISCUSSION

Describe how one target capability from each of the five tables (Tables 24-4 to 24-8) can influence these upstream and downstream activities:

- Upstream activities involving prevention, promotion, and protection
- Downstream activities involving the provision of care

REFERENCES

1. Keim M. *Disaster Planning: A Practical Guide to Effective Health Outcomes*. Cambridge, UK: Cambridge University Press; 2021.

2. US Department of Homeland Security. *Target Capabilities List: A Companion to the National Preparedness Guidelines*. 2007:5–7.
3. Frieden T. A framework for public health action: the health impact pyramid. *Am J Public Health*. 2010;100(4):590–595.

25

The Role of Public Health Professionals

LEARNING OBJECTIVES

Upon completion, the reader will be able to

1. Recognize key public health professions associated with major disciplines of public health.
2. Recognize the multidisciplinary role of public health professionals in emergency health.
3. Recognize the need for emergency health as a programmatic focus of public health.
4. Recognize the need for "emergency health in all policies."
5. Recognize the role of public health as the community-based convener and catalyst for emergency health.

THE MULTIDISCIPLINARY ROLE OF EMERGENCY HEALTH PROFESSIONALS

In addition to being multisectoral across society, emergency health is multidisciplinary within the field of public health. A wide range of disciplines perform the study and practice of emergency health. For example, the role of public health has been described to include the following core disciplines: biostatistics and informatics; congenital and developmental disabilities; clinical practice; communications; community health; prevention and control of infectious disease, noninfectious disease, and injury; emergency management; environmental health; epidemiology and surveillance; global health; immunization; laboratory; mental health; public policy and administration; public health education; and social and behavioral science. Table 25-1 offers an example of public health professions listed according to these core public health disciplines.

THE PROGRAMMATIC FOCUS OF EMERGENCY HEALTH PROFESSIONALS

Emergency health is intended to convene a broad set of public health capabilities within an organizational framework for action. For this reason, Table 25-1 could just as easily represent the role of public health disciplines in emergency health. All these disciplines (and associated professional roles) are involved in emergency health functions. In the

Table 25-1. Examples of Public Health Professions Listed According to Core Discipline

Public Health Discipline	Public Health Professional
Birth defects and developmental disabilities	Epidemiologist
	Geneticist
	Laboratorian
	Risk communication specialist
Clinical practice	Physician
	Nurse
	Nutritionist
	Pharmacist
Communications	Risk communication specialist
	Public health information officer
	Media spokesperson
Community health	Community health worker
	Outreach specialist
	Social worker
	Community service officer
	Director of family health services
Disease control	Communicable disease specialist
	Noncommunicable disease specialist
	Health care administrator
	Safety manager
Emergency management	Emergency manager
	Emergency preparedness specialist
	Emergency operations center staff
	Field logistics and supply chain
Environmental health	Environmental scientist
	Toxicologist
	Environmental lawyer
	Public health engineer
	Occupational physician
Epidemiology and surveillance	Epidemiologist
	Health information technician
	Database administrator
	Statistician

(Continued)

Table 25-1. (Continued)

Public Health Discipline	Public Health Professional
Global health	Global health security specialist
	Refugee health scientist
	Disease analyst
	Epidemiologist
Immunization	Immunologist
	Vaccinologist
	Microbiologist
Laboratory	Laboratorian
	Laboratory technician
	Laboratory director
	Biosafety specialist
Mental health	Health and wellness manager
	Behavioral scientist
	Intervention researcher
	Mental health clinician
Public policy and administration	Policy advisor
	Public health administrator/director
	Health care administrator
	Health services manager
Public health education	Nurse educator
	Health teacher
	Public health journalist
Social and behavioral science	Behavioral scientist
	Social scientist
	Monitoring and evaluation specialist
	Intervention researcher

past many of these capabilities were delivered within an "all of the agency" approach by periodically convening public health professionals from various disciplines to address an emergency incident. However, the ecosocial nature of disaster-related health effects necessitates a sustained programmatic effort across disciplines to address upstream and downstream determinants of health, wellness, and equity (DoHWE). Emergency health calls for integrating public health disciplines to address hazards' causes and effects, rather than integrating hazards to fit one specific discipline. As such, the role of emergency health professionals is best circumscribed within the scope of their collective mandate—namely, to lower disaster-related morbidity and mortality. This effort requires a wide range of disciplines and specialties that converge on the mutual goal of identifying and intervening in disaster-related DoHWE. The goal of emergency health is population-based health, wellness, and equity. This goal is best served by a long-term approach for capability maturity intended to impart affordable and sustainable reductions in morbidity and mortality.

THE MULTISECTORAL ROLE OF EMERGENCY HEALTH PROFESSIONALS

Effective emergency health interventions require a multisectoral approach that is often beyond the influence of public health or medicine. (See Tables 24-4 to 24-8.) Many decisions that affect disaster-related health risk extend beyond the traditional role of public health to include stakeholders within other sectors (e.g., policy, emergency management, environment, governance, industry, finance, security, and transportation).

Public health is uniquely positioned at the community level to serve as the convener and the catalyst for addressing the multisectoral DoHWE. The tenet of emergency health in all policies (EHiAP) recognizes that many factors and societal sectors create health. In many cases, health outcomes are determined by the actions of sectors beyond public health. EHiAP addresses the key drivers of health, wellness outcomes, and equity. EHiAP recognizes the model for "public health 3.0" in which leaders serve as chief health strategists, partnering across multiple sectors and leveraging resources to address the entire range of DoHWE.[1] Public health 3.0 focuses on innovative clinical interventions and total population-wide prevention that engages multiple sectors and community partners to generate collective impact that measurably improves DoHWE.[1]

These multilateral efforts are intended to promote health and equity through intersectoral collaboration, resulting in co-benefits for multiple stakeholders across multiple sectors. EHiAP provides a process for integrating emergency health into population-based decision-making, including upstream and downstream interventions. This joint effort also allows for aligning emergency health decisions with sustainable development goals.[2]

TOPICS FOR DISCUSSION

1. Discuss the role of emergency health professionals for each of the core public health disciplines listed in Table 25-1, according to the following disaster scenarios:
   - Flood
   - Chemical release
   - Epidemic

2. Compare the role of public health professionals for each of the four pillars of emergency health:
    - Prevention of societal risk factors
    - Promotion of individual protective factors
    - Protection of health
    - Provision of care

REFERENCES

1. DeSalvo K, Wang Y, Harris A, Auerbach J, Koo D, O'Carroll P. Public health 3.0: a call to action for public health to meet the challenges of the 21st century. *Prev Chronic Dis*. 2017;14:170017.
2. World Health Organization (WHO). Promoting health in the SDGs: report on the 9th Global Conference for Health Promotion, Shanghai, China. 2017. Available at: https://www.who.int/publications/i/item/promoting-health-in-the-sdgs. Accessed November 23, 2022.

26

Performance Management

LEARNING OBJECTIVES

Upon completion, the reader will be able to

1. Define the following terms and phrases:
   - Ability
   - Accountability
   - Activity
   - Egalitarian
   - Key performance indicators
   - Management by objectives
   - Operational objective
   - Operations
   - Operations management
   - Operations plan
   - Performance
   - Performance management
   - Performance measurement
   - Productivity
   - Resource
   - Responsible party
   - Satisfaction
   - Six Sigma
   - SOARR planning format
   - Strategic goal
   - Systems theory
2. Recognize the five cascading elements of the SOARR format for planning.
3. Compare the order of the SOARR format with that of a program logic model.
4. Recall that the SOARR format and Six Sigma model may be used to define and improve emergency health intervention processes.
5. Given an example of process definition, identify the strategic goal, operational objective, activities, and responsible parties.
6. Recall that performance measurement refers to data collection regarding key performance indicators.

7. Recall the fundamental role of performance measurement.
8. Describe one way to monitor and evaluate progress toward health equity.

DEFINITION

Principles of **performance management** can be used to guide interventions that most efficiently and effectively organize emergency health professionals during public health interventions that address target capabilities related to health, wellness, and equity.

These interventions involve a series of coordinated, multisectoral operations. **Operations** are a group of processes implemented by an organization to accomplish an objective or goal.[1] For example, emergency operations typically involve an organized system for incident **management by objectives. Operations management** is the administration of management science to create the highest level of efficiency possible within an organization. It is concerned with converting materials and labor into goods and services as efficiently as possible to maximize the impact of an organization.[1]

Operations management uses **systems theory** to support managerial decision-making. Systems are groups of processes (i.e., tactics) that transform **inputs** (i.e., resources) into outputs (products and services) and outcomes (i.e., objectives). Program logic models are schematic diagrams that represent the logic underlying a program's design, indicating how various components are expected to interact with the services they produce and how they generate desired results.[2]

Figure 26-1 depicts a generic program logic model with the three components of operations: resources, processes, and performance.[1] In this model, **inputs** of resources

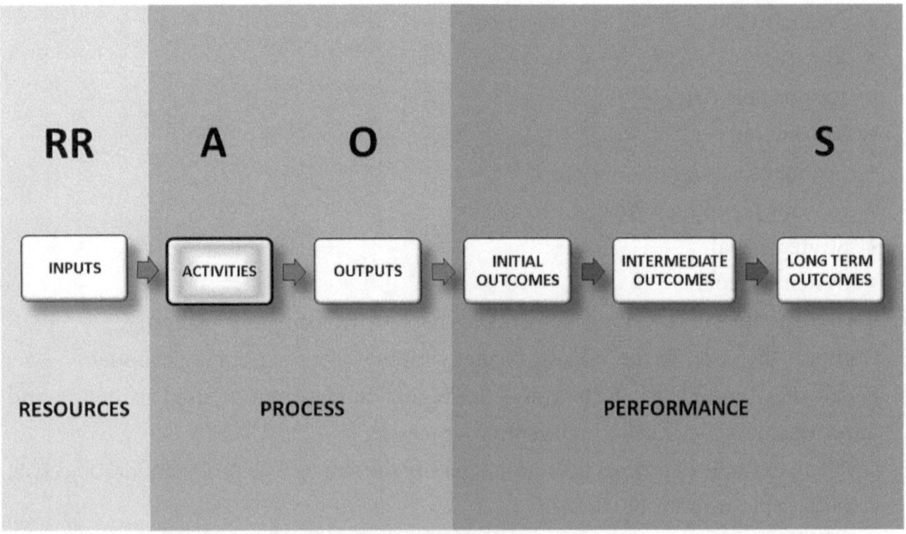

Source: Keim.[1] Adapted with permission of Cambridge University Press. © Cambridge University Press 2021.

Figure 26-1. Framework for a Generic Program Logic Model

Table 26-1. Relationship Between Measures of Resource, Process, and Performance

System Component	Inputs	Outputs	Outcomes
Program Component	Resources	Processes	Performance
Key Performance Indicator	Utilization	Efficiency	Effectiveness
Performance Measure	Time Staffing Materials Information Cost	Unit-cost ratio **Productivity** rate Cycle time Variability	Completeness Cost-effectiveness Completion time Stakeholder **satisfaction**

are used to perform activities that create measurable outputs. These activities and outputs accomplish initial, intermediate, and long-term outcomes.

Operations management includes resource management, process management, and performance management. Processes are groups of activities that accomplish an objective according to predetermined outputs. Performance management is the collection and use of performance measurement to support decisions that achieve predetermined outcomes

Table 26-1 depicts the relationship between inputs, outputs, and outcomes.

PLANNING FOR PERFORMANCE

Operations plans (e.g., public health intervention plans) draw directly from strategic plans to describe an operation's goals, objectives, and activities. This information is best organized according to a cascading network of planning elements under each capability. The five elements that accomplish a capability have been described as the SOARR cascading format for planning and are outlined as follows[1]:

Capability,

- Strategic goals,
  - Operational objectives,
    - Activities,
      - Responsible parties, and
      - Resources.

It should be noted that the **SOARR planning format** is considered in reverse order of the program logic model, as depicted in Figure 26-1. Where the logic model begins with resources, moves to processes, and then ends with outcomes, the SOARR format is intended to begin with outcomes (e.g., target capabilities lists and outcome statement as in Tables 24-4 to 24-8) and move in the opposite direction to address processes and resources that will accomplish this goal. The approach recognizes a planning hierarchy of **strategic goals, operational objectives, activities**, and tactical **resources.** For every strategic goal of the plan, there is a set of corresponding operational objectives that accomplish the goal. In turn, there is also a set of activities that accomplish the operational objective. And for each activity, there is an assigned **responsible party**. Finally, other resource requirements are identified besides primary responsibility for completing the activity (e.g., time, labor, cost, materials, and information).[1]

As such, the SOARR format can be used to define the outcomes for each emergency health capability and the processes intended to achieve those outcome statements. Tables 24-4 to 24-8 represent a list of target capabilities and outcome statements identified for the ecosocial determinants of health, wellness, and equity. Within a model of performance management, these tables represent the capabilities and strategic objectives (i.e., measurable outcomes) for emergency health. These outcomes may be evaluated as a candidate reference standard for measuring and managing the performance of emergency health interventions (i.e., measures of intended outputs and outcomes).

PERFORMANCE MANAGEMENT

Figure 26-2 represents one approach to performance management using SOARR and Six Sigma.[1] The **Six Sigma** method is summarized by the acronym DMAIC, which stands for definition, measurement, analysis, improvement, and control of a process.

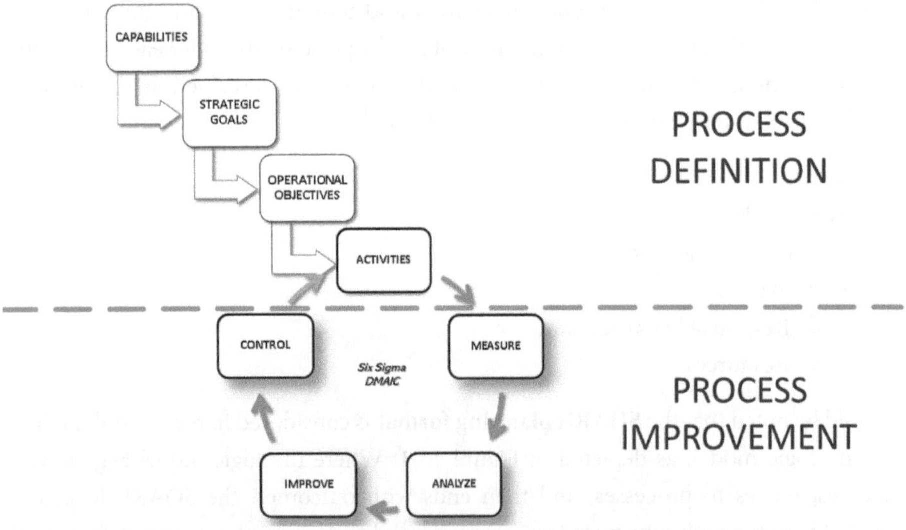

Source: Keim.[1] Adapted with permission of Cambridge University Press. © Cambridge University Press 2021.

Figure 26-2. The Six Sigma DMAIC Cycle Applied to Performance Management

This approach is also repeated as an iterative cycle until the intended results are achieved.

The SOARR planning cascade integrates with the iterative cycles of process improvement that are involved in managing the performance of operations. This connection allows for process definitions developed in the operations plan to inform a process improvement plan. This iterative process is intended to continuously improve the quality of performance for emergency health capabilities.

PERFORMANCE MANAGEMENT FOR EMERGENCY HEALTH

Let us now consider an example from Table 24-4, the Target Capabilities List and Outcome Statement for Individual (Personal) Determinants of Health and Wellness. This table lists a target capability for water, along with the following statement that describes the intended outcome: All people have safe and equitable access to a sufficient quantity of water.

This intended outcome is treated as the strategic goal for water. Under this strategic goal are four operational objectives (i.e., measures of success). This SOARR cascade could include the following elements: strategic goal, operational objectives, activities, responsible parties, and other resources. See Table 26-2, which serves to define the process. The next step is to improve it by measuring, analyzing, improving, and controlling the process during implementation.

Table 26-2. Example of Process Definition for the Capability of Water

Strategic Goal	Operational Objective	Activities	Responsibility	Resources
All people have safe and equitable access to a sufficient quantity of water[3]	Average water used in any house is at least 15 liters per person per day.[3]	1. Assess household needs. 2. Report needs. 3. Monitor water distribution. 4. Monitor ongoing needs.	Public health	1 survey 2 FTE 8 hours
	Maximum distance from any household to the nearest water point is 500 meters.[3]	1. Assess population location. 2. Identify distribution points. 3. Publicize distribution points. 4. Distribute water. 5. Monitor needs.	Water department	2 FTE Website 8 hours
	Queuing time at a water source is no more than 30 minutes.[3]	1. Calculate queuing time per distribution point. 2. Distribute water. 3. Monitor queuing time. 4. Adjust delivery as needed.	NGO	1 volunteer 8 hours

Note: FTE = fulltime employee; NGO = nongovernmental organization.

PERFORMANCE MEASUREMENT

Peter Drucker, one of the fathers of modern quality improvement, once said, "If you can't measure it, you can't manage it." For this reason, performance management begins with performance measurement. Performance measurement is "the regular measurement of the results and efficiencies of services or programs."[2]

The ability to quantitatively measure performance is critical for achieving desired performance goals. These measures of performance may include steps of a process as well as measures of outcome.[4] Performance measurement refers to data collection regarding key performance indicators. (See Table 26-1.)

The fundamental role of performance measurement is to help hold the various agents to account by enabling stakeholders to make informed decisions.[5] Establishing **accountability** is an effective use of performance information. This accountability has been described according to five dimensions: transparency, liability, control, **ability**, responsibility, and responsiveness.[2]

In many respects, performance information is what economists refer to as a "public good" that is unlikely to develop optimally without the guidance and encouragement of governments.[5] Setting targets for the attainment of improvement goals expresses a commitment to achieve specified outputs in a defined period and helps monitor progress toward realizing broader goals and objectives. Targets are viewed as a means of defining and setting priorities, creating high-level political and administrative commitments to outputs, and providing a basis for the follow-up and evaluation. In short, they can become central to the governance system.[5]

Measuring Equity

Health systems should be evaluated against the goal of ensuring that all people in need receive effective emergency health services (e.g., prevention, health promotion, health protection, and provision of care). One way to measure progress toward this goal is to measure the extent to which access and quality of resources are based on need rather than ability to pay or some other ecosocial determinants of health, wellness, and equity.[5] This **egalitarian** principle of equity or fairness is the primary motivation for health systems' efforts to separate individual financing from the production of health and wellness.[5]

TOPICS FOR DISCUSSION

Referring to Figure 26-2, describe an example of the environmental target capability of "home health and safety" that includes strategic goals, operational objectives, activities, and responsible parties for each activity.

REFERENCES

1. Keim M. *Disaster Planning: A Practical Guide to Effective Health Outcomes*. Cambridge, UK: Cambridge University Press; 2021.
2. Poister T, Aristigueta M, Hall J. *Managing and Measuring Performance in Public and Nonprofit Organizations*. San Francisco, CA: Josey Bass; 2015.
3. The Sphere Project. *Humanitarian Charter and Minimum Standards in Disaster Response*. Geneva, Switzerland: The Sphere Project; 2008.
4. Harbour J. *The Basics of Performance Measurment*. 2nd ed. New York, NY: Taylor & Francis Group; 2009.
5. Smith P, Mossialos E, Papanicolas I, Leatherman S. *Performance Measurement of Health System Improvement*. New York, NY: Cambridge University Press; 2009.

VII. OPPORTUNITIES FOR EMERGENCY HEALTH

27

Opportunities for Research, Education, Intervention, and Integration

LEARNING OBJECTIVES

Upon completion, the reader will be able to

1. Define the following terms and phrases:
   - Competency
   - Competency-based learning
   - Information exchange
   - Task analysis
2. Recognize that the Great Acceleration of the mid-20th century has created challenges and opportunities for public health impact.
3. Recognize examples of long-standing research needs that now represent opportunities.
4. Recall that opportunities remain for the development of standardized education for a broad range of public health and medical professionals.
5. Recall the opportunities for public health as the convenor and the catalyst for multi-sectoral community-based interventions.
6. Recognize the range of national and international opportunities for integration with public policies and strategy.

OPPORTUNITIES FOR IMPACT

Figure 1-1 set the stage for our discussion of emergency health. It brought to our attention the remarkable increase in disaster frequency that closely aligns with the simultaneous rise in human development, known as the "Great Acceleration."[1] This phrase represents the rapid increase of humanity's impact on planetary ecology that is characteristic of this period. But of course, this impact has not been limited to the planet but extends to its inhabitants. The socioeconomic impacts of the great acceleration also appear to correlate with the growing annual incidence of both natural and human-made disasters.[2] There is an increased awareness of the connection between human development and disasters. And with this awareness comes the opportunity for human development to affect health positively and productively, lessening the risk of disaster-related morbidity and mortality, preserving wellness, and ensuring health equity.

These opportunities for emergency health are no longer limited to downstream interventions. Public health can apply a range of practical public health principles that address the upstream factors (i.e., personal, social, environmental, societal factors as well as beliefs) known to influence disaster-affected populations' health outcomes. Perhaps the most unmistakable sign of capability maturity for public health is the growing recognition that measures of process must also be connected to measures of outcome. It is no longer sufficient to report the laurels of disaster-related public health accomplishments in terms of "number of persons treated" or "number of meals delivered" when the most important questions remain unanswered: How many lives were saved? How many illnesses and injuries were averted?

> It's not good enough to just "do good." We must do good well.

OPPORTUNITIES FOR RESEARCH

Over 30 years ago the Centers for Disease Control published a special monograph entitled "The Public Health Consequences of Disasters, 1989."[3] One of the first collections of public health information related to disasters, this early monograph described the research needs that existed at the time. Now, decades later and well into the 21st century, while disappointing, it is also quite enlightening to review the status of these research needs as they existed several decades ago. Many, if not most, of the identified essential public health needs remain wholly unanswered to this day. Of the following research topics introduced in the 1989 monograph, many have yet to be attained:

1. Risk Assessment
   - Hazard identification, monitoring and forecasting
   - Dose response modeling for disaster hazards
   - Multivariate risk analysis
     - Risk assessment for chemical disasters
     - Risk mapping at the county level
     - Disaster-related injuries, including building occupant behavior (i.e., exposure data)
     - Risk assessment validation and accuracy
2. Impact Assessment
   - Disaster epidemiology
   - Basic capabilities
     - Accurate assessment of disaster-related deaths and injuries
     - Emphasis on descriptive and analytical epidemiology as compared with case reports

    - Standardization of case definitions for disaster-related disease
    - Risk factors for morbidity and mortality
    - Health consequences of disasters among multiple populations
    - Techniques for rapid needs assessment
    - Surveillance
        - Data systems for disaster-related health surveillance
        - Psychosocial impacts
3. Risk management
    - Vulnerability reduction
4. Prevention
    - Preventive health and safety
    - Prevention strategies
5. Protection
    - Protection from disaster hazards
    - Public education, alert, and warning
    - Population protective measures
    - Occupational health outcomes for responders
6. Provision of care
    - Planning for emergency operations
    - Techniques for locating and rescuing disaster victims

These research topics represent questions from the disaster literature that have gone unanswered for decades despite billions of dollars in disaster-related public allocations in the United States alone. And yet, many of these subjects relate to core principles and the fundamental capabilities of public health practice. For example, the list of research needs includes the basic building blocks of public health, such as case definition, risk analysis, needs assessment, and accurate reporting of disaster-related morbidity and mortality. It is notably distressing to find the use of descriptive and analytical epidemiology (not subjective case reports) as research needs that, in many examples, remain pertinent today.[4–6] The controversy regarding the number of deaths that occurred because of Hurricane Maria in Puerto Rico exemplifies the unresolved research needs.[7–9] However, these basic needs also represent opportunities to make dramatic strides by simply updating our approach in a way commensurate with other public health fields.

EDUCATIONAL OPPORTUNITIES

Just as there are research opportunities, there are many corresponding opportunities for education and learning related to emergency health. These opportunities include the public health and medical disciplines of epidemiology, environmental health, injury prevention, disaster medicine, and humanitarian assistance.

As was the research case, educational opportunities simply require the development of essential public health capabilities. For example, in contrast to the curriculum in place for emergency management agencies, there is no standardized curriculum for public health emergency managers. There is also a general lack of professional knowledge related to exposure science and other essential environmental health principles that would be best served by inclusion in future disaster education opportunities. And as for public health, there exists no standardized curriculum or set of competencies for disaster medical care providers. Beyond care, there remains no clear scope of practice for disaster medicine, which is often described as performing both clinical and public health activities. At the same time, most training programs focus on clinical care. Finally, the practice of humanitarian assistance is also sorely in need of modernization and applications that take advantage of societal capability involving networking, big data, and **information exchange**. In summary, most educational opportunities regarding disaster-related professions remain underdeveloped and, therefore, ripe for substantial improvement with minimal public investments.

While prevention is a foundational principle of public health, much still needs to be done with respect to education of the public and of the professional community for preventing disaster-related disease. In addition, tremendous opportunities abound for growth related to emergency health education and competency-based learning grounded on task analysis. Opportunities for health education related to health promotion and health protection are also growing. Finally, there are many opportunities for developing evidence-based **competency** standards for public health responders, emergency managers, and disaster-related clinical care.

OPPORTUNITIES FOR INTERVENTION

The ecosocial nature of these factors aligns with many of the strengths of public health. Understanding the broad range of ecosocial determinants of health-related to disasters, public health offers an expanding array of potential opportunities for intervention. Opportunities abound for public health officials to serve as the conveners and the catalysts for a wide variety of multisectoral, community-based interventions.[10] Public health is uniquely positioned at the community level to ensure immersive levels of community engagement. As the saying goes, "All disasters are local."[11] So too is public health.

There are opportunities for environmental justice and health equity at the community and family levels, which are the most proximal health determinants. Also positioned at the community level are many of the same disaster hazards that threaten a population's health, wellness, and equity. These hazards are not randomly dispersed but rather exist within an inequitable distribution that places an unequal burden on some populations while sparing others. Many of the upstream principles of public health, risk management, and preventive control of hazards are also the foundations of models for long-term adaption to the health impacts of climate change. Public health is also uniquely suited to facilitate multisectoral interventions related to climate change adaptation.

OPPORTUNITIES FOR INTEGRATION

Recall that emergency health is a subdiscipline of environmental health and, as such, is typically characterized by multisectoral collaborations. These collaborations require close integration to accomplish the intended outcome. One valuable means for integration involves partnerships grounded on more extensive and comprehensive national and international strategies. Examples of such opportunities for emergency health include integration and standardization of processes according to international standards like Sphere and ISO 31000 for risk management.[12,13] Using this integrative approach, collaborators work together to develop practice standards for humanitarian assistance, human development, and international policy supporting the UN Sustainable Development Goals and the Sendai Framework for Disaster Risk Reduction.[12,14,15] The proactive, upstream approach to emergency health also aligns with US national strategies like the US National Prevention Strategy and Healthy People 2030 program.[16] As is frequently the case, integration is too often considered an end when it more often serves as the means for sustainable multisectoral accomplishments.

> "The function of the well-intentioned individual, acting in isolation, is to formulate or disseminate theoretical truths. The function of the well-intentioned individuals in association is to live in accordance with those truths, to demonstrate what happens when theory is translated into practice, to create small-scale working models of the better form of society to which the speculative idealist looks forward."[17]
>
> –Aldous Huxley, *Ends and Means*

TOPICS FOR DISCUSSION

It can be said that integration often represents the biggest challenge and the most significant opportunity for public health activities. Referring to Table 24-3, describe barriers to integration that may occur in terms of personal, social, environmental, societal, and cultural factors.

REFERENCES

1. Steffen W, Broadgate W, Deutsch L, Gaffney O, Ludwig C. The trajectory of the Anthropocene: the Great Acceleration. *Anthropocene Rev.* 2015;2(1):81–98.
2. Keim ME, Smith TM, Burkle FM. The annual global incidence rate of extreme weather event disasters appears positively correlated with world GDP, 1961–2020. *Prehosp Disaster Med.* 2022;37(4):431–436.

3. Centers for Disease Control and Prevention (CDC). *Public Health Consequences of Disasters.* Atlanta, GA: Centers for Disease Control and Prevention; 1989.
4. Birnbaum M, Adibhatla S, Dudek O, Ramsel-Miller J. Categorization and analysis of disaster health publications: an inventory. *Prehosp Disaster Med.* 2017;32(5):473–482.
5. Zorrilla CD. The view from Puerto Rico: Hurricane Maria and its aftermath. *New Engl J Med.* 2017;377(19):1801–1803.
6. Yordan-Lopez N, Hernandez-Suarez DF, Marrero-Ortiz W, Marshall-Perez L, Lopez-Candales A. Challenges and opportunities after Hurricane Maria: University of Puerto Rico medical students' perspectives. *J Grad Med Educ.* 2018;10(4):382–384.
7. Verma AA, Murray J, Mamdani MM. Mortality in Puerto Rico after Hurricane Maria. *New Engl J Med.* 2018;379(17):e30.
8. Santos-Lozada AR. In Puerto Rico, counting deaths and making deaths count. *Health Aff* (Millwood). 2018;37(4):520–522.
9. Santos-Burgoa C, Sandberg J, Suarez E, et al. Differential and persistent risk of excess mortality from Hurricane Maria in Puerto Rico: a time-series analysis. *Lancet Planet Health.* 2018;2(11):e478–e488.
10. DeSalvo K, Wang Y, Harris A, Auerbach J, Koo D, O'Carroll P. Public health 3.0: a call to action for public health to meet the challenges of the 21st century. *Prev Chronic Dis.* 2017;14:170017.
11. AlertMedia. How FEMA helps businesses and communities navigate disasters. *Emerg Manage.* 2021. Available at: https://www.alertmedia.com/blog/fema-disaster-response. Accessed November 23, 2022.
12. The Sphere Project. *Humanitarian Charter and Minimum Standards in Disaster Response.* Geneva, Switzerland: The Sphere Project; 2008.
13. International Standards Organization. ISO 31000:2009: Risk management: principles and guidelines. 2009. Revised by ISO 31000:2018. https://www.iso.org/standard/65694.html. Accessed November 23, 2022.
14. World Health Organization (WHO). Promoting health in the SDGs: report on the 9th Global Conference for Health Promotion, Shanghai, China. 2017. Available at: https://www.who.int/publications/i/item/promoting-health-in-the-sdgs. Accessed November 23, 2022.
15. United Nation Office for Disaster Risk Reduction (UNDRR). *Sendai Framework for Disaster Reduction, 2015–2030.* New York, NY: United Nations; 2015.
16. Srinivasan S. Creating healthy communities, healthy homes, healthy people: initiating a research agenda on the built environment and public health. *Am J Public Health.* 2003;93(9):1446–1450.
17. Huxley, A. *Ends and Means: An Inquiry Into the Nature of Ideals and Into the Methods Employed for Their Realization*. London, UK: Harper & Brothers Publishers; 1937.

VIII. APPENDICES

APPENDIX A

The Etiology of Disaster-Related Disease

Table A-1. Etiology of Disease Associated With Cold Waves and Storm Disasters

Health Hazard	Health Effect	Etiology
Motor vehicle accident	Blunt trauma	Ice and snow create hazardous driving conditions. Icy conditions result in motor vehicle accidents. Accidents cause mostly blunt trauma.
Heating and cooking stoves	Burns Carbon monoxide poisoning	Ice and windy conditions cause power line breaks. Widespread line breaks cause power failures. People use unfamiliar/unsafe alternatives for cooking and heating. Unsafe alternatives cause burns and emit carbon monoxide. Persons who inhale stove emissions are poisoned. Persons who use a stove incorrectly are burned.
Power generators	Carbon monoxide poisoning	Generators are improperly operated within an enclosed space. Persons who inhale generator exhaust are poisoned.
Increased physical exertion	Exacerbation of cardiovascular disease	Ice and snow impede walkways and entrap vehicles. Persons not normally accustomed to strenuous exercise attempt to shovel snow. Increased exertion and cold stress exacerbate coronary artery disease.
Cold ambient air and wind	Hypothermia Cold injuries	Cold ambient temperatures and wind chill effect lower body temperatures. Low body temperatures cause cardiac dysrhythmias.
Precipitation	Cold injuries	Soft tissues are frozen by air, ice, and snow.

Source: The tables in this appendix are based on the following publications.[1-261]

Table A-2. Etiology of Disease Associated With Cyclone Disasters

Health Hazard	Health Effect	Etiology
Ballistic projectiles	Blunt and penetrating trauma	High winds create structural collapse and ballistic projectiles. Persons are hit by flying or falling debris.
Cooking stoves and lanterns	Burns Carbon monoxide poisoning	Windy conditions cause power line breaks. Widespread line breaks cause power failures. People use unfamiliar/unsafe alternatives for cooking and lighting. Unsafe alternatives cause burns and emit carbon monoxide. Persons who inhale stove emissions are poisoned. Persons who use a stove incorrectly are burned.
Power generators	Carbon monoxide poisoning	Generators are improperly operated within an enclosed space. Persons who inhale generator exhaust are poisoned.

(*Continued*)

Table A-2. (Continued)

Health Hazard	Health Effect	Etiology
Floodwater	Drowning Immersion injuries	Cyclones create storm surge in coastal areas. Heavy precipitation causes inland flooding. Floodwaters inundate populated areas. Persons are immersed in water. Persons are submerged under water.
Rooftop activity	Falls	High winds create roof and tree damage. Persons attempt rooftop repairs and fall from roof.
Power lines	Electrocution	High winds damage power lines. Persons are electrocuted while performing tree removal and home repairs.
High ambient air temperature	Heat illness Cardiovascular disease	Seasonal temperatures are typically high during cyclone season. Persons are exposed to heat during rescue and cleanup operations. Cardiovascular disease is exacerbated by heat.
Airborne particulates	Allergic reactions Asthma and COPD Pneumonitis	Floodwaters contaminate drywall in buildings. Mold grows inside structures. Home repair activities cause mold to become airborne. Persons inhale mold particulates.
Poor sanitation and hygiene	Diarrheal illness Food poisoning Skin infections Diarrheal illness Upper respiratory infections	Persons are displaced from their homes. Displacement results in limited access to sanitation and hygiene. Unsanitary conditions cause increase in endemic diseases.
Toxic chemicals	Toxic exposures and poisoning	Chemicals kept in the home and workplace are released during the storm. Persons are exposed to chemicals during cleanup.

Source: The tables in this appendix are based on the following publications.[1-261]

Note: COPD = chronic obstructive pulmonary disease.

Table A-3. Etiology of Disease Associated With Drought Disasters

Health Hazard	Health Effect	Etiology
Food insecurity	Malnutrition Developmental diseases	Drought causes widespread agricultural failure. Agricultural losses exacerbate social dysfunction. Food production, distribution and availability are constrained. Persons become malnourished.
Conflict	Blunt and penetrating trauma Burns	Socioeconomic losses increase competition for limited resources and exacerbate political crisis. Conflict results in violence.
Unsafe drinking water	Diarrheal illness	Water is scarce. Sources are overutilized and contaminated. Persons are displaced from their homes. Displacement results in limited access to sanitation and hygiene. Scarcity causes increased risk of drinking unsafe water.

(*Continued*)

Table A-3. (Continued)

Health Hazard	Health Effect	Etiology
Poor sanitation and hygiene	Diarrheal illness	Water is scarce. Persons are displaced from their homes. Displacement results in limited access to sanitation and hygiene. Unsanitary conditions cause increase in endemic diseases.
Waterborne pathogens	Diarrheal illness	Water sources become contaminated by infectious pathogens. Scarcity causes increased risk of drinking unsafe water.
Traumatic stress	Anxiety disorders PTSD Suicide Violence	Chronic nature of drought creates unresolved long-term stress. Drought-related damage result in socioeconomic losses. Socioeconomic losses create long-term stress. Stress results in maladaptive behaviors.

Source: The tables in this appendix are based on the following publications.[1-261]

Note: PTSD = post-traumatic stress disorder.

Table A-4. Etiology of Disease Associated With Earthquake Disasters

Health Hazard	Health Effect	Etiology
Structural collapse	Blunt and penetrating trauma	Persons are injured by falling debris.
Structure fires	Burns	Rupture of gas and electrical lines results in structure fires. Persons are burned by the fire.
	Inhalational injuries	Persons are injured by fire smoke inhalation.
Airborne particulates		Structural damage generates dust particulates. Persons inhale respirable components of dust, causing airway and lung injury.
Entrapment	Asphyxia, crush injury, renal failure	Persons become entrapped by falling structural debris. Chest compression results in traumatic asphyxia. Extremity crush injuries result in cardiac dysrhythmias and rhabdomyolysis. Dehydration and rhabdomyolysis trigger renal failure.
Hazardous materials	Poisoning Toxic exposures	Persons inhale or come into direct contact with toxic substances.
Traumatic stress	Anxiety disorders PTSD	Traumatic event results in acute psychological injury. Acute psychological injuries progress to anxiety and stress disorders or exacerbate existing mental illness.
Inadequate wound care	Wound infections	Persons injured during the earthquake do not have access to adequate wound care. Contaminated wounds become infected.
Poor sanitation and hygiene	Diarrheal illness	Water is scarce. Persons are displaced from their homes. Displacement results in limited access to sanitation and hygiene. Unsanitary conditions cause increase in endemic diseases.

Source: The tables in this appendix are based on the following publications.[1-261]

Note: PTSD = post-traumatic stress disorder.

Table A-5. Etiology of Disease Associated With Epidemic Disasters

Health Hazard	Health Effect	Etiology
Infectious pathogens	Communicable disease	Susceptible populations are exposed to pathogens by direct contact, inhalation, or ingestion.
Health care overutilization	Other communicable and non-communicable diseases	Resources become scarce as they are rapidly consumed and diverted to epidemic response. Persons are unable to access health care and/or postpone nonurgent care.

Table A-6. Etiology of Disease Associated With Flood Disasters

Health Hazard	Health Effect	Etiology
Debris cleanup	Blunt and penetrating trauma	Persons are injured during cleanup phase after flooding.
Heating and cooking stoves Lanterns	Burns Carbon monoxide poisoning	Flood conditions cause power line breaks. Widespread line breaks cause power failures. People use unfamiliar/unsafe alternatives for heating, cooking, and lighting. Unsafe alternatives cause burns and emit carbon monoxide. Persons who inhale stove emissions are poisoned. Persons who use stove incorrectly are burned.
Power generators	Carbon monoxide poisoning	Generators are improperly operated within an enclosed space. Persons who inhale generator exhaust are poisoned.
Floodwater	Drowning Immersion injuries	Heavy precipitation causes inland flooding. Floodwaters inundate populated areas. Persons are immersed in water. Persons are submerged under water. Submersions result in fatal and nonfatal drowning.
Power lines	Electrocution	Floodwater reaches damaged power lines. Persons are electrocuted while performing cleanup.
High ambient air temperature	Heat illness Cardiovascular disease	During seasonal floods, persons are exposed to heat during rescue and cleanup operations. Cardiovascular disease is exacerbated by heat.
Airborne particulates	Allergic reactions Asthma and COPD Pneumonitis	Floodwaters contaminate drywall in buildings. Mold grows inside structures. Home repair activities cause mold to become airborne. Persons inhale mold particulates.
Poor sanitation and hygiene	Diarrheal illness, Food poisoning Skin infections Diarrheal illness and Upper respiratory infections	Persons are displaced from their homes. Displacement results in limited access to sanitation and hygiene. Unsanitary conditions increase exposures to endemic diseases.

(*Continued*)

Table A-6. (Continued)

Health Hazard	Health Effect	Etiology
Toxic chemicals	Toxic exposures and poisoning	Chemicals kept in the home and workplace are released during the storm. Persons are exposed to chemicals during cleanup.
Traumatic stress	Anxiety disorders PTSD	Traumatic event results in acute psychological injury. Acute psychological injuries progress to anxiety and stress disorders or exacerbate existing mental illness.

Source: The tables in this appendix are based on the following publications.[1-261]

Note: COPD = chronic obstructive pulmonary disease; PTSD = post-traumatic stress disorder.

Table A-7. Etiology of Disease Associated With Heat Wave Disasters

Health Hazard	Health Effect	Etiology
High ambient air temperature	Heat illness	Exposed persons are more likely to become dehydrated and overheated.
High levels of endemic chronic disease	Exacerbations of chronic disease	Cardiovascular disease is exacerbated by heat.

Source: The tables in this appendix are based on the following publications.[1-261]

Table A-8. Etiology of Disease Associated With Landslide Disasters

Health Hazard	Health Effect	Etiology
Structural collapse	Blunt and penetrating trauma	Persons are injured by falling debris.
Airborne particulates	Inhalational injuries	Structural damage generates dust particulates. Persons inhale respirable components of dust, causing airway and lung injury.
Entrapment	Asphyxia, crush injury, renal failure	Persons become entrapped by falling structural debris. Chest compression results in traumatic asphyxia. Extremity crush injuries result in cardiac dysrhythmias and rhabdomyolysis. Dehydration and rhabdomyolysis trigger renal failure.
Hazardous materials	Toxic exposures and poisoning	Persons inhale or come into direct contact with toxic substances.
Traumatic stress	Anxiety disorders PTSD	Traumatic event results in acute psychological injury. Acute psychological injuries progress to anxiety and stress disorders or exacerbate existing mental illness.
Inadequate wound care	Wound infections	Persons injured during the earthquake cannot access care. Contaminated wounds become infected.

Source: The tables in this appendix are based on the following publications.[1-261]

Note: PTSD = post-traumatic stress disorder.

Table A-9. Etiology of Disease Associated With Tornadoes and Convective Storm Disasters

Health Hazard	Health Effect	Etiology
Ballistic projectiles	Blunt and penetrating trauma	High winds create structural collapse and ballistic projectiles. Persons are hit by flying or falling debris.
Structural collapse	Blunt and penetrating trauma	Persons are injured by falling debris.
Insects, pets, and wild animals	Bites, envenomation, and stings	Storms disrupt the environment. This disruption causes increased stress among wild and domestic animals. It also increases exposure to insects and wild animals.

Source: The tables in this appendix are based on the following publications.[1-261]

Table A-10. Etiology of Disease Associated With Tsunami Disasters

Health Hazard	Health Effect	Etiology
Structural collapse	Blunt and penetrating trauma	Persons are injured by falling debris.
Airborne particulates	Airborne particulates	Structural damage generates dust particulates. Persons inhale respirable components of dust, causing airway and lung injury.
Inundation	Drowning Pneumonia	Persons become submerged by the tsunami inundation.
Entrapment	Asphyxia	Persons become entrapped by structural debris. Chest compression results in traumatic asphyxia.
Hazardous materials	Poisoning and toxic exposures	Environmental damage releases toxic household and industrial materials. People inhale or come into direct contact with toxic substances.
Traumatic stress	Anxiety disorders PTSD	Traumatic event results in acute psychological injury. Acute psychological injuries progress to anxiety and stress disorders or exacerbate existing mental illness.
Wound contamination	Wound infections	Injured persons cannot access wound care. Contaminated wounds become infected. Tetanus immunoglobulin is overutilized, creating scarcity.
Poor sanitation and hygiene	Diarrheal illness	Water is scarce. People are displaced from their homes. Displacement limits access to sanitation and hygiene. Unsanitary conditions promote endemic disease.

Source: The tables in this appendix are based on the following publications.[1-261]
Note: PTSD = post-traumatic stress disorder.

Table A-11. Etiology of Disease Associated With Volcano Disasters

Health Hazard	Health Effect	Etiology
Ballistic projectiles and avalanches	Blunt and penetrating trauma	Explosive eruptions create ballistic projectiles, rockfalls, and avalanches. Persons are hit by flying or falling debris.
Pyroclastic flows	Blunt trauma Burns	Explosive eruptions create large clouds of superheated gases and debris that collapse and flow downhill at very high speeds. People living at the foot of the volcano are engulfed by superheated flows.
Lahars	Blunt trauma Drowning	Eruptions and tephra melt snowcaps or disturb volcanic lakes to create slurries that flow downhill at very high speeds. People living in low-lying areas downhill from the volcano are inundated by lahars.
Tephra	Asthma and COPD	Explosive eruptions create large clouds of superheated gases and debris. These clouds are carried by atmospheric winds, contaminating the air quality. People living downwind inhale airborne gases and particulates. Chronic respiratory disease is exacerbated.
Structural collapse	Blunt and penetrating trauma	Tephra buildup causes failure of large, roofed structures Persons are injured by falling debris.
Chemical and radioactive substances	Poisoning	Explosive eruptions create large clouds of superheated gases and debris. These clouds are carried by atmospheric winds, contaminating downwind air quality, agriculture, and surface water. People living downwind inhale toxins in the air and ingest toxic particulates in food and water.

Source: The tables in this appendix are based on the following publications.[1-261]

Note: COPD = chronic obstructive pulmonary disorder.

Table A-12. Etiology of Disease Associated With Wildfire Disasters

Health Hazard	Health Effect	Etiology
High ambient air temperature	Heat illness	Heat from fire combines with seasonal temperatures to create high ambient temperatures. People are exposed to high temperatures.
Fire	Burns	Wildfires extend into populated areas, resulting in structural fires. Escape routes become impassable as people are trapped and directly exposed to fire.
Airborne particulates	Inhalational injury Asthma and COPD	Fires create large clouds of smoke and gases. These clouds are carried by atmospheric winds. People located downwind inhale airborne gases and particulates. Inhalational injuries occur. Chronic respiratory disease is exacerbated.
Toxic chemicals	Toxic exposures and poisoning	People located downwind inhale toxic airborne gases and inhale or ingest particulates in water or food. Toxic exposures occur. People are poisoned.

Source: The tables in this appendix are based on the following publications.[1-261]

Note: COPD = chronic obstructive pulmonary disease.

Table A-13. Etiology of Disease Associated With Explosion Disasters

Health Hazard	Health Effect	Etiology
Ballistic projectiles and structural collapse	Blunt and penetrating trauma	Explosions create ballistic projectiles and structural damage. Persons are hit by flying or falling structural debris.
Pressure wave	Blunt trauma	Explosions create high pressure waves. People are hit by the pressure wave. Pressure waves injure hollow organs and soft tissues.
Fire	Burns	Explosions cause structural fires. People are directly exposed to fire.
Hazardous materials	Poisoning	People located downwind inhale toxic airborne gases and inhale or ingest particulates in water or food. Toxic exposures occur. People are poisoned.

Source: The tables in this appendix are based on the following publications.[1-261]

Table A-14. Etiology of Disease Associated With Fire Disasters

Health Hazard	Health Effect	Etiology
Fire	Burns	Structure fires directly expose people to fire.
Airborne particulates and hot, toxic gases	Inhalational injury Asthma and COPD Poisoning	Fires create large clouds of smoke and gases These clouds are carried by atmospheric winds People located downwind inhale airborne gases and particulates Inhalational injuries and poisonings occur. Chronic respiratory disease is exacerbated
High-intensity large-scale firestorms	Mortality	Large-scale high-intensity firestorms create high-speed wind circulation. High-speed winds fuel high-intensity large-scale fires. High-intensity fires kill unusually large numbers of people.

Source: The tables in this appendix are based on the following publications.[1-261]
Note: COPD = chronic obstructive pulmonary disease.

Table A-15. Etiology of Disease Associated With Hazardous Material Disasters

Health Hazard	Health Effect	Etiology
Pressurized gas	Blunt trauma	Explosions create high-pressure waves. People are hit by the pressure waves. Pressure waves injure hollow organs and soft tissues.
Airborne particulates	Inhalational injury	Atmospheric plume of gas and/or particulates appear. Persons inhale respirable components of plume, causing airway and lung injury.
Biological pathogens	Communicable disease	Biological pathogens are released as a result of an intentional act or laboratory incident. People are directly exposed to pathogens and develop an infection. The infectious disease may or may not be transmissible from person to person.

(Continued)

Table A-15. (Continued)

Health Hazard	Health Effect	Etiology
Chemical or radioactive substances	Toxic exposures and poisoning	An atmospheric release of hazardous material occurs. People inhale or come into direct contact with toxic substances.
Fire	Burns	Some hazardous material releases are associated with fire.
Ballistic projectiles and structural collapse	Blunt and penetrating trauma	Explosions create ballistic projectiles and structural damage. Persons are hit by flying or falling structural debris.

Source: The tables in this appendix are based on the following publications.[1-261]

Table A-16. Etiology of Disease Associated With Mass Gathering Disasters

Health Hazard	Health Effect	Etiology
Stampede	Blunt trauma	Events occur that cause high-density crowds to move abruptly. Impediments to abrupt movement result in crowd stampede. Stampedes result in people being crushed by foot traffic or pushed against structural barriers.
Fire	Burns and inhalation injury	Fires occur at mass gathering events. People become directly exposed to fire or smoke.
Structural collapse	Blunt and penetrating trauma	Collapses occur involving structures associated with mass gatherings (e.g., stages, seating stands, and light towers). People are injured by falls and debris.
Contaminated food	Foodborne infection	Food safety is not maintained during a mass gathering. Biological pathogens are transmitted through food. People become exposed to foodborne pathogens while attending the event. Illness may occur during the event or afterward.
High ambient air temperature	Heat illness	Sun exposures, extending periods of standing, and poor air circulation combine with high seasonal temperatures to create high ambient air temperatures in the crowd. People are exposed to high temperatures.
Violence	Blunt and penetrating trauma, Burns, Gender-based violence	Violence occurs as a result of social rivalry (e.g., sports team), political conflict, and crime.

Source: The tables in this appendix are based on the following publications.[1-261]

Table A-17. Etiology of Disease Associated With Mining Disasters

Health Hazard	Health Effect	Etiology
Structural collapse	Blunt and penetrating trauma	Collapses create structural damage and debris. Persons are hit by flying or falling structural debris.
Entrapment	Asphyxia	Persons become entrapped by structural debris. Lack of ventilation results in anoxic asphyxia.
Explosion	Blunt trauma	Enclosed space amplifies the effect of any high-pressure waves generated by explosion, especially on hollow organs.
Fire	Burns and inhalation injury	Fires occur within the mine or in its surface structures. People become directly exposed to fire and/or smoke.
Airborne particulates	Inhalational injury	Mining releases airborne particulates and gases. People in the mine inhale airborne gases and particulates. Inhalational injuries occur.
	Asthma and COPD	Chronic respiratory disease is exacerbated.
Toxic chemicals	Toxic exposures and poisoning	People inhale or ingest particulates in water or food. Toxic exposures occur. People are poisoned.

Source: The tables in this appendix are based on the following publications.[1-261]

Note: COPD = chronic obstructive pulmonary disorder.

Table A-18. Etiology of Disease Associated With Poisoning Disasters

Health Hazard	Health Effect	Etiology
Adulterated commercial products	Poisoning	Commercial products are contaminated with toxic substances. People are poisoned when they inhale or ingest the substance.
Contaminated air, food, and/or water		
Toxic chemicals	Burns	People are exposed to toxic chemicals or radioactive materials through direct contact, inhalation, or ingestion. These exposures result in soft tissue burns.
Radioactive substances	Cancer Birth defects	People are exposed to radioactive materials and sustain genetic damage. Genetic damage results in cancer and/or birth defects.

Source: The tables in this appendix are based on the following publications.[1-261]

Table A-19. Etiology of Disease Associated With Structural Collapse

Health Hazard	Health Effect	Etiology
Structural debris	Blunt and penetrating trauma	Persons are injured by falling debris.
Structure fires	Burns	Rupture of gas and electrical lines results in structure fires. Persons are burned by the fire.
	Inhalational injuries	Persons are injured by fire smoke inhalation.
Airborne particulates		Structural damage generates dust particulates. Persons inhale respirable components of dust, causing airway and lung injury,
Entrapment	Asphyxia, crush injury and renal failure	Persons become entrapped by falling structural debris. Chest compression results in traumatic asphyxia. Extremity crush injuries result in cardiac dysrhythmias and rhabdomyolysis. Dehydration and rhabdomyolysis trigger renal failure.
Hazardous materials	Poisoning and toxic exposures	Persons inhale or come into direct contact with toxic substances.
Traumatic stress	Anxiety disorders PTSD	Traumatic event results in acute psychological injury. Acute psychological injuries progress to anxiety and stress disorders or exacerbate existing mental illness.

Source: The tables in this appendix are based on the following publications.[1-261]

Note: PTSD = post-traumatic stress disorder.

Table A-20. Etiology of Disease Associated With Transportation

Health Hazard	Health Effect	Etiology
Downing, crashes and derailment	Blunt and penetrating trauma	Failure occurs, resulting in aviation, ground transportation, or rail crash. People are injured during the crash.
Violence		Some failures may be attributable to violence.
Explosions		Some failures may be associated with fires or explosions.
Fires	Burns	
Sinking	Drowning	Failures involving marine vessels result in sinking.
Hazardous material release	Poisoning	Some failures may be associated with release of hazardous materials during transport. People are exposed to the release of hazardous materials and become poisoned.

Source: The tables in this appendix are based on the following publications.[1-261]

REFERENCES

1. Floret N, Viel JF, Mauny F, Hoen B, Piarroux R. Negligible risk for epidemics after geophysical disasters. *Emerg Infect Dis*. 2006;12(4):543–548.
2. Cattamanchi S, Curcio A. winter storm. In: Ciottone G, ed. *Disaster Medicine*. 2nd ed. Philadelphia, PA: Elsevier; 2016:592–597.
3. Kilbourne E. Cold environments. In: Noji E, ed. *Public Health Consequences of Disasters*. New York, NY: Oxford University Press; 1997:270–286.
4. Rocklov J, Forsberg B, Ebi K, Bellander T. Susceptibility to mortality related to temperature and heat and cold wave duration in the population of Stockholm County, Sweden. *Global Health Action*. 2014;7:22737.
5. Bunker A, Wildenhain J, Vandenbergh A, et al. Effects of air temperature on climate-sensitive mortality and morbidity outcomes in the elderly; a systematic review and meta-analysis of epidemiological evidence. *EBioMed*. 2016;6:258–268.
6. Ageev FT, Smirnova MD, Svirida ON, et al. Impact of a cold wave on disease course, hemodynamics, carbohydrate metabolism, and blood rheological properties in cardiac patents. Article in Russian. *Ter Arkh*. 2015;87(9):11–16.
7. Chen TH, Du XL, Chan W, Zhang K. Impacts of cold weather on emergency hospital admission in Texas, 2004–2013. *Environ Res*. 2019;169:139–146.
8. Tang ZY, Zhu QY, Xu LJ, et al. Artificial cold wave–induced cerebral infarction in rats with carotid atherosclerosis. *J Mol Neurosci*. 2012;47(2):278–285.
9. Chak Ho H, Chan TC, Xu Z, Huang C, Li C. Individual- and community-level shifts in mortality patterns during the January 2016 East Asia cold wave associated with a super El Niño event: empirical evidence in Hong Kong. *Sci Total Environ*. 2020;711:135050.
10. Chan EY, Goggins WB, Yue JS, Lee P. Hospital admissions as a function of temperature, other weather phenomena and pollution levels in an urban setting in China. *Bull World Health Organ*. 2013;91(8):576–584.
11. Grimsley LF, Chulada PC, Kennedy S, et al. Indoor environmental exposures for children with asthma enrolled in the HEAL study, post-Katrina New Orleans. *Environ Health Perspect*. 2012;120(11):1600–1606.
12. Park KJ, Moon JY, Ha JS, et al. Impacts of heavy rain and typhoon on allergic disease. *Osong Public Health Res Perspect*. 2013;4(3):140–145.
13. Malilay J. Tropical cyclones. In: Noji E, ed. *The Public Health Consequences of Disasters*. New York, NY: Oxford University Press; 1997:207–227.
14. Panda S, Pati KK, Bhattacharya MK, Koley H, Pahari S, Nair GB. Rapid situation & response assessment of diarrhoea outbreak in a coastal district following tropical cyclone AILA in India. *Indian J of Med Res*. 2011;133:395–400.
15. Guill CK, Shandera WX. The effects of Hurricane Mitch on a community in northern Honduras. *Prehosp Disaster Med*. 2001;16(3):166–171.
16. Mendoza MT, Roxas EA, Ginete JK, et al. Clinical profile of patients diagnosed with leptospirosis after a typhoon: a multicenter study. *Southeast Asian J Trop Med Public Health*. 2013;44(6):1021–1035.

17. Sergienko E. Hurricanes, cyclones, and typhoons. In: Ciottone G, Darling R, Anderson P, et al., eds. *Disaster Medicine*. 3rd ed. Philadelphia, PA: Mosby-Elsevier; 2006:475–478.
18. Harville EW, Xiong X, Smith BW, Pridjian G, Elkind-Hirsch K, Buekens P. Combined effects of Hurricane Katrina and Hurricane Gustav on the mental health of mothers of small children. *J Psychiatr Ment Health Nurs*. 2011;18(4):288–296.
19. Kolves K, Kolves KE, De Leo D. Natural disasters and suicidal behaviours: a systematic literature review. *J Affective Disord*. 2013;146(1):1–14.
20. Fussell E, Lowe SR. The impact of housing displacement on the mental health of low-income parents after Hurricane Katrina. *Soc Sci Med*. 2014;113:137–144.
21. Rando RJ, Lefante JJ, Freyder LM, Jones RN. Respiratory health effects associated with restoration work in post–Hurricane Katrina New Orleans. *J Environ Public Health*. 2012;2012:462478.
22. Sengul H, Santella N, Steinberg LJ, Cruz AM. Analysis of hazardous material releases due to natural hazards in the United States. *Disasters*. 2012;36(4):723–743.
23. Eriksson J, Adelman H, Borton J, et al. The international response to conflict and genocide: lessons from the Rwanda experience. 1996. Available at: www.oecd.org/countries/rwanda/50189495.pdf. Accessed November 26, 2022.
24. Selbya J, Dahib O, Fröhlich C, Hulmee M. Climate change and the Syrian civil war revisited. *Polit Geogr*. 2017;60:232–244.
25. Stanke C, Kerac M, Prudhomme C, Medlock J, Murray V. Health effects of drought: a systematic review of the evidence. *PLoS Curr*. 2013;5.
26. Kim JJ, Guha-Sapir D. Famines in Africa: is early warning early enough? *Global Health Action*. 2012;5.
27. Arlappa N, Venkaiah K, Brahmam GN. Severe drought and the vitamin A status of rural pre-school children in India. *Disasters*. 2011;35(3):577–586.
28. Davis L. Famines and droughts. In: *Natural Disasters*. New York, NY: Checkmark Books; 2008:105–136.
29. Smith LT, Aragao LE, Sabel CE, Nakaya T. Drought impacts on children's respiratory health in the Brazilian Amazon. *Sci Rep*. 2014;4:3726.
30. Bernstein AS, Rice MB. Lungs in a warming world: climate change and respiratory health. *Chest*. 2013;143(5):1455–1459.
31. Hanigan IC, Butler CD, Kokic PN, Hutchinson MF. Suicide and drought in New South Wales, Australia, 1970–2007. *PNAS*. 2012;109(35):13950–13955.
32. Rigby CW, Rosen A, Berry HL, Hart CR. If the land's sick, we're sick: the impact of prolonged drought on the social and emotional well-being of Aboriginal communities in rural New South Wales. *Australian J Rural Health*. 2011;19(5):249–254.
33. Carnie TL, Berry HL, Blinkhorn SA, Hart CR. In their own words: young people's mental health in drought-affected rural and remote NSW. *Australian J Rural Health*. 2011;19(5):244–248.
34. AlKhadi K. Earthquake. In: Ciottone G, ed. *Disaster Medicine*. Philadelphia, PA: Elsevier; 2016:572–574.
35. Raines A, Lees J, Fry W, Parks A, Tuggle D. Field amputation: response planning and legal considerations inspired by three separate amputations. *Ame J Disaster Med*. 2014;9(1):53–58.

36. Bolin R, Stanford L. *The Northridge Earthquake: Vulnerability and Disaster*. London, UK: Routledge; 2003.
37. Ogawa S, Ishiki M, Nako K, et al. Effects of the Great East Japan Earthquake and huge tsunami on glycaemic control and blood pressure in patients with diabetes mellitus. *BMJ Open*. 2012;2(2):e000830.
38. Schultz C. Earthquakes. In: Hogan D, Burstein J, eds. *Disaster Medicine*. Philadelphia, PA: Lippincott Williams & Wilkins; 2002:163–170.
39. Shiga H, Miyazawa T, Kinouchi Y, et al. Life-event stress induced by the Great East Japan Earthquake was associated with relapse in ulcerative colitis but not Crohn's disease: a retrospective cohort study. *BMJ Open*. 2013;3(2).
40. Moriyama K, Kaga M. Mental healthcare efforts for the public after the Great East Japan Earthquake: "Guide to Good Mental Health for Those Affected by Natural Disasters" published by the Cabinet Office. *Brain Dev*. 2013;35(3):201–208.
41. Valenti M, Masedu F, Mazza M, et al. A longitudinal study of quality of life of earthquake survivors in L'Aquila, Italy. *BMC Public Health*. 2013;13:1143.
42. Shultz JM, Forbes D, Wald D, et al. Trauma signature analysis of the great East Japan disaster: guidance for psychological consequences. *Disaster Med Public Health Prep*. 2013;7(2):201–214.
43. Sugiura H, Akahane M, Ohkusa Y, et al. Prevalence of insomnia among residents of Tokyo and Osaka after the great East Japan earthquake: a prospective study. *Interact J Med Res*. 2013;2(1):e2.
44. World Health Organization (WHO). Top epidemic-prone diseases without sufficient counter-measures. 2018. Available at: https://www.preventionweb.net/news/top-epidemic-prone-diseases-without-sufficient-counter-measures. Accessed November 26, 2022.
45. Frost WH. Some conceptions of epidemics in general. *Am J Epidemiol*. 1976;103(2):141–151.
46. Zell R. Global climate change and the emergence/re-emergence of infectious diseases. *Int J Med Microbiol*. 2004;293(suppl 37):16–26.
47. Centers for Disease Control and Prevention (CDC). Epidemic disease occurrence. Introduction to epidemiology. 2022. Available at: https://www.cdc.gov/csels/dsepd/ss1978/lesson1/section11.html. Accessed November 26, 2022.
48. Davis L. Plagues and epidemics. In: *Natural Disasters*. New York, NY: Checkmark Books; 2008:203–230.
49. Bompangue D, Giraudoux P, Piarroux M, et al. Cholera epidemics, war and disasters around Goma and Lake Kivu: an eight-year survey. *PLoS Negl Trop Dis*. 2009;3(5):e436.
50. Kim SH. Flood. In: Ciottone G, Darling R, Anderson P, et al., eds. *Disaster Medicine*. 3rd ed. Philadelphia, PA: Mosby-Elsevier; 2006:489–491.
51. Malilay J. Floods. In: Noji E, ed. *The Public Health Consequences of Disasters*. New York, NY: Oxford University Press; 1997:207–227.
52. Waite T, Murray V, Baker D. Carbon monoxide poisoning and flooding: changes in risk before, during and after flooding require appropriate public health interventions. *PLoS Curr*. 2014;6.
53. Chaturongkasumrit Y, Techaruvichit P, Takahashi H, Kimura B, Keeratipibul S. Microbiological evaluation of water during the 2011 flood crisis in Thailand. *Sci Total Environ*. 2013;463–464:959–967.

54. Vanasse A, Cohen A, Courteau J, et al. Association between floods and acute cardiovascular diseases: a population-based cohort study using a geographic information system approach. *Int J Environ Res Public Health.* 2016;13(2):168.
55. Alderman K, Turner LR, Tong S. Floods and human health: a systematic review. *Environ Int.* 2012;47:37–47.
56. Tempark T, Lueangarun S, Chatproedprai S, Wananukul S. Flood-related skin diseases: a literature review. *Int J Dermatol.* 2013;52(10):1168–1176.
57. Diaz JH. Superficial and invasive infections following flooding disasters. *Am J Disaster Med.* 2014;9(3):171–181.
58. Bei B, Bryant C, Gilson KM, et al. A prospective study of the impact of floods on the mental and physical health of older adults. *Aging Ment Health.* 2013;17(8):992–1002.
59. Nahar N, Blomstedt Y, Wu B, Kandarina I, Trisnantoro L, Kinsman J. Increasing the provision of mental health care for vulnerable, disaster-affected people in Bangladesh. *BMC Public Health.* 2014;14(1):708.
60. Kolves K, Kolves KE, De Leo D. Natural disasters and suicidal behaviours: a systematic literature review. *J Affective Disord.* 2013;146(1):1–14.
61. Kettaneh A, Fardet L, Mario N, et al. The 2003 heat wave in France: hydratation status changes in older inpatients. *Eur J Epidemiol.* 2010;25(7):517–524.
62. Brunetti ND, Amoruso D, De Gennaro L, et al. Hot spot: impact of July 2011 heat wave in southern Italy (Apulia) on cardiovascular disease assessed by emergency medical service and telemedicine support. *Telemed J E Health.* 2014;20(3):272–281.
63. Bustinza R, Lebel G, Gosselin P, Bélanger D, Chebana F. Health impacts of the July 2010 heat wave in Québec, Canada. *BMC Public Health.* 2013;13:56–56.
64. Tian Z, Li S, Zhang J, Guo Y. The characteristic of heat wave effects on coronary heart disease mortality in Beijing, China: a time series study. *PloS One.* 2013;8(9):e77321.
65. Shaposhnikov D, Revich B, Bellander T, et al. Mortality related to air pollution with the Moscow heat wave and wildfire of 2010. *Epidemiol.* 2014;25(3):359–364.
66. Sherbakov T, Malig B, Guirguis K, Gershunov A, Basu R. Ambient temperature and added heat wave effects on hospitalizations in California from 1999 to 2009. *Environ Res.* 2018;160:83–90.
67. Zheng S, Wang M, Shang K, et al. A case-crossover analysis of heat wave and hospital emergency department visits for cardiovascular diseases in three hospitals in Beijing. Article in Chinese. *Wei Sheng Yan Jiu.* 2016;45(2):246–251.
68. Tian Z, Li S, Zhang J, Guo Y. The characteristic of heat wave effects on coronary heart disease mortality in Beijing, China: a time series study. *PloS One.* 2013;8(9):e77321.
69. Chen K, Bi J, Chen J, Chen X, Huang L, Zhou L. Influence of heat wave definitions to the added effect of heat waves on daily mortality in Nanjing, China. *Sci Total Environ.* 2015;506-507:18–25.
70. Kue R, Dyer KS. The impact of heat waves on transport volumes in an urban emergency medical services system: a retrospective review. *Prehosp Disaster Med.* 2013;28(6):610–615.
71. Turner L, Connell D, Tong S. The effect of heat waves on ambulance attendances in Brisbane, Australia. *Prehosp Disaster Med.* 2013;28(5):482–487.
72. Sun X, Sun Q, Zhou X, et al. Heat wave impact on mortality in Pudong New Area, China in 2013. *Sci Total Environ.* 2014;493:789–794.

73. Yang J, Liu HZ, Ou CQ, et al. Impact of heat wave in 2005 on mortality in Guangzhou, China. *Biomed Environ Sci.* 2013;26(8):647–654.
74. D'Ippoliti D, Michelozzi P, Marino C, et al. The impact of heat waves on mortality in 9 European cities: results from the EuroHEAT project. *Environ Health.* 2010;9:37.
75. Azhar G, Mavalankar D, Nori Sarma A, et al. Heat-related mortality in India: excess all-cause mortality associated with the 2010 Ahmedabad heat wave. *PloS One.* 2014;9(3):e91831.
76. Ricco M. Air temperature exposure and agricultural occupational injuries in the Autonomous Province of Trento (2000–2013, North-Eastern Italy). *Int J Occup Med Environ Health.* 2018;31(3):317–331.
77. Josseran L, Fouillet A, Caillere N, et al. Assessment of a syndromic surveillance system based on morbidity data: results from the Oscour network during a heat wave. *PloS One.* 2010;5(8):e11984.
78. Hartz DA, Golden JS, Sister C, Chuang WC, Brazel AJ. Climate and heat-related emergencies in Chicago, Illinois (2003–2006). *Int J Biometeorol.* 2012;56(1):71–83.
79. Kim E, Kim H, Kim YC, Lee JP. Association between extreme temperature and kidney disease in South Korea, 2003–2013: Stratified by sex and age groups. *Sci Total Environ.* 2018;642: 800–808.
80. Hausfater P, Megarbane B, Fabricatore L, et al. Serum sodium abnormalities during nonexertional heatstroke: incidence and prognostic values. *Am J Emerg Med.* 2012;30(5):741–748.
81. Pereira BM, Morales W, Cardoso RG, Fiorelli R, Fraga GP, Briggs SM. Lessons learned from a landslide catastrophe in Rio de Janeiro, Brazil. *Am J Disaster Med.* 2013;8(4):253–258.
82. Homma Y, Watari T, Baba T, et al. Injury patterns after the landslide disaster in Oshima, Tokyo, Japan on October 16, 2013. *Disaster Med Public Health Prep.* 2016;10(2):248–252.
83. Uddin T, Islam MT, Gosney JE. 2017 Bangladesh landslides: physical rehabilitation perspective. *Disabil Rehabil.* 2019:1–8.
84. Sanchez C, Lee TS, Young S, Batts D, Benjamin J, Malilay J. Risk factors for mortality during the 2002 landslides in Chuuk, Federated States of Micronesia. *Disasters.* 2009;33(4):705–720.
85. Keim M. Landslides. In: Ciottone G, Darling R, Anderson P, et al., eds. *Disaster Medicine.* 3rd ed. Philadelphia, PA: Mosby; 2006:509–513.
86. Sette P, Carlini M, Berti D, et al. Complex alpine extrication: case report of mountain and speleological rescue cooperation. *Wilderness Environ Med.* 2015;26(2):180–184.
87. Arango-Granados MC, Cruz Mendoza DF, Salcedo Cadavid AE, García Marin AF. Amputation in crush syndrome: a case report. *Int J Surg Case Rep.* 2020;72:346–350.
88. Jones MD, Pfaff J. Tornado. In: Ciottone G, Darling R, Anderson P, et al., eds. *Disaster Medicine.* 3rd ed. Philadelphia, PA: Mosby-Elsevier; 2006:484–488.
89. Regens JL, Mould N. Prevention and treatment of traumatic brain injury due to rapid-onset natural disasters. *Frontiers Public Health.* 2014;2:28.
90. Deng Q, Lv Y, Zhao F, Yu W, Dong J, Zhang L. Factors associated with injuries among tornado victims in Yancheng and Chifeng, China. *BMC Public Health.* 2019;19(1):1556.
91. Niederkrotenthaler T, Parker EM, Ovalle F, et al. Injuries and post-traumatic stress following historic tornados: Alabama, April 2011. *PloS One.* 2013;8(12):e83038.
92. Zhao F, Hu C, Xu Z, Deng Q, Wu Y, Zhang L. Injury patterns and memdical evacuation of patients in Chifeng tornado in China, August 11, 2017. *Disaster Med Public Health Prep.* 2019:1–6.

93. Chern JJ, Miller JH, Tubbs RS, et al. Massive pediatric neurosurgical injuries and lessons learned following a tornado disaster in Alabama. *J Neurosurg Pediatr.* 2011;8(6):588–592.
94. Neblett Fanfair R, Benedict K, Bos J, et al. Necrotizing cutaneous mucormycosis after a tornado in Joplin, Missouri, in 2011. *New Engl J Med.* 2012;367(23):2214–2225.
95. Mu GH, Li X, Hou SS, Lu ZQ, Deng YJ. Injury patterns and outcomes of victims after the 2016 Jiangsu tornado in China: a retrospective analysis of injuries treated at a teaching hospital. *Disaster Med Public Health Prep.* 2020;14(2):208–213.
96. Niederkrotenthaler T, Parker EM, Ovalle F, et al. Injuries and post-traumatic stress following historic tornados: Alabama, April 2011. *PloS One.* 2013;8(12):e83038.
97. Adams ZW, Sumner JA, Danielson CK, et al. Prevalence and predictors of PTSD and depression among adolescent victims of the spring 2011 tornado outbreak. *J Child Psychol Psychiatry.* 2014;55(9):1047–55.
98. Houston JB, Spialek ML, Stevens J, First J, Mieseler VL, Pfefferbaum B. 2011 Joplin, Missouri tornado experience, mental health reactions, and service utilization: cross-sectional assessments at approximately 6 months and 2.5 years post-event. *PLoS Curr.* 2015;7.
99. Danielson CK, Sumner JA, Adams ZW, et al. Adolescent substance use following a deadly US tornado outbreak: a population-based study of 2,000 families. *J Clin Child Adolesc Psychol.* 2017;46(5):732–745.
100. Xu W, Fu G, An Y, Yuan G, Ding X, Zhou Y. Mindfulness, posttraumatic stress symptoms, depression, and social functioning impairment in Chinese adolescents following a tornado: mediation of posttraumatic cognitive change. *Psychiatry Res.* 2018;259:345–349.
101. Xu W, Yuan G, Liu Z, Zhou Y, An Y. Prevalence and predictors of PTSD and depression among adolescent victims of the summer 2016 tornado in Yancheng City. *Arch Psychiatr Nurs.* 2018;32(5):777–781.
102. Resnick H, Zuromski KL, Galea S, et al. Prior interpersonal violence exposure and experiences during and after a disaster as predictors of posttraumatic stress disorder and depression among adolescent victims of the spring 2011 tornadoes. *J Interpers Violence.* 2020 Nov;35(23–24):5179–5197.
103. Cluster of rare fungal infections identified after tornado. *BMJ.* 2012;345:e8382.
104. Lastra TJ, Guzmán CG, Conejeros RC, Suárez VG, Chávez FO. Epidemiological profile of deaths after the 2010 earthquake in Chile. Article in Spanish. *Rev Med Chil.* 2012;140(6): 732–739.
105. Guha-Sapir D, van Panhuis WG. Health impact of the 2004 Andaman Nicobar earthquake and tsunami in Indonesia. *Prehosp Disaster Med.* 2009;24(6):493–499.
106. Matsuzawa G, Sano H, Ohnuma H, et al. Patient trends in orthopedic traumas and related disorders after tsunami caused by the Great East Japan Earthquake: an experience in the primary referral medical center. *J Orthop Sci.* 2016;21(4):507–511.
107. Yamanda S, Kobayashi S, Hanagama M, et al. Two cases of tsunami dust pneumonia: organizing pneumonia caused by the inhalation of dried tsunami sludge after the 2011 Great East Japan Earthquake. *Intern Med.* 2016;55(24):3645–3653.
108. Nagamatsu S, Maekawa T, Ujike Y, Hashimoto S, Fuke N; Japanese Society of Intensive Care Medicine. The earthquake and tsunami—observations by Japanese physicians since the 11 March catastrophe. *Crit Care.* 2011;15(3):167.

109. Li X, Aida J, Hikichi H, Kondo K, Kawachi I. Association of postdisaster depression and posttraumatic stress disorder with mortality among older disaster survivors of the 2011 Great East Japan Earthquake and tsunami. *JAMA Netw Open.* 2019;2(12):e1917550.
110. Ishiura Y, Fujimura M, Yamamoto H, et al. Asthma exacerbations after the East Japan disaster. *J Med Invest.* 2013;60(1–2):61–65.
111. Nakamura M, Tanaka F, Nakajima S, et al. Comparison of the incidence of acute decompensated heart failure before and after the major tsunami in Northeast Japan. *Am J Cardiol.* 2012;110(12):1856–1860.
112. Morita T, Nomura S, Tsubokura M, et al. Excess mortality due to indirect health effects of the 2011 triple disaster in Fukushima, Japan: a retrospective observational study. *J Epidemiol Community Health.* 2017;71(10):974–980.
113. Schwab FD, Zettler EK, Moh A, Schotzau A, Gross U, Gunthert AR. Predictive factors for preterm delivery under rural conditions in post-tsunami Banda Aceh. *J Perinat Med.* 2016;44(5):511–515.
114. Shibata Y, Ojima T, Tomata Y, et al. Characteristics of pneumonia deaths after an earthquake and tsunami: an ecological study of 5.7 million participants in 131 municipalities, Japan. *BMJ Open.* 2016;6(2):e009190.
115. Ebisawa K, Yamada N, Okada S, et al. Combined Legionella and Escherichia coli lung infection after a tsunami disaster. *Intern Med.* 2011;50(19):2233–2236.
116. Kawakami Y, Tagami T, Kusakabe T, et al. Disseminated aspergillosis associated with tsunami lung. *Respir Care.* 2012;57(10):1674–1678.
117. Daito H, Suzuki M, Shiihara J, et al. Impact of the Tohoku earthquake and tsunami on pneumonia hospitalisations and mortality among adults in northern Miyagi, Japan: a multicentre observational study. *Thorax.* 2013;68(6):544–550.
118. Kawano T, Tsugawa Y, Nishiyama K, Morita H, Yamamura O, Hasegawa K. Shelter crowding and increased incidence of acute respiratory infection in evacuees following the Great Eastern Japan Earthquake and tsunami. *Epidemiol Infect.* 2016;144(4):787–795.
119. Kuwabara H, Araki T, Yamasaki S, Ando S, Kano Y, Kasai K. Regional differences in posttraumatic stress symptoms among children after the 2011 tsunami in Higashi-Matsushima, Japan. *Brain Dev.* 2015;37(1):130–136.
120. Isaranuwatchai W, Coyte PC, McKenzie K, Noh S. The 2004 tsunami and mental health in Thailand: a longitudinal analysis of one-and two-year post-disaster data. *Disasters.* 2017;41(1):150–170.
121. Sitdhiraksa N, Piyasil V, Pariwatcharakul P, et al. Association of adolescent substance use: behavioral problems and family background among school students in tsunami affected area in southern Thailand. *J Med Assoc Thai.* 2014;97(suppl 6):58–65.
122. Dyb G, Jensen TK, Nygaard E. Children's and parents' posttraumatic stress reactions after the 2004 tsunami. *Clin Child Psychol Psychiatry.* 2011;16(4):621–634.
123. Terayama T, Shigemura J, Kobayashi Y, et al. Mental health consequences for survivors of the 2011 Fukushima nuclear disaster: a systematic review. Part 2: emotional and behavioral consequences. *CNS Spectr.* 2020:1–13.
124. Irwanto, Faisal, Zulfa H. Posttraumatic stress disorder among indonesian children 5 years after the tsunami. *Southeast Asian J Trop Med Public Health.* 2015;46(5):918–923.

125. Doocy S, Daniels A, Dooling S, Gorokhovich Y. The human impact of volcanoes: a historical review of events 1900–2009 and systematic literature review. *PLoS Curr.* 2013;5.
126. Tam E, Miike R, Labrenz S, et al. Volcanic air pollution over the Island of Hawaiʻi: emissions, dispersal, and composition. Association with respiratory symptoms and lung function in Hawai'i Island school children. *Environ Int.* 2016;92-93:543–552.
127. Gudmundsson G. Respiratory health effects of volcanic ash with special reference to Iceland: a review. *Clin Respir J.* 2011;5(1):2–9.
128. Zabert I, Benitez S, Maldonado C, Uribe Evhevarría L, Zabert GE. Prevalence of asthma at-risk symptoms in adolescents exposed to volcanic ash, in two Patagonian cities. Article in Spanish. *Rev Fac Cien Med Univ Nac Cordoba.* 2020;77(2):61–67.
129. Carlsen HK, Hauksdottir A, Valdimarsdottir UA, et al. Health effects following the Eyjafjallajokull volcanic eruption: a cohort study. *BMJ Open.* 2012;2(6).
130. Cadelis G, Tourres R, Molinie J, Petit RH. Exacerbations of asthma in Guadeloupe (French West Indies) and volcanic eruption in Montserrat (70 km from Guadeloupe). Article in French. *Rev Mal Respir.* 2013;30(3):203–214.
131. Baxter PJ, Jenkins S, Seswandhana R, et al. Human survival in volcanic eruptions: thermal injuries in pyroclastic surges, their causes, prognosis and emergency management. *Burns.* 2017;43(5):1051–1069.
132. Trisnawati I, Budiono E, Sumardi, Setiadi A. traumatic inhalation due to Merapi volcanic ash. *Acta Med Indones.* 2015;47(3):238–243.
133. Camarinho R, Garcia PV, Choi H, Rodrigues AS. Chronic exposure to non-eruptive volcanic activity as cause of bronchiolar histomorphological alteration and inflammation in mice. *Environ Pollut.* 2019;253:864–871.
134. Jones T, Bérubé K. The bioreactivity of the sub-10 mum component of volcanic ash: Soufrieìre Hills volcano, Montserrat. *J Hazard Mat.* 2011;194:128–134.
135. Nguyen HT, Wijayanti LW, Kim K, Lee WK, Lee CH, Shin K. High prevalence of cognitive impairment among students near Mount Merapi: a case study. *J Exerc Rehabil.* 2018;14(4): 573–580.
136. Giacoppo S, Galuppo M, Calabro RS, et al. Heavy metals and neurodegenerative diseases: an observational study. *Biol Trace Elem Res.* 2014;161(2):151–160.
137. Balsa AI, Caffera M, Bloomfield J. Exposures to particulate matter from the eruptions of the Puyehue volcano and birth outcomes in Montevideo, Uruguay. *Environ Health Perspect.* 2016;124(11):1816–1822.
138. Warsini S, Buettner P, Mills J, West C, Usher K. Post-traumatic stress disorder among survivors two years after the 2010 Mount Merapi volcano eruption: a survey study. *Nurs Health Sci.* 2015;17(2):173–180.
139. Gan RW, Liu J, Ford B, et al. The association between wildfire smoke exposure and asthma-specific medical care utilization in Oregon during the 2013 wildfire season. *J Expo Sci Environ Epidemiol.* 2020;30(4):618–628.
140. Reid CE, Considine EM, Watson GL, Telesca D, Pfister GG, Jerrett M. Associations between respiratory health and ozone and fine particulate matter during a wildfire event. *Environ Int.* 2019;129:291–298.

141. Schranz CI, Castillo EM, Vilke GM. The 2007 San Diego wildfire impact on the emergency department of the University of California, San Diego hospital system. *Prehosp Disaster Med.* 2010;25(5):472–476.
142. Glass DC, Del Monaco A, Pircher S, Vander Hoorn S, Sim MR. Mortality and cancer incidence among male volunteer Australian firefighters. *Occup Environ Med.* 2017;74(9):628–638.
143. Navarro KM, Kleinman MT, Mackay CE, et al. Wildland firefighter smoke exposure and risk of lung cancer and cardiovascular disease mortality. *Environ Res.* 2019;173:462–468.
144. Alman BL, Pfister G, Hao H, et al. The association of wildfire smoke with respiratory and cardiovascular emergency department visits in Colorado in 2012: a case crossover study. *Environ Health.* 2016;15(1):64.
145. Stowell JD, Geng G, Saikawa E, et al. Associations of wildfire smoke $PM_{2.5}$ exposure with cardiorespiratory events in Colorado, 2011–2014. *Environ Int.* 2019;133(part A):105151.
146. DeFlorio-Barker S, Crooks J, Reyes J, Rappold AG. Cardiopulmonary effects of fine particulate matter exposure among older adults, during wildfire and non-wildfire periods, in the United States, 2008–2010. *Environ Health Perspect.* 2019;127(3):37006.
147. Raines J, Snow R, Nichols D, Aisbett B. Fluid intake, hydration, work physiology of wildfire fighters working in the heat over consecutive days. *Ann Occup Hyg.* 2015;59(5):554–565.
148. Holstius DM, Reid CE, Jesdale BM, Morello-Frosch R. Birth weight following pregnancy during the 2003 Southern California wildfires. *Environ Health Perspect.* 2012;120(9):1340–1345.
149. O'Donnell MH, Behie AM. Effects of wildfire disaster exposure on male birth weight in an Australian population. *Evol Med Public Health.* 2015;2015(1):344–354.
150. Kim YH, Tong H, Daniels M, et al. Cardiopulmonary toxicity of peat wildfire particulate matter and the predictive utility of precision cut lung slices. *Part Fibre Toxicol.* 2014;11:29.
151. Santos LR, Alves-Correia M, Cámara M, et al. Multiple victims of carbon monoxide poisoning in the aftermath of a wildfire: a case series. *Acta Med Port.* 2018;31(3):146–151.
152. Papadatou D, Giannopoulou I, Bitsakou P, Bellali T, Talias MA, Tselepi K. Adolescents' reactions after a wildfire disaster in Greece. *J Trauma Stress.* 2012;25(1):57–63.
153. Brown MRG, Agyapong V, Greenshaw AJ, et al. After the Fort McMurray wildfire there are significant increases in mental health symptoms in grade 7–12 students compared to controls. *BMC Psychiatry.* 2019;19(1):18.
154. Marshall GN, Schell TL, Miles JN. All PTSD symptoms are highly associated with general distress: ramifications for the dysphoria symptom cluster. *J Abnorm Psychol.* 2010;119(1): 126–135.
155. McAlister CN, Marble AE, Murray TJ. The 1917 Halifax explosion: the first coordinated local civilian medical response to disaster in Canada. *Can J Surg.* 2017;60(6):372–374.
156. Romolo FS, Aromatario M, Bottoni E, Cappelletti S, Fiore PA, Ciallella C. Accidental death involving professional fireworks. *Forensic Sci Int.* 2014;234:e5–e9.
157. Sanghi A, Ambrose RPK. Analysis of the effect of prevailing weather conditions on the occurrence of grain dust explosions. *J Agric Safety Health.* 2016;22(3):187–197.
158. Ramasamy A, Hill AM, Hepper AE, Bull AM, Clasper JC. Blast mines: physics, injury mechanisms and vehicle protection. *J R Army Med Corps.* 2009;155(4):258–264.
159. Ramasamy A, Hill AM, Masouros S, Gibb I, Bull AM, Clasper JC. Blast-related fracture patterns: a forensic biomechanical approach. *J R Soc Interface.* 2011;8(58):689–698.

160. Karimi H, Montevalian A, Motabar AR, Safari R, Parvas MS, Vasigh M. Epidemiology of paediatric burns in Iran. *Ann Burns Fire Disasters.* 2012;25(3):115–120.
161. Qin FJ, Chen Z, Zhao YH, et al. Analysis of effects of discipline cooperation on rescue and treatment of severe mass burn patients involved in August 2nd Kunshan factory aluminum dust explosion accident. Article in Chinese. *Zhonghua Shao Shang Za Zhi.* 2018;34(6):349–353.
162. Shao F, Ren WJ, Meng WZ, Wang GZ, Wang TY. Burn wound bacteriological profiles, patient outcomes, and tangential excision timing: a prospective, observational study. *Ostomy Wound Manage.* 2018;64(9):28–36.
163. Roeder RA, Schulman CI. An overview of war-related thermal injuries. *J Craniofac Surg.* 2010;21(4):971–975.
164. Jiang H, Xue C, Gao Y, Wang Y. Analysis of ocular injury characteristics in survivors of the 8.12 Tianjin Port explosion, China. *J Ophthalmol.* 2019;2019:1360805.
165. Zhang Y, Zhang MN, Jiang CH, Qiu HY. Analysis on characteristics of ocular trauma caused by military affairs in soldiers. Article in Chinese. *Zhonghua Yan Ke Za Zhi.* 2011;47(10):920–926.
166. Kalayci M, Er S, Tahtabasi M. Bomb explosion: ocular effects of primary, secondary and tertiary mechanisms. *Clin Ophthalmol.* 2020;14:1145–1151.
167. Tian LQ, Guo ZH, Meng WZ, et al. The abnormalities of coagulation and fibrinolysis in acute lung injury caused by gas explosion. *Kaohsiung J Med Sci.* 2020;36(suppl 6).
168. Arch-Tirado E, Garnica-Escamilla MA, Delgado-Hernández A, Campos-Muñoz T, Rodríguez-Rodríguez L, Verduzco-Mendoza A. Acoustic trauma generated by exposure to gun powder. Article in Spanish. *Cir Cir.* 2014;82(5):528–536.
169. Peng LH, Guo GH. Advances in the research of blast lung injury. Article in Chinese. *Zhonghua Shao Shang Za Zhi.* 2016;32(3):156–159.
170. Zhang YH, Guo GH, Shen GL, et al. Analysis on treatment of extremely severe burn patients with severe inhalation injury in August 2nd Kunshan factory aluminum dust explosion accident. Article in Chinese. *Zhonghua Shao Shang Za Zhi.* 2018;34(7):455–458.
171. Liu W. An accident of trichlorosilane explosion. Article in Chinese. *Zhonghua Lao Dong Wei Sheng Zhi Ye Bing Za Zhi.* 2011;29(3):175.
172. O'Neill TB, Rawlins J, Rea S, Wood F. Complex chemical burns following a mass casualty chemical plant incident: how optimal planning and organisation can make a difference. *Burns.* 2012;38(5):713–718.
173. Xing Y, Chen S, Zhu S, Zhang Y, Lu J. Exploring risk factors contributing to the severity of hazardous material transportation accidents in China. *Int J of Environ Res Public Health.* 2020;17(4).
174. Hansen MB, Birkeland MS, Nissen A, Blix I, Solberg O, Heir T. Prevalence and course of symptom-defined PTSD in individuals directly or indirectly exposed to terror: a longitudinal study. *Psychiatry.* 2017;80(2):171–183.
175. Su YJ. Prevalence and predictors of posttraumatic stress disorder and depressive symptoms among burn survivors two years after the 2015 Formosa Fun Coast Water Park explosion in Taiwan. *Eur J Psychotraumatol.* 2018;9(1):1512263.
176. Su YJ, Chow CC. PTSD, depression and posttraumatic growth in young adult burn survivors: three-year follow-up of the 2015 Formosa Fun Coast Water Park explosion in Taiwan. *J Affect Disord.* 2020;274:239–246.

177. Williams G, O'Malley M. Surgical considerations in the management of combined radiation blast injury casualties caused by a radiological dirty bomb. *Injury*. 2010;41(9):943–947.
178. Kobeissy F, Mondello S, Tumer N, et al. Assessing neuro-systemic & behavioral components in the pathophysiology of blast-related brain injury. *Front Neurol*. 2013;4:186.
179. Perez-Arredondo A, Cazares-Ramirez E, Carrillo-Mora P, et al. Baclofen in the therapeutic of sequele of traumatic brain injury: spasticity. *Clin Neuropharmacol*. 2016;39(6):311–319.
180. Cernak I. Blast injuries and blast-induced neurotrauma: overview of pathophysiology and experimental knowledge models and findings. In: Cernak I, Kobeissy FH, eds. *Brain Neurotrauma: Molecular, Neuropsychological, and Rehabilitation Aspects*. Boca Raton, FL: CRC Press/Taylor & Francis; 2015:chap. 15.
181. Li BC, Li Y, Xu C, et al. Blast-induced traumatic brain injury of goats in confined space. *Neurol Res*. 2014;36(11):974–982.
182. Manning WA. *The World Trade Center Bombing: Report and Analysis*. USFA-TR-076. New York, NY: US Fire Administration, Dept of Homeland Security; 1993.
183. Sanderson L. Fires. In: Noji ER, ed. *The Public Health Consequences of Disasters*. New York, NY: Oxford University Press; 1997:373–396.
184. Geldner G, Koch EM, Gottwald-Hostalek U, et al. Report on a study of fires with smoke gas development: determination of blood cyanide levels, clinical signs and laboratory values in victims. *Der Anaesthesist*. 2013;62(8):609–616.
185. Dumestre D, Nickerson D. Use of cyanide antidotes in burn patients with suspected inhalation injuries in North America: a cross-sectional survey. *J Burn Care Res*. 2014;35(2): e112–e117.
186. Guidotti T. Acute cyanide poisoning in prehospital care: new challenges, new tools for intervention. *Prehosp Disaster Med*. 2006;21(2):s40–s48.
187. Laugharne J, van der Watt G, Van de Watt G, Janca A. After the fire: the mental health consequences of fire disasters. *Curr Opin Psychiatry*. 2011;24(1):72–77.
188. Trinh NH, Nadler DL, Shie V, et al. Psychological sequelae of the Station Nightclub fire: comparing survivors with and without physical injuries using a mixed-methods analysis. *PloS One*. 2014;9(12):e115013.
189. Sanderson L. Toxicologic disasters: natural and technologic. In: Sullivan J, Krieger G, eds. *Hazardous Materials Toxicology: Clinical Principles of Environmental Health*. Philadelphia, PA: Lippincott Williams & Wilkins; 1992.
190. Berry L, Perera TB. EMS, hazardous waste response. In: *StatPearls* [Internet]. Treasure Island, FL: StatPearls Publishing; 2020. Available at: https://www.ncbi.nlm.nih.gov/books/NBK482193. Accessed November 26, 2022.
191. Keim M, Humphrey A, Dreyfuss A. *Situation Assessment Report Involving the Hazardous Material Disaster Site at LaGuaira Port, Venezuela*. CDC Report to Office of Disaster Assistance, US Agency for International Development; 2000.
192. Choi KH, Park MS, Ha M, Hur JI, Cheong HK. Cancer incidence trend in the Hebei Spirit oil spill area, from 1999 to 2014: an ecological study. *Int J Environ Res Public Health*. 2018;15(5):1006.
193. Diaz JH. The legacy of the Gulf oil spill: analyzing acute public health effects and predicting chronic ones in Louisiana. *Am J Disaster Med*. 2011;6(1):5–22.

194. Hildur K, Templado C, Zock JP, et al. Follow-up genotoxic study: chromosome damage two and six years after exposure to the Prestige oil spill. *PloS One*. 2015;10(7):e0132413.
195. Rispens JR, Jones SA, Clemmons NS, et al. Anhydrous ammonia chemical release—Lake County, Illinois, April 2019. *MMWR*. 2020;69(4):109–113.
196. Culley JM, Richter J, Donevant S, Tavakoli A, Craig J, DiNardi S. Validating signs and symptoms from an actual mass casualty incident to characterize an irritant gas syndrome agent (IGSA) exposure: a first step in the development of a novel IGSA triage algorithm. *J Emerg Nurs*. 2017;43(4):333–338.
197. Melnikova N, Wu J, Yang A, Orr M. Acute chemical incidents with injured first responders, 2002–2012. *Disaster Med Public Health Prep*. 2018;12(2):211–221.
198. Grainge C, Rice P. Management of phosgene-induced acute lung injury. *Clin Toxicol* (Phila). 2010;48(6):497–508.
199. Meselson M, Guillemin J, Hugh-Jones M, et al. The Sverdlovsk anthrax outbreak of 1979 *Science*. 1994;266(5188):1202–1208.
200. Čobeljić M. Smallpox outbreak in Yugoslavia in 1972. *Vojnosanitetski Pregl*. 2004;61(5): 569–573.
201. Michaels D, Howard J. Review of the OSHA-NIOSH response to the Deepwater Horizon oil spill: protecting the health and safety of cleanup workers. *PLoS Curr*. 2012;4: e4fa83b7576b7576e.
202. Harville EW, Shankar A, Zilversmit L, Buekens P. Self-reported oil spill exposure and pregnancy complications: the GROWH study. *Int J Environ Res Public Health*. 2017;14(7).
203. Harville EW, Shankar A, Zilversmit L, Buekens P. The Gulf oil spill, miscarriage, and infertility: the GROWH study. *Int Arch Occup Environ Health*. 2018;91(1):47–56.
204. Nugent N, Gaston SA, Perry J, Rung AL, Trapido EJ, Peters ES. PTSD symptom profiles among Louisiana women affected by the 2010 Deepwater Horizon oil spill: a latent profile analysis. *J Affect Disord*. 2019;250:289–297.
205. Généreux M, Maltais D, Petit G, Roy M. Monitoring adverse psychosocial outcomes one and two years after the Lac-Mégantic train derailment tragedy (Eastern Townships, Québec, Canada). *Prehosp Disaster Med*. 2019;34(3):251–259.
206. Osofsky JD, Osofsky HJ, Weems CF, Hansel TC, King LS. Effects of stress related to the Gulf oil spill on child and adolescent mental health. *J Pediatr Psychol*. 2016;41(1):65–72.
207. Bromet E. Mental health consequences of the Chernobyl disaster. *J Radiol Prot*. 2012; 32(1):N71–N75.
208. Collins D. Human responses to the threat of or exposure to ionizing radiation at Three Mile Island, Pennsylvania, and Goiania, Brazil. *Mil Med*. 2002(suppl 2);167:137–138.
209. Molloy MS, Sherif Z, Natin S, McDonnel J. Management of mass gatherings. In: Koenig K, Schultz C, eds. *Disaster Medicine: Comprehensive Principles and Practices*. New York, NY: Cambridge University Press; 2010:228–252.
210. Hsieh YH, Ngai KM, Burkle FM, Jr., Hsu EB. Epidemiological characteristics of human stampedes. *Disaster Med Public Health Prep*. 2009;3(4):217–223.
211. El Warea M, Sasso R, Bachir R, El Sayed M. Riots in Beirut: Description of the impact of a new type of mass casualty event on the emergency system in Lebanon. *Disaster Med Public Health Prep*. 2019;13(5-6):849–852.

212. Tsouros AD, Efstathiou PA, eds. *Mass Gatherings and Public Health: The Experience of the Athens 2004 Olympic Games*. World Health Organization Europe; 2007. Available at: https://www.researchgate.net/publication/233387448_Mass_Gatherings_and_Public_Health. Accessed November 26, 2022.
213. Turris SA, Lund A, Bowles RR. An analysis of mass casualty incidents in the setting of mass gatherings and special events. *Disaster Med Public Health Prep*. 2014:1–7.
214. Tavakoli H, Khashayar P, Amoli HA, et al. Firework-related injuries in Tehran's Persian Wednesday Eve Festival (Chaharshanbe Soori). *J Emerg Med*. 2011;40(3):340–345.
215. Brennan RJ, Keim ME, Sharp TW, et al. Medical and public health services at the 1996 Atlanta Olympic Games: an overview. *Med J Aust*. 1997;167(11–12):595–598.
216. Aleeban M, Mackey TK. Global health and visa policy reform to address dangers of Hajj during summer seasons. *Front Public Health*. 2016;4:280.
217. Andrews T. Riots, deaths, sexual assault: maybe Woodstock was always a nightmare. *Washington Post*. August 13, 2019.
218. Ozer E, Yilmaz R, Evcuman D, et al. Autopsy evaluation of coal mining deaths in the city of Zonguldak, Turkey. *Med Sci Monit*. 2014;20:438–443.
219. Jafari H, Jafari AJ, Nekoei-Moghadam M, Goharinezhad S. Morbidity and mortality from technological disasters in Iran: a narrative review. *J Educ Health Promot*. 2019;8:147.
220. Luo X, Lin F, Zhu S, et al. Mine landslide susceptibility assessment using IVM, ANN and SVM models considering the contribution of affecting factors. *PloS One*. 2019;14(4):e0215134.
221. Thrush P. *A Dictionary of Mining, Mineral and Related Terms*. Washington, DC: US Bureau of Mines; 1968.
222. Orecka B, Sikora L, Misiołek M, et al. The quality of voice in coal-miners after burn/inhalation injury due to methane explosion. Article in Polish. *Otolaryngol Pol*. 2012;66(2):102–108.
223. Bolaños-Álvarez Y, Alonso-Hernández CM, Morabito R, Díaz-Asencio M, Pinto V, Gómez-Batista M. Mercury contamination of riverine sediments in the vicinity of a mercury cell chlor-alkali plant in Sagua River, Cuba. *Chemosphere*. 2016;152:376–382.
224. Hall HI, Dhara R, Price-Green PA, Kaye W. Surveillance for emergency events involving hazardous substances—United States, 1990–1992 *MMWR*. 1994;43(SS-2):1–6.
225. Wang X, Liu G, Hu R, Zhang H, Zhang M, Zhang F. Distribution, sources, and health risk assessment of volatile organic compounds in Hefei City. *Arch Environ Contam Toxicol*. 2020;78(3):392–400.
226. James AK, Nehzati S, Dolgova NV, et al. Rethinking the Minamata tragedy: what mercury species was really responsible? *Environ Sci Technol*. 2020;54(5):2726–2733.
227. Kloske M, Witkiewicz Z. Novichoks—the A group of organophosphorus chemical warfare agents. *Chemosphere*. 2019;221:672–682.
228. Worek F, Wille T, Koller M, Thiermann H. Toxicology of organophosphorus compounds in view of an increasing terrorist threat. *Arch Toxicol*. 2016;90(9):2131–2145.
229. Sawano T, Kambe T, Seno Y, et al. High internal radiation exposure associated with low socio-economic status six years after the Fukushima nuclear disaster: a case report. *Medicine* (Baltimore). 2019;98(47):e17989.
230. Li Q, Song P, Wen J. Melamine and food safety: a 10 year review. *Curr Opin Food Sci*. 2019;30:79–84.

231. Hanna-Attisha M. Lead poisoning in the 21st century: the silent epidemic continues. *Am J Public Health.* 2018;108:1430.

232. Cruz M, Keim M, Schier J, Gonzalez R, Valencia A, Telfer J. Organizational and command aspects for coordinating the public health response to an outbreak of acute renal failure, Republic of Panama, 2006. *Prehosp Disaster Med.* 2011;26(3):217–223.

233. Campos AMS, Bucaretchi F, Fernandes LCR, Fernandes CB, Capitani EM, Beck ARM. Toxic exposures in children involving legally and illegally commercialized household sanitizers. *Rev Paul Pediatr.* 2017;35(1):11–17.

234. Li Y, Gao Y, Yu X, Peng J, Ma F, Nelson L. Tetramine poisoning in China: changes over a decade viewed through the media's eye. *BMC Public Health.* 2014;14:842.

235. Desel H. Mass poisoning events. Article in German. *Med Klin Intensivmed Notfmed.* 2015;110(1):15–20.

236. Deng X, Li G, Mei R, Sun S. Long term effects of tetramine poisoning: an observational study. *Clin Toxicol* (Phila). 2012;50(3):172–175.

237. Jaworowski Z. Observations on the Chernobyl disaster and LNT. *Dose-Response.* 2010;8(2):148–171.

238. Hatch M, Cardis E. Somatic health effects of Chernobyl: 30 years on. *Eur J Epidemiol.* 2017;32:1047–1054.

239. Park AS, Ritz B, Ling C, Cockburn M, Heck JE. Exposure to ambient dichloromethane in pregnancy and infancy from industrial sources and childhood cancers in California. *Int J Hyg Environ Health.* 2017;220(7):1133–1140.

240. Kruger D, Cupal S, Franzen S, et al. Toxic trauma: household water quality experiences predict posttraumatic stress disorder symptoms during the Flint, Michigan, water crisis. *J Community Psychol.* 2017;45(7):957–962.

241. Oshima T, Yoshikawa H, Ohtani M, Mimasaka S. Three cases of suprachoroidal hemorrhage associated with chest compression or asphyxiation and detected using postmortem computed tomography. *Leg Med* (Tokyo). 2015;17(3):188–191.

242. Colville-Ebeling B, Freeman M, Banner J, Lynnerup N. Autopsy practice in forensic pathology—evidence-based or experience-based? A review of autopsies performed on victims of traumatic asphyxia in a mass disaster. *J Forensic Leg Med.* 2014;22:33–36.

243. US Occupatonal Safety and Health Administration. Structural collapse guide. Emergency preparedness guides. 2022. Available at: https://www.osha.gov/emergency-preparedness/guides/structural-collapse. Accessed December 5, 2022.

244. Ingrassia P, Geddo A, Lombardi F, Della Corte F. Events associated with structural collapse/crashing/crushing. In: Ciottone G, Darling R, Anderson P, et al., eds. *Disaster Medicine.* 3rd ed. Philadelphia, PA: Mosby-Elsevier; 2006:817–859.

245. Holtz TM, Leighton J, Balter S, Weiss D, Blank S, Weisfuse I. The public health response to the World Trade Center disaster. In: Levy BS, Sidel VS, eds. *Terrorism and Public Health.* New York, NY: Oxford University Press; 2003:19–48.

246. Boodram B, Torian L, Thomas P, et al. Rapid assessment of injuries among survivors of the terrorist attack on the World Trade Center—New York City, September 2001. *MMWR.* 2002;51(1):1–5.

247. Perritt KR, Herbert R, Levin SM, Moline J. Work-related injuries and illnesses reported by World Trade Center response workers and volunteers. *Prehosp Disaster Med.* 2011;26(6): 401–407.
248. Boffetta P, Hall C, Todd A, et al. Cancer risk among World Trade Center rescue and recovery workers: a review. *CA Cancer J Clin.* 2022;72(4):308–314.
249. Beusse R, Hatfield J, Fabirkiewicz S, et al. *EPA's Response to the World Trade Center Collapse: Challenges, Successes, and Areas of Improvement.* EPA Report No. 2003-P-00012. Environmental Protection Agency (EPA); 2003.
250. Postma IL, Weel H, Heetveld MJ, et al. Mass casualty triage after an airplane crash near Amsterdam. *Injury.* 2013;44(8):1061–1067.
251. Postma IL, Winkelhagen J, Bloemers FW, et al. February 2009 airplane crash at Amsterdam Schiphol Airport: an overview of injuries and patient distribution. *Prehosp Disaster Med.* 2011;26(4):299–304.
252. Centers for Disease Control and Prevention (CDC). Fatal and nonfatal injuries involving fishing vessel winches—southern shrimp fleet, United States, 2000–2011. *MMWR.* 2013;62(9):157–160.
253. Doohan I, Bjornstig U, Ostlund U, Saveman BI. Exploring injury panorama, consequences, and recovery among bus crash survivors: a mixed-methods research study. *Prehosp Disaster Med.* 2017;32(2):165–174.
254. Postma IL, Winkelhagen J, Bijlsma TS, Bloemers FW, Heetveld MJ, Goslings JC. Delayed diagnosis of injury in survivors of the February 2009 crash of flight TK 1951. *Injury.* 2012;43(12):2012–2017.
255. Goers M, Leidman E, Sultan AS, Hassan A, Bilukha O. Injury-related deaths before and during the Islamic State insurgency—Baghdad, Iraq, 2010–2015. *Confl Health.* 2020;14:8.
256. Morita S, Omata A, Yoshizaki C, Miura N, Inokuchi S. The fatal fire accident of the Japanese high-speed railway lines (Shinkansen). *Burns.* 2016;42(1):232–233.
257. Khodadadizadeh A, Jahangiri K, Khorasani-Zavareh D, Vazirinejad R. Epidemiology of vehicle fire fatalities of road traffic injuries in Kerman Province, Iran: a cross-sectional study. *Open Access Maced J Med Sci.* 2019;7(12):2036–2043.
258. Zakrevskii YN, Shevchenko AG, Peretechikov AV, Serdyuk VI, Arkhangelskii DA. Combined mechanical-cold and mechanical-burn injuries in patients injured in maritime disasters. Article in Russian. *Voen Med Zh.* 2015;336(6):34–40.
259. Lincoln JM, Lucas DL. Occupational fatalities in the United States commercial fishing industry, 2000–2009. *J Agromed.* 2010;15(4):343–350.
260. Doohan I, Gyllencreutz L, Bjornstig U, Saveman BI. Survivors' experiences of consequences and recovery five years after a major bus crash. *Scand J Caring Sci.* 2018;32(3):1179–1187.
261. Lenferink LIM, de Keijser J, Smid GE, Djelantik A, Boelen PA. Prolonged grief, depression, and posttraumatic stress in disaster-bereaved individuals: latent class analysis. *Eur J Psychotrauma.* 2017;8(1):1298311.

APPENDIX B

Glossary of Key Terms

ability: Possessing the means to accomplish a goal.

accountability: The acceptance of responsibility for performance or outcomes.

accuracy: The degree to which a measurement conforms to the correct value or standard. Accuracy measures the validity of a measurement or test. It describes systemic errors and is measured as statistical bias.

activity: An action (or task) taken by an individual or group to achieve their aims.

agent: A factor whose presence, excessive presence, or in the case of deficiency diseases, relative absence is essential for the occurrence of a disease or other adverse health outcome.

all-hazard approach: The design and implementation of emergency management strategies for the full range of likely emergencies or disasters, including those caused by all (e.g., natural and technological) hazards.

analysis: The process of breaking a complex system into smaller parts to better understand it.

analytical risk assessment: A standard process for estimating risk on the basis of an analysis of its components related to hazard, exposure, and impacts.

Anthropocene Epoch: An interval of geologic time characterized as the time in which activities of human beings began to substantially alter Earth's surface, atmosphere, oceans, and nutrient-cycling systems.

approach: A perspective or method intended to improve the likelihood of success.

assumption: A fact or statement assumed to be true when uncertainty exists.

biohazardous materials (i.e., biohazards): Hazardous biologic materials that present a risk or potential risk to the health of humans, animals, or the environment.

biological: Pertaining to living organisms.

Bronfenbrenner's ecosocial model for human development: A theory of human development that describes how interactions between individuals and their environment form the basis for human development.

BS 11200: An international standard for crisis management that summarizes the defining features of a crisis before making specific recommendations for successful crisis management.

candidate cause: A factor considered during causal assessments that could be the source of stressors causing a biological impairment.

capability: The ability to achieve a desired operational effect under specified standards and conditions through various ways to perform a set of tasks.

capability-based planning: Planning to provide capabilities suitable for a wide range of circumstances while working within an economic framework that necessitates a choice.

case: An occurrence of disease that meets a set of uniform criteria used for public health surveiallance.

case fatality rate (i.e., death-to-case ratio): The proportion of deaths from a specified disease among all individuals diagnosed over a certain period.

catastrophe: A sudden and usually unforeseen disruption that exceeds the ability of the affected community to cope even using outside resources.

causal assessment: A standard process for assessing and inferring event causation.

causal factors: A major unplanned, unintended contributor to an incident (an adverse condition) that if eliminated would have either prevented the incident or reduced its severity or frequency.

causal pathway of disease: Models that link sources of disease to the cause that serve as supplementary or surrogate indicators of the biological effect.

climatological: Pertaining to the climate—that is, to long-term atmospheric phenomena.

clinical: Involving direct observation of the patient, usually in a healthcare setting.

clinical disease: A disease that has recognizable clinical signs and symptoms.

cold wave disaster: A disaster caused by cold wave hazards. These are characterized by a rapid fall in temperature within 24 hours.

cold weather disaster: A disaster caused by cold waves and winter storm hazards.

collapse disaster: A disaster caused by the collapse of a large structure.

common cause variation: A fluctuation caused by unknown factors resulting in a random distribution of output around the average of the data. Common cause variation is considered a natural pattern, whereas special causes are unusual, not previously observed, and nonquantifiable variations.

communicable disease: An infectious disease that can be passed (i.e., transmitted) from person to person.

community-based: An activity that is organized and takes place locally.

community engagement: The process of working collaboratively with people affiliated by geographic proximity to address issues affecting the well-being of those people.

competency: A modern management theory that relates the resources and capabilities that compose the strategic advantage of an organization. As applied to education, core competencies describe the demonstrable knowledge, skills, and abilities to complete a strategic goal.

competency-based learning: An approach to education that focuses on the student's demonstration of desired learning outcomes (i.e., competencies) as central to the learning process.

consequence: The result or effect when a vulnerable asset is exposed to a disaster hazard.

consequence management: Measures taken to protect populations affected by the consequences of a disaster incident.

control: A management function that involves measuring and correcting processes to ensure that activities accomplish the goals of a group.

convective storm disaster: A disaster caused by convective storm hazards—that is, by atmospheric storms caused by convective movement (i.e., when warmer parts move up and the cooler parts move down).

crisis management: Measures that manage resources needed to anticipate, prevent, or resolve a credible or imminent threat.

cyclone disaster (i.e., tropical cyclone, hurricane, and typhoon): A disaster caused by a tropical cyclone, which is a rotating, organized system of clouds and thunderstorms that originates over tropical or subtropical waters and has a closed low-level circulation.

decision tree: A decision support tool that models decisions and their possible consequences, including chance event outcomes, resource costs, and utility.

defects: Attributes that indicates that the product or service failed to meet one of the desired specifications.

determinants of clinical outcome (DoO): Factors that influence health outcomes of clinical care.

determinants of disease (DoD): Factors that influence the development of disease.

determinants of disparity (DoD): Factors that influence the development of health disparity.

determinants of equity (DoEq): Factors that influence the development of health equity.

determinants of exposure (DoEx): Factors that influence the likelihood of exposure to health hazards.

determinants of health (DoH): Also know as health determinants, these are factors that influence the production of health.

determinants of health, wellness, and equity (DoHWE): Factors that influence the production of health, wellness, and equity.

determinants of wellness (DoW): Factors that influence the production of wellness.

deterministic: Effects that are dose-dependent.

disability: Any impairment that makes it more difficult for persons to do certain activities and interact with the world around them.

disaster: A severe disruption of the functioning of a society involving widespread human, material, economic, or environmental losses and impacts, which exceeds the ability of the affected community or society to cope using its resources.

disaster management: Measures involved in preparing for, mitigating the effects of, responding to, and recovering from disasters.

disaster medicine: The delivery of health care to disaster victims.

disaster pathway: A model that conceptualizes five sequential stages in disaster development: hazards, incidents, consequences, needs, and resources.

disaster-related disease: Diseases (including injury) that are caused by exposure to disaster-related hazards.

disaster-related health risk: An adverse event or negative health consequence caused by a disaster-related hazard.

disaster risk: The probability that a disaster will occur.

disaster risk management: The systematic process of strategies, policies, and improved coping capacities to reduce the adverse impacts and the possibility of disaster.

disaster risk reduction (DRR): The practice of reducing disaster risks through systematic efforts to analyze and manage the causal factors of disasters.

disease: A deviation from normal health that derives from an identifiable pathological process and which the patient experiences as an illness.

disease management: A system of coordinated interventions and communications for populations with conditions in which patient self-care efforts are significant.

disease prevention: The deferral or elimination of specific illnesses and conditions by one or more interventions.

displacement: The act of being compelled to leave a place of residence.

distal health determinants: Factors situated farthest from a reference point of hazardous exposure that are known to influence health outcomes.

dose: A measure of the quantity of exposure to a hazard.

dose rate: A measure of the rate of exposure to a hazard.

dose-response modeling: A modeling of the relationship between the magnitude of the response of an organism as a function of exposure to a hazard after a specific exposure time (i.e., dose rate).

drought disaster: A disaster caused by drought hazard, which is a period of abnormally dry weather sufficiently long enough to cause a severe water imbalance.

early warning system (EWS): System that generates and disseminates warnings to enable those threatened to prepare and act appropriately to minimize losses.

earthquake disaster: A disaster caused by earthquake hazard—that is, by radiated seismic energy and ground shaking caused by the sudden slip of a geological fault, volcanic activity, or other sudden stress changes in the earth.

ecosocial model of health: A model that conceptualizes health broadly in terms of how people interact with each other and their environment.

effectiveness: The degree to which objectives accomplish the desired outcome.

efficiency: The ratio of the resources expended per activity accomplished by a process.

effusive eruption: Volcanic eruptions that are associated with pouring flows of lava.

egalitarian: Relating to or believing that all people are equal and deserve equal rights and opportunities.

emergency: A sudden event that calls for immediate measures to minimize its adverse consequences.

emergency health: The science and practice of preventing disaster-related human disease and promoting wellness by (1) evaluating environmental sources and hazardous agents and (2) limiting exposures to hazardous agents in environmental media or settings that may adversely affect human health.

emergency management: The managerial function for creating the framework within which communities reduce vulnerability to hazards and cope with disasters.

endemic: The presence or usual prevalence of a disease or infectious agent in a population within a geographic area.

environment: External physical conditions that influence the growth, development, behavior, and survival of organisms.

environmental health: The practice of preventing human disease and promoting wellness by (1) identifying and evaluating environmental sources and hazardous agents and (2) limiting exposures to hazardous physical, chemical, and biological agents in air, water, soil, food, and other environmental media or settings that may adversely affect human health.

environmental impact assessment: The assessment of the environmental consequences of an activity prior to the decision to move forward with the proposed action.

environmental justice: The fair treatment and meaningful involvement of all people regardless of race, color, or national origin or income risk concerning the development, implementation, and enforcement of environmental laws, regulations, and policies.

epidemic: Increases in disease that often occur suddenly, with an increase above what is typically expected in that population in that area.

epidemiological triad: The standard model of disease causation that involves (1) an external agent, (2) a susceptible host, and (3) an environment that brings the host and agent together for disease to occur.

epidemiology: The study of disease factors relating to health.

equity: A state in which all people have a fair and just opportunity to attain their highest level of accomplishment.

eruption cloud: A cloud of gases, ash, and large rock fragments that form downwind of an erupting volcano.

etiology of disease: The branch of medicine that deals with the causes or origins of disease.

evacuation: A population protection measure intended to remove occupants from hazardous areas during an emergency.

evaluation: The systematic determination of a project's or program's merit, worth, and significance, using criteria governed by standards.

event: The occurrence of an incident that meets a set of uniform criteria used for public health surveiallance.

event-based surveillance (EBS): The organized collection, monitoring, assessment, and interpretation of mainly unstructured ad hoc information regarding health events or risks, which may represent an acute health risk.

evidence-based decision-making: Using scientific evidence to inform or guide decisions.

explosion disaster: A disaster caused by explosion hazards.

explosive eruption: Volcanic eruptions that are associated with explosive fragmentation of lava.

exposure: To come into contact with a cause of, or possessing a characteristic that is a determinant of, a particular health problem.

exposure science: The study of our contact with environmental factors and their effects on the human body.

fire disaster: A disaster caused by fire hazards—that is, by rapid, persistent chemical changes that release heat and light and are accompanied by flame.

flood disasters: Disasters caused by flood hazards—that is, by water overflowing the usual confines of a stream or other body of water or by water accumulating over areas that are not usually submerged.

forest fire: An unplanned fire burning in natural forests.

function: Any group of related actions contributing to a more significant action (especially if it is specifically designed to accomplish the more extensive action).

functional ability: The actual or potential means to perform expected activities.

geophysical: Pertaining to the earth's physical phenomena.

good governance: A governmental system founded in justice and peace that protects individuals' human rights and civil liberties.

governance: The processes of interaction and decision-making among the actors involved in a collective problem that lead to the creation, reinforcement, or reproduction of social norms and institutions.

Great Acceleration: The dramatic, continuous, and simultaneous surge in growth rate across an extensive range of measures of human activity, first recorded in the mid-20th century and continuing to this day.

hazard: A dangerous phenomenon, substance, human activity, or condition.

hazard analysis: The process of determining which hazards are significant for health and should therefore be addressed in mission area planning.

hazard characterization: A description of the relationship between levels of hazard exposure (dose) and the probability and severity of adverse health outcomes (response).

hazard identification: The initial step of risk assessment is identifying the hazards for further investigation.

hazard-impact matrix: Also known as a hazard prioritization matrix, this is a visual representation of the risks presented as a graph, rating them by category of hazard probability (i.e., likelihood) and impact (i.e., the severity of consequences).

hazardous exposure: A situation in which a person comes in contact with a dangerous phenomenon, substance, human activity, or condition.

hazardous materials (i.e., hazmat): Articles or substances that can pose a risk to health, safety, property, or the environment.

hazardous material release: A disaster hazard caused by the release of hazardous materials into the environment.

hazardous substance: Any disease-causing agent (i.e., noninfectious and infectious hazardous materials) that after release into the environment and upon exposure will result in health risk.

hazmat: See **hazardous materials**.

health: A state of complete physical, mental, and social well-being.

health determinants (i.e., determinants of health, DoH): Factors that influence the production of health.

health effects: The causation, promotion, facilitation, or exacerbation of a structural or functional abnormality with the implication that the abnormality produced has the potential of lowering the quality of life, contributing to a disabling illness or leading to premature death.

health equality: The state in which all people have a fair and equal health outcome across an entire population.

health equity: The state in which all people have a fair and equal opportunity to attain their optimum health outcome.

health hazard: Chemical, physical, biological, or environmental factors that can negatively affect short- or long-term health.

health impact assessment: A combination of procedures, methods, and tools by which an intervention may be evaluated according to potential health effects.

health in all policies (HiAP): An approach to public policy development across sectors that systematically considers the health implications of decisions, seeks synergies, and avoids harmful health impacts to improve population health and health equity.

health literacy: Personal knowledge and competencies that accumulate through daily activities and social interactions and across generations.

health promotion: An approach for empowering people to improve their health.

health protection: The protection of individuals, groups, and populations through expert advice and effective collaboration to prevent and mitigate the impact of infectious disease and environmental, chemical, and radiological hazards.

health risk: An adverse event or negative health consequence resulting from a specific event, disease, or condition.

healthy settings: An approach for creating healthy and supportive environments that emphasize a comprehensive strategy for health promotion.

heat index: A measurement of severity that factors in the effect of relative humidity, used as an indicator of the perceived air temperature.

heat wave disaster: A disaster caused by heat wave hazards—that is, by periods of abnormally hot and humid weather.

hierarchy of process control: The management approach (based on the hierarchy of objectives) that applies a layered approach to integrate process control at various levels (e.g., elimination, substitution, engineering, administration, resource allocation).

holistic: An approach that emphasizes the importance of the whole and the interdependence of its parts.

homeostasis: The tendency for a physiological process (e.g., health) to maintain a relatively stable equilibrium.

hormesis: The effects of a given acute dose that differ from those of an equal fractionated dose.

household goods: Products used within households (e.g., apparel, furniture, appliances).

humanitarian assistance: All acts, activities, and human and material resources for the provision of goods and services of an exclusively humanitarian character, indispensable for the survival and the fulfillment of the essential needs of the victims of disasters.

Humanitarian Charter: The foundation document stating the ethical and legal principles that inspired the creation of the Sphere movement by recognizing the human rights of disaster victims.

hurricane disaster (i.e., cyclone, tropical cyclone, and typhoon): A disaster caused by a tropical cyclone—that is, by a rotating, organized system of clouds and thunderstorms that originates over tropical or subtropical waters and has a closed low-level circulation.

hydrological: Pertaining to water in the atmosphere and on the earth.

hydrometeorological: Pertaining to both hydrological and meteorological phenomena.

illness: The subjective sense of feeling unwell that often motivates a patient to consult a physician.

impact: A measure of the severity of consequences caused by disaster hazards.

impact analysis: The component of risk assessment that involves quantifying the degree of damage or losses (e.g., disease) that may be expected when a vulnerable population is exposed to a hazard.

incidence: The occurrence, rate, or frequency of an event of interest.

incident: An event or occurrence.

incident command system (ICS): An organizational system for managing emergency incidents that integrates response capabilities within a standard organizational structure.

incident continuum: A model that illustrates how emergencies and disasters are part of a relative continuum of incidents that extend from routine events to catastrophes.

incubation period: The time elapsed between an exposure to a disease-causing organism and the appearance of signs and symptoms.

index: A figure in a system or scale representing the average value of specified values and other items compared with some reference figure. It is a measurement constructed by summarizing different, more straightforward measures.

indicator-based surveillance (IBS): The organized collection, monitoring, assessment, and interpretation of structured information regarding the frequency, origin, and distribution of reportable diseases.

indivisible self: An evidence-based wellness model based on factor analytic studies.

industrial disaster: A disaster caused by hazards related to the manufacturing industry.

infectious disease: A disease caused by pathogenic microorganisms.

infectious dose: The amount of pathogen (measured in the number of microorganisms) required to cause an infection in the host.

information exchange: The bidirectional transmission or transfer of information, usually through electronic means.

injury: Disease caused by acute exposure to physical agents in amounts or at rates that exceed the threshold of human tolerance.

inputs: That which is put in, taken in, or operated on by a process or system.

investment in health: The concept that focused attention by health systems on delivering powerful but often inexpensive interventions can lead to dramatic improvements in health at a modest cost.

ISO 31000: An international standard that provides businesses with guidelines and principles for risk management from the International Organization for Standardization.

justice: A legal structure or system that is designed to judge in a general sense which should be accorded, a benefit or a burden, when the law is applied to a person's factual circumstance.

key performance indicator (KPI): A quantifiable measure used to evaluate the success in meeting objectives for performance.

kinetic: Pertaining to motion.

lahar: Mixtures of water (e.g., molten snow, rainfall, or a crater lake) and volcanic debris that move rapidly downhill.

land fire: An unplanned burning in shrublands, grasslands, prairies, or peatlands.

landslide: The abrupt down-slope movement of bedrock, loose soil, and rock particles.

latency period: The time elapsed between an exposure to a chemical, radiological, thermal, or kinetic hazard and the appearance of signs and symptoms.

lethal dose (LD_{50}): The amount of material administered all at once that causes the death of 50% of those exposed.

management: The designing and maintaining of a system wherein individuals work together efficiently to accomplish selected aims.

management by objectives: A strategic management model wherein employees have a say in planning and aligning objectives across the organization.

mass care: The capability to provide congregate sheltering, feeding, emergency supplies, and reunification of families.

mass casualty incident (MCI): Any event that creates many casualties that exceed the resources usually available from local resources.

mass gathering: A planned or spontaneous event where the number of people attending could strain the planning and response resources of the community or country hosting the event.

mass movement (i.e., mass-wasting): The down-slope movement of loose soil and rock particles by the force of gravity.

measures of effectiveness: Often expressed as probabilities, these measures are designed to correspond to the accomplishment of mission objectives and achievement of the desired outcome (i.e., objectives).

measures of efficiency: Often expressed as a rate, these measures relate to performance quality in terms of resources used per outcome accomplished.

measures of process: Measures used to assess the accomplishment of a process (e.g., health-related intervention or treatment).

measures of success: Quantifiable expressions of successful performance collected during the execution of a process.

meteorological: Pertaining to weather—that is, to short-term atmospheric phenomena.

mining disaster: A disaster caused by mining hazards, which include activities that produce, extract, leach, and refine mineral resources.

mitigation: The lessening or limiting of the adverse impacts of hazards and related disasters.

modeling: Using a mathematical model that embodies a set of statistical assumptions concerning sample data (and similar data) from a larger population.

modifiable risk factor: Any changeable characteristic that increases or decreases the likelihood of developing a disease or disorder.

monitoring and evaluation: A method used to assess performance by continuously examining activities according to objectives.

morbidity: Any departure from a state of well-being. In practice, morbidity encompasses disease, injury, and disability.

mortality: The state of being subject to death.

multisectoral: An approach to emergency preparedness that involves input from the entire society (public and private) across all sectors.

natural hazards: Natural processes or phenomena that may cause loss of life, injury, or other health impacts.

natural history of disease: A model that considers the progression of a disease process as occurring in distinct stages if left untreated.

noncommunicable disease (NCD): A chronic disease that cannot be passed person to person.

normative safety: All measures and practices taken to preserve the life, health, and bodily integrity of individuals that are based on applicable norms and standards regardless of safety history.

objective: The object of an effort. It is the aim or desired result of work activity.

operational objective: Short-term aim or desired result whose achievement brings an organization closer to its long-term strategic goals.

operations: An organization implements a group of processes according to a strategy.

operations management: A subdiscipline of management science concerned with designing and controlling the production of goods or services.

operations plan: A plan that describes accomplishing short-term objectives in activities.

ordinal scale: An index representing the ordinal ranking of the differences in intensity regarding one attribute of the same variable.

Ottawa Charter: A global document for health promotion developed from the social model of health.

outbreak: The occurrence of disease cases above average expectancy.

outcome: The intended goal or objective.

outcome measures: Measures used to assess the effect of a process (e.g., health-related intervention or treatment).

outputs: Actions or items that contribute to achieving an outcome (i.e., an intended goal or objective).

pandemic: An international event in which a disease spreads to infect many people.

pathological: Related to or caused by disease. Pertaining to a disordered physiological process associated with disease or injury.

perceived safety: All measures and practices taken to preserve the life, health, and bodily integrity of individuals that are based on the perception of safety regardless of actual safety history.

performance: The process of accomplishing an activity, process, or operation.

performance indicators: A type of measurement used to evaluate the successful performance of a particular activity according to measurable standards.

performance management: Ensuring that activities and outputs accomplish an organization's goals effectively and efficiently.

performance measurement: An objective quantification of performance over time.

pillars of emergency health: A model for producing disaster-related health, wellness, and equity by application of four basic public health practices: prevention, health promotion, health protection, and provision of care.

plan: A design for achieving goals.

planetary health: A multidisciplinary field focused on addressing the human impacts to Earth's natural systems on human health and all life on Earth.

planning: The process of creating plans.

poisoning disaster: A disaster caused by poisoning hazards—that is, by harmful effects that occur when a toxic substance is swallowed, inhaled, or comes in contact with an affected person.

population: A particular selection, group, or type of people living in a specific area.

population health: The health outcomes of a population, including the distribution of such outcomes within the group; this includes health outcomes, patterns of health determinants, and policies and interventions that link these two.

predictability: The ability to make a correct prediction or forecast of a system's future state.

preparedness: Activities taken in advance to ensure an effective response to the impact of hazards.

Presidential Decision Directive 39 (PDD-39): A 1995 order by President Bill Clinton setting US policy for counterterrorism.

prevalence: Sometimes referred to as prevalence rate, it is the proportion of persons who have a particular attribute over a specified period.

prevention: The outright avoidance of adverse impacts of hazards and related disasters.

preventive control: One of three types of control (i.e., detective, preventive, and corrective), this type of internal control is put in place to avert an adverse event from occurring.

primary health care: Health care that is provided in a patient's first contact with the health care system.

primary prevention: A group of prevention activities intended to avoid hazardous exposures.

primordial prevention: A group of prevention activities intended to avoid the adverse ecosocial determinants of health.

principle: A basic assumption that serves as the foundation for a chain of reasoning.

process: A set of activities (i.e., tasks) that are interrelated or that interact with one another.

process control: The management function of actively changing the process based on process-monitoring results.

process management: The aligning of processes with an organization's strategic goals.

process-person-context-time (PPCT) model: An approach that recognizes that human development occurs within an ecosocial context and changes with life stage.

productivity: A measure of process efficiency calculated by measuring the relative number of inputs required to produce outputs or outcomes.

program: A set of related measures with a particular long-term objective.

program logic model: Schematic diagrams representing the logic underlying the program's design, indicating how various components interact with the goods or services they produce and how they generate the desired results.

promotion: One of the four pillars of emergency health involves modifying personal health determinants.

protection: One of emergency health's four pillars involves protection from hazardous exposures.

protective factors: Attributes that when present mitigate or eliminate risk in families and communities and increase health, wellness, and equity.

provision of care: One of the four pillars of emergency health involving the provision of care intended to (1) terminate or cease and prevent exposures and (2) treat existing disease (e.g., mass care and medical care).

proximate cause of disease: An event, in a natural and continuous sequence, that when unbroken by any efficient intervening cause produces disease and without which the injury would not have occurred.

public health: The science of preventing disease, prolonging life, and promoting health through organized efforts and informed choices.

public health impact: The measurable effect of a public health intervention is usually represented in terms of morbidity and mortality.

pyroclastic flow: A fluidized volcanic mixture of hot rock fragments and hot gases that moves at high speed in thick, gray-to-black, turbulent clouds that hug the ground.

quality: The features and characteristics of a product or service that bear on its ability to satisfy given needs.

quality of life: An individual's perception of their position in life.

quaternary prevention: A group of prevention activities intended to identify patients at risk of overmedicalization, protect them from new medical invasion, and suggest ethically acceptable interventions.

recovery: The restoration, and improvement, where appropriate, of facilities, livelihoods, and living conditions of disaster-affected communities, including efforts to reduce disaster risk factors.

relative frequency: The number of observations in a statistical category compared to the total number of observations.

reliability: The degree to which repeated measurements (under unchanged conditions) show the same results. Reliability describes the degree of random errors and is measured as statistical variability. In other words, precision measures the reproducibility of a test as compared to itself.

residual risk (i.e., accepted risk): Risk that is not prevented, or transferred, thus assuming some or all the consequences.

resilience: The ability of a system to resist, absorb, accommodate, and recover from the effects of a hazard.

resource: A stock or supply of assets (e.g., money, materials, or staff) that can be drawn on to function effectively.

resource allocation: The assignment of available resources to various uses.

resource management: When needed, efficient and effective development of an organization's resources.

response: Activities that address an incident's short-term, direct effects (consequences).

responsible party: A person or group that should accomplish a particular activity.

Ring of Fire (i.e., Circum-Pacific Belt): A group of tectonic borders around the Pacific Ocean.

risk: The probability of harmful consequences.

risk acceptance: Accepting some or all the consequences of a risk.

risk assessment: A methodology to determine the extent of risk by analyzing potential hazards and evaluating existing conditions of vulnerability.

risk characterization: Estimating the probability of occurrence and severity of potential adverse health effects based on the preceding steps of hazard and impact analysis.

risk communication: A process involving the exchange of information and expert opinion about risks and the decisions taken to combat them.

risk equation: A simplified mathematical formula used to represent the interaction between hazards and their impact in terms of the probability of harmful consequences or losses.

risk factor: Attributes in individuals, families, communities, or the larger society that when present mitigate or eliminate risk in families and communities that decrease health, wellness, and equity.

risk index: A relative scale that broadly characterizes risk using a semi-quantitative index.

risk management: An international standard (ISO 31000) for forecasting and evaluating risks and identifying procedures to avoid or minimize their impact.

risk perception: The subjective judgment about a risk's characteristics and severity.

risk ratio scale: An interval scale that characterizes risk using quantitative measures.

risk reduction: Reducing the negative effect of the risk.

risk transfer: Transferring the risk to another party (i.e., risk-sharing/pooling).

risk treatment: Measures put into place to control risk.

routes of human exposure: Pathways by which health hazards may come in contact with the body.

safety: All measures and practices taken to preserve the life, health, and bodily integrity of individuals.

safety standards: Standards designed to ensure safety.

sanitation: The study of measures designed to ensure provision of clean water and the disposal of sewage and waste.

satisfaction: A customer-focused measure of quality regarding how well products and services supplied meet or surpass customer expectations.

scenario: An expected or supposed situation or sequence of events.

secondary prevention: A group of prevention activities intended to avoid disease, given that a hazardous exposure has already occurred.

security: All measures and practices taken to preserve the function and integrity of social safety.

sediment flow: A form of landslide involving materials that flow downhill when mixed with water or air.

Sendai Framework for Disaster Risk Reduction: The first major world agreement with concrete actions to protect development gains from the risk of disaster.

Shanghai Declaration: Outcome documents of an international conference promoting health in the 2030 UN Agenda for Sustainable Development.

shelter in place: a population protection measure that directs people to stay in the indoor place or building they already occupy and not leave unless absolutely necessary.

Six Sigma: A quality control method used to improve the capability of business processes by increasing performance and decreasing process variation. This leads to improvement in outcomes, employee morale, and quality of products or services.

slope failure: A form of landslide involving a sudden collapse of a slope resulting in the transport of debris downhill by sliding, rolling, falling, or slumping.

SOARR planning format: Organizational structure for planning that includes strategic goals, operational objectives, activities, responsible parties, and resources.

social safety: All measures and practices (e.g., public safety and security) taken to preserve the life, health, and bodily integrity of individuals from intentional harm.

socio-politicization of risk: A process for unequal risk of environmental pollution occurring among different social classes, racial/ethnic groups and countries.

special cause variation: A cause of variation that is assignable to a defect, fault, mistake, delay, breakdown, accident, or shortage in the process.

stakeholder: An entity with an interest in something.

standard: A measurable norm for acceptability of quality.

stochastic: Effects that are not dose-dependent.

storm surge: Ocean coastal flooding that occurs during tropical cyclones.

strategic goal: Long-term aims or desired results whose achievement brings an organization closer to its intended outcome.

strategic plan: A type of plan that describes the accomplishment of long-term goals in terms of objectives.

strategy: A plan to achieve a major overall goal.

structural collapse: A disaster hazard created by the collapse of large built structures.

subclinical disease: A disease that does not have recognizable clinical signs and symptoms.

subduction zone: A location where two of the planet's tectonic plates collide and one dives, or subducts, beneath the other.

substantive safety: All measures and practices taken to preserve the life, health, and bodily integrity of individuals that are based on actual safety history that is substantial or acceptable regardless of whether standards are met.

supportive environment for health: One of the five action areas of the Ottawa Charter that calls for the creation of environments that support health.

susceptibility: The state of being likely to be harmed by a particular hazard.

sustainable development: Development that meets present needs without compromising those of future generations.

sustainable development goal (SDG): A United Nations-led collection of 17 interlinked global goals designed for peace and prosperity now and into the future.

syndrome: A group of symptoms that indicate or characterize a disease, disorder, or other condition considered abnormal.

systems theory: The interdisciplinary study of systems.

target capability: An ability that will be required to accomplish a set of predetermined (i.e., targeted) objectives.

task analysis: The process of observing what steps it takes to perform a task for which there is a goal.

technological hazards: Hazards originating from technological or industrial conditions.

tectonic plate: In the theory of plate tectonics, one of the sections of the earth's lithosphere is constantly moving concerning the other sections.

tephra: Rock fragments and dust produced by a volcanic eruption regardless of composition, fragment size, or emplacement mechanism.

Terrorism Incident Annex: An annex to the Federal Response Plan created by Presidential Decision Directive 39.

tertiary prevention: A group of prevention activities intended to avoid disease progression, disability, or death, given that disease has already occurred.

thermal: Pertaining to heat.

tornado disaster: A disaster caused by tornado hazards, which are created by the tornado's rapidly rotating column of air extending from the ground to the base of a cloud.

toxic: Pertaining to poison.

transportation disaster: A disaster caused by transportation hazards—that is, by the movement of goods and persons and the various means by which such activity is accomplished.

tropical cyclone disaster (i.e., cyclone, hurricane, and typhoon): A disaster caused by a tropical cyclone, which is a rotating, organized system of clouds and thunderstorms that originates over tropical or subtropical waters and has a closed low-level circulation.

tsunami disaster: A disaster caused by tsunami hazards. Tsunamis involve a series of ocean waves generated by the displacement of a large mass of water.

typhoon disaster (i.e., cyclone, hurricane, and tropical cyclone): A disaster caused by tropical cyclone hazards. Typhoons involve a rotating, organized system of clouds and thunderstorms that originates over tropical or subtropical waters and has a closed low-level circulation.

uncertainty: A state of limited knowledge where it is impossible to describe a future outcome exactly. In statistics, it is the amount of measurable error associated with the estimation of an unknown value.

unified command: An organizational authority structure in which the role of an incident commander is shared by the authority in different responding agencies.

utility: The condition of helping accomplish a task.

validity: The degree to which the result of a measurement conforms to the actual or correct value. In other words, validity measures the consistency of a test as compared to an external standard. Validity describes systemic errors and is measured as statistical bias.

variability: A statistical value that measures the spread of a dataset around the mean.

volcanic eruption: The expulsion of gases, rock fragments, or molten lava from within the earth through a vent onto the earth's surface or into the atmosphere.

vulnerability: The state of possibility for being harmed. It is typically represented as the slope of the hazard dose-human response curve.

well-being: A subjective state of wellness.

wellness: An active process through which people identify options and make choices toward a more successful existence.

wildfire disaster: A disaster caused by wildfire hazards—that is, by unplanned fire burning in natural (wildland) areas such as forests, shrub lands, grasslands, or prairies and peatland.

wildland: Wilderness containing natural areas such as forests, shrub lands, grasslands, or prairies and peatland.

winter storm disaster: A disaster caused by winter storm hazards—that is, by atmospheric storms characterized by cold ambient temperatures accompanied by wind and precipitation.

Afterword

Today, our vulnerabilities are widespread, more so than at any time in our fragile world's history. I measure those vulnerabilities in terms of public health's capacity to perform daily—to bring expected safety to everyday life. But equally critical is public health's capacity to surge across the entire disaster cycle to protect humankind during local or global crises.

At no time in my history have public health survival capacities been more threatened. Significant and often frightening global challenges to public health unfolded daily during the COVID-19 pandemic, resulting in stark losses in vital public health leadership and immeasurable preventable human losses worldwide. Like you, I am frightened that a new global crisis will be more catastrophic.

We must ensure a new international response capacity that supports a global "one health" approach with public health infrastructure capacity at the forefront, meeting global expectations for all. This capacity requires new international educational, training, and performance requirements, with public health protections at the forefront of all our research and writings.

We must also heed concerns regarding our ability to provide basic preventive measures critical to health systems and population health. I contend that this weakness can no longer be tolerated and will reveal its ugly head again in future global crises. We must all fast-track our learning curves to understand our essential roles. The backbone of understanding and response to future crises lies in our ability to ensure a public health framework for future studies. We must consider this framework essential for survival and apply it in our multidisciplinary research, decision-making, and teaching.

Frederick M. Burkle, Jr., MD, MPH, DTM, PhD (Hon.)
Global Fellow, Woodrow Wilson International Center for Scholars
Washington, DC

About the Author

Mark Keim, MD, MBA, is Chief Executive Officer for DisasterDoc LLC, an international firm specializing in consultation, education, and research related to public health emergencies. He is also Adjunct Professor at Emory University, Rollins School of Public Health, and Guest Faculty at Beth Israel Deaconess Medical Center, Harvard Medical School, Disaster Medicine Fellowship.

Dr. Keim is residency trained in emergency medicine (Albany, NY) and fellowship trained in disaster medicine (Emory University). He most recently earned an MBA at Emory University Goizueta Business School in 2014.

Dr. Keim is retired from a career at the US Centers for Disease Control and Prevention (CDC), where he served as Associate Director for Science for the CDC Office for Environmental Health Emergencies. He also served on the White House Subcommittee for Disaster Reduction from 2006 to 2015.

He was twice commended with the US Secretary of Health Secretary's Award for Distinguished Service as CDC's incident manager for both the Anthrax letter emergency and Hurricane Katrina. He also received the CDC Special Service Award for leading field response after the Indonesia tsunami. As well, he led regional pandemic planning efforts during the H5N1 bird flu outbreaks in Vietnam, Cambodia, Thailand, and Laos.

Dr. Keim published his first sentinel study documenting the health effects of climate change and sea level rise in 2007. He served as a review editor for the 2012 UN Intergovernmental Panel on Climate Change (IPCC) Special Report on Exposures. He was also a contributing author for the 2016 US Global Change Research Program's Climate and Health Assessment.

In 2015 Dr. Keim received the prestigious United Nations Sasakawa Certificate of Merit recognizing global impact on disaster risk reduction. In 2016 he spoke at former US vice president Al Gore's Climate and Health Summit in Atlanta, Georgia.

Dr. Keim is the author of 58 journal publications and 24 book chapters, and one textbook entitled *Disaster Planning: A Practical Guide for Effective Health Outcomes*. He has served as a peer review consultant for 21 scientific journals and on the editorial board of 2 scientific journals. His press interviews have appeared on CNN and PBS and in *USA Today*, *Chicago Tribune*, *LA Times*, *Washington Post*, *The Lancet*, and *Scientific American*. He has more than 30,000 followers on LinkedIn. His YouTube channel receives more than 3,000 views per month.

About the Author

Index

Note: Italicized page references indicate Figures, Tables, or Illustrations.

A

ability, 311. *See also* functional ability
  in performance measurement, 272
  for prevention, 333
accepted risk. *See* residual risk
accountability, 311
  good governance and, 226
  HiAP and, 225
  in performance measurement, 272
accuracy, 311
  disaster risk assessment and, 195
  of uncertainty, 38
acid rain, 74
activity, 269, 311
Adler, A., 167
Agency for Healthcare Research and Quality, 210
agents, 311. *See also* biological agents
  emergency health for, 15
  environmental health and, 14
  in epidemiological triad, *32*
  of health hazards, 48
  heath promotion and, *19*
air pollution
  from heat wave disasters, 67
  from wildfire disasters, 75
all-hazard approach, 135, 311
American Chemical Society, 82
analysis, 311. *See also specific types*
  in environmental health, 14
analytical risk assessment, 192, 311
Anthropocene Epoch, 38, 153, 311
  investment in health and, 227
approach, 311
  all-hazard, 135, 311
  to disaster risk assessment, 195–199, *197, 199*
  in health promotion, 18
assumption, 311
  causal pathways of disease and, 126
avalanches, *48, 50,* 68, *68,* 72

B

ballistic effect
  in cyclone disasters, *285*
  in explosion disaster, *50,* 83, *106, 292*
  in hazardous material release disasters, *293*
  in tornadoes and convective storms, *50, 105, 290*
  in volcanic eruptions, 73, *291*
Belt of Fire, 63
biological, 311
biological agents
  emergency health for, 15
  hazardous material release disasters of, 86
biological disasters, *43*
biological hazards (biohazards), 41, 48, *48,* 52, 311
  epidemics from, 64
blast effect, in explosion disaster, 82, 83
boiling liquid-expanding vapor explosion (BLEVE), 82–83
Bronfenbrenner's ecosocial model for human development, 28–29, *29,* 31, 311
Brundtland Report, 227
BS 11200, 188, 312
Burkle, Frederick (Skip), 247, 333

C

candidate cause, 126, 312
capability, 312
  of disaster hazards, 47
  DoH and, 177
  target capability, 175, 253, 329
capability-based planning, 253–258, *254–258,* 312
Carr, M., 247
case, 312
  in provision of care, *243,* 243–245
case fatality rate (death-to-case ratio), 157, 312
catastrophe, 312
  in drought disasters, 61
  incident continuum and, 39–41, *40*
Causal Analysis/Diagnosis Decision Information System (CADDIS), 126
causal assessment, 126, 312
causal factors, 312
  for disease, *32,* 32–33
causal pathway of disease, 102–103, *103,* 312
  for disaster-related disease, 126–128
  downstream, 128–129, *129,* 131–137, *133, 135, 136*
  in heat wave disaster, 129, *129, 136,* 136–137
  upstream, 125–128, *127*
Centers for Disease Control and Prevention, 14
  on biological agents, 86
  on DoH, *30,* 30–31
  on provision of care, 246–247
chemical explosions, 82
Chernobyl, 42

climatological disasters, *42, 43,* 312
clinical, 26, 312
clinical disease, 27, 133, 312
cold wave disaster, 312
  disaster-related disease in, *104*
  etiology of diseases in, *285*
  health hazards of, *48, 49*
cold weather disaster, *43,* 58–59, 312
  mortality from, 159
collapse disaster, 81–82, 312. *See also* structural collapse disasters
common cause variation, 26, 28, 38, 312
communicable disease, 34, 313
  as disaster-related disease, *108*
community-based, 313
  HiAP, 208
community engagement, 313
  in environmental health, 14
competency, 313
  standards for, 280
competency-based learning, 280, 313
consequence, 313
  of cold weather disasters, 59
  of convective storm disasters, 70
  crisis management and, 188, *188*
  of cyclone disasters, 60
  of disaster hazards, 47, *52,* 141–147, *142–144*
  in disaster pathway, 38
  of drought disasters, 61
  of earthquake disasters, 63
  of epidemic, 65
  of explosion disasters, 83–84
  of fire disasters, 85
  of flood disasters, 66
  of hazardous exposure, 46
  of hazardous material release disasters, 87–88
  of heat wave disasters, 67
  of industrial disasters, 89–90
  of landslide disasters, 68–69
  of mass gathering disasters, 91
  of mine disasters, 92–93
  on public health, *148*
  resilience and, 9
  of structural collapse disasters, 81–82
  of technological disasters, *80*
  of tornado disasters, 70
  of transportation disasters, 95
  of tsunami disasters, 72
  uncertainty and, 38
  of volcanic eruptions, 73–74
  of wildfire disasters, 75
consequence management, 188–189, 313
control, 313. *See also* preventive control; process control
  DoW and, 177
  good governance and, 226
  in health promotion, 18
convective storm disaster, 69–70, 313. *See also* cyclone disaster; tornado disaster
  disaster-related disease in, *105*
  etiology of diseases in, *290*
  fire disasters and, 84
  health hazards of, *48*
Coriolis effect, 59
Covello, V., 203
crisis management, *188,* 188–189, 313
  risk communication and, 201–202
cyclone disasters, *43,* 59–60, 313
  disaster-related disease in, *104*
  etiology of diseases in, *285–286*
  health hazards of, 47, 48, *48, 49*

D

Dahlgren, G., 30
Davies, S. E., 235
deaths. *See* mortality
death-to-case ratio (case fatality rate), 157, 312
decision tree, *197,* 198, 313
defects, 182, 313
Department of Energy, 212
Department of Health and Human Services (HHS), 4, 211
Department of Health and Human Services, Office of the Assistant Secretary for Preparedness and Response (HHS/ASPR), 8, 9
Department of Homeland Security, 4
Department of Transportation, 86
DesInventar database, 152
determinants of clinical outcome (DoO), 313
  disease prevention and, *217*
  tertiary prevention and, 220
determinants of disease (DoD), 313
  disease prevention and, *217*
determinants of disparity (DoD), 314
  disease prevention and, *217*
  quaternary prevention and, 221
determinants of equity (DoEq), 314
determinants of exposure (DoEx), 314
  disease prevention and, *217*
  environmental justice and, 237
  health protection and, 234
  primary prevention and, 218
determinants of health (DoH), 29–32, *30, 32,* 175–177, *176,* 314, 318
  causal pathways of disease and, 126–129, *127*
  disaster-related disease and, 102–103
  in disease management, 33
  in disease prevention, 16, *217*
  in emergency health, 19, 21
  health equity and, 169, 212
  in health promotion, 18
  health promotion and, 19
  HiAP and, 208
  in outcomes, 27
  population heath and, 210
  prevention and, 213
  social machinery for, 4
  underfunding of, 7
determinants of health, wellness, and equity (DoHWE), 217, 314
  capability-based planning and, 254–258, *255–259*

emergency health professionals and, 263–264
in health promotion, 224
determinants of wellness (DoW), 166, 177, 314
quaternary prevention and, 221
deterministic, 314
health effects, 27
disability, 314
disease prevention and, 18
heath equity and, 211
tertiary prevention and, 220
disaster. *See also specific types and topics*
defined, 37–43, 314
from development, 5–6
displacement from, 159
ecosocial models of health for wellness in, 167–168
emergency health for, 15
in environment, 41
etymology of, 37–38
incidence of, 38, 153
incident continuum in, 39–41, *40*
increased frequency of, *6*, 6–7, *7*
key characteristics of, 38
mortality from, 4, 9, *154*, 155–157, *156*, 159
outdated understanding of, 8–9
provision of care in, 246–248
public health and, *148*
relative frequency of, 153, *153*, 326
risk reduction of, 9
typology of, 41–43, *42*, *43*
underdeveloped science of, 8
wellness and, 178–179
disaster hazards
consequence of, 47, *52*, 141–147, *142–144*
disaster-related diseases and, 103, *104–107*
disaster risk and, *193*, 193–194
health hazards and, *48–51*
disaster management, 183, 314
safety and, 237
disaster medicine, 314
provision of care for, 21
disaster pathway, 38, 314
disaster-related disease, 101–109, *105–107*, 314
causal pathways of disease for, 126–128
etiology of disease of, 109, *285–295*
evidence-based decision-making for, 211
global patterns of, 151
health effects and, 103, *104–108*, 107–109
outcome of, 107–108, *108*
disaster-related health risk, 314
disaster risk and, 194
risk assessment and, 192
Disaster Relief Act of 1974, 246
disaster risk, 184–186, *193*, 193–194, 314
disaster-related health risk and, 194
health risk and, 194
risk retention and, 187
disaster risk assessment
approach to, 195–199, *197*, *199*
evidence-based decision-making for, *187*, 196–199, *199*
disaster risk management, 181–188, *185*, 314
prioritization in, 193
twilight zone of, 195
disaster risk reduction (DRR), 9, 314
disease, 314. *See also specific types and topics*
categories of, 34
causal factors for, *32*, 32–33
defined, 25–34, 314
DoW and, 177
environmental health and, 14
prevention of, risk reduction and, 187
protective factors for, 32
provision of care for, 20
disease management, 315
natural history of, *33*, 33–34
disease prevention
in emergency health, 16–18, *17*, 315
stages of, 215–221, *216*, *217*
displacement, 315
in convective storm disasters, 70
from disasters, 159
in drought disasters, 61
from earthquake disasters, 63
from epidemic, 65
from hazardous material release disasters, 88
from mine disasters, 92
provision of care for, 20
from structural collapse disasters, 82
in volcanic eruptions, 74
distal health determinants, 218–219, 315
dose, 53, 315
of hazardous exposure, 46–47
dose rate, 315
exposure science and, 53
of hazardous exposure, 47
dose-responsive modeling, 54, *54*, 315
drought disasters, *43*, 60–61, 315
disaster-related disease in, *104*
etiology of diseases in, *286–287*
food insecurity in, 42, 61
health hazards of, *48*, *49*
mortality from, 156
Drucker, Peter, 272

E

early warning system (EWS), 315
for drought disasters, 61
for flood disasters, 219
earthquake disasters, *43*, *62*, 62–64, 315
disaster-related disease in, *104*
etiology of diseases in, *287*
health hazards of, *48*, *49*
mine disasters and, 92
mortality from, 63, 156, 159
structural collapse disasters and, 81
tsunami disasters from, 70–72
ecosocial model of health, 28–29, *29*, 315
DoH and, 31, *31*
for emergency heath, 212–213
for health equity, 169–172, *170–172*

for primordial prevention, 218
for risk communication, 203–204
for wellness, *164*, 164–165
in disasters, 167–168
Eddy, D., 210
effectiveness, 315
on disaster mortality, 4
measures of, 210, 322
of outcomes, 8
risk management and, *186*
efficiency, 315
HiAP and, 225
measures of, 210, 322
of outcomes, 8
effusive eruption, 72, 73, 315
egalitarian, 272, 315
EM-DAT, 86, 88, 152
emergency, 315
incident continuum and, 39, *40*
safety in, 235
emergency health, 13–21, *15*, 315, 316
determinants of health (DoH) in, 19
disease prevention in, 16–18, *17*
ecosocial model of health for, 212–213
educational opportunities in, 279–280
framework for, 21, *21*
health promotion in, 18–20, *19*
health protection in, 20
impact in, 277–278
integration opportunities in, 281
intervention opportunities in, 280–281
outcome in, 208–210, *209*
performance management for, 271
prevention and, 213–214
professionals in, 261–264, *262–263*
provision of care in, 15, *15*
research in, 278–279
risk and, 213–214
tenets of, 207–214
wellness and, 179, 213–214
emergency management, 316
crisis management and, 189
endemic, 64, 316
Enhanced Fujita scale, 70
environment, 316
causal pathways of disease and, *127*
disaster in, 41
in epidemiological triad, *32*
hazard in, 41
health promotion and, 19, *19*
mine disasters and, 93
safety in, primary prevention and, 219
environmental health, 14
in emergency health, 316
environmental impact assessment, 14, 316
environmental justice, 212, 237–238, 280
Environmental Protection Agency, 237
epidemic, *43*, 64–65, 316
disaster-related disease in, *104*
disease prevention for, 16
in drought disasters, 61
emergency health for, 21
etiology of diseases in, 288
from hazardous material release disasters, 86, 88
health hazards of, *48*, *49*
mortality from, 65, 159
risk avoidance in, 186
epidemiological triad, *32*, 316
epidemiology, 316
primary prevention and, 219
tertiary prevention and, 220
equity, 211–212, 316. *See also* determinants of health, wellness, and equity; health equity
measurement of, 272
eruption cloud, 73, 316
etiology of disease, 316
of disaster-related disease, 109, *285–295*
evacuation, 316
from fire disasters, 85
from flood disasters, 219
from wildfire disasters, 75
evaluation, 316
in health protection, 20
event, 317
provision of care in, 244, 245
event-based surveillance (EBS), 242–243, 317
evidence-based decision-making, 210–211, 317
for disaster risk assessment, *187*, 196–199, *199*
good governance and, 226
excess heat factor (EHF), 67
explosion disasters, *43*, 82–84, 317
disaster-related disease in, *106*
from earthquake disasters, 62, 63
etiology of diseases in, *292*
health hazards of, *48*, *50*
industrial disasters from, 89
from mine disasters, 92
mortality from, 84, 159
from structural collapse disasters, 81, 82
transportation disasters and, 94, 95
explosive volcanic eruptions, 72–73, 74
exposure, 52, 317. *See also* determinants of exposure; hazardous exposure
causal pathways of disease and, 126
disaster-related disease from, 102–103
disaster risk and, 194
to disease, 32
disease prevention and, 16, 18
in emergency health, 21, *209*
in epidemic, 64
to hazmat, 86
incidence and, 54
in poisoning disaster, 94
provision of care for, 20
risk avoidance and, 186
exposure science, 53, 317
extreme weather events (EWEs), 5. *See also* *specific types*
mass gathering disasters and, 91
mine disasters and, 92
structural collapse disasters and, 81

F

Federal Emergency Management Administration (FEMA), 248
fire disaster, *43,* 84–86, 317. *See also* wildfire disaster
  disaster-related disease in, *106*
  from earthquake disasters, 63
  etiology of diseases in, *292*
  explosion disasters from, 83
  in flood disasters, 66
  health hazards of, *48, 50*
  mass gathering disasters and, 91
  from mine disasters, 92
  from structural collapse disasters, 82
  transportation disasters and, 94
fireline intensity, 75
flash floods, 66
flood disasters, 65–66, 317
  in convective storm disasters, 70
  from cyclone disasters, 60
  disaster-related disease in, *104–105*
  disease prevention in, 16–17
  etiology of diseases in, *288–289*
  health hazards of, 47, *48, 49*
  health promotion in, 18–19
  mortality from, 32–33, 159
  primordial prevention for, 218–219
  risk avoidance in, 186
  from structural collapse disasters, 82
  wellness in, 178
food insecurity
  in drought disasters, 42, 61
  in flood disasters, 66
forest fire, 74, 317
fracking, 62
function, 317
  in health promotion, 18
  healthy settings and, 226
  tertiary prevention and, 220
functional ability, 33, 317
  causal pathways for disaster-related disease and, 128, 129, 136
  DoH and, *256*
  recovery of, 253

G

geophysical, *42,* 47, 317
geophysical disasters, *42, 43,* 108–109
global health security, 235, *236*
global warming, 5
good governance, 225, 226, 317
governance, 317. *See also* good governance
  in drought disasters, 61
  incident continuum and, 40
Great Acceleration, 5–6, 153, 317
  planetary health and, 228
gross domestic product (GDP), 6–7, *7*
Grumbach, K., 173
Gunn, S. W. A., 246–247

H

Haddon, W., 246
hazard, 318. *See also specific types and topics*
  disaster-related disease from, 102–103
  disease prevention for, 16
  in environment, 41
  environmental health and, 14
  healthy settings and, 226
  risk avoidance and, 186
  vulnerability to, 9
hazard analysis, 318
  in disaster risk management, *185*
  in risk assessment, 192
hazard characterization, 318
  in risk assessment, 192, 193
hazard identification, 318
  in environmental health, 14
  research for, 278
  in risk assessment, 192
hazard-impact matrix, 199, *199,* 318
hazardous exposure, 45–55, 318
  capability-based planning and, 253
  causes and effects of, 55
  health promotion and, 234
  impact of, 46–47
hazardous material release disasters, 86–89, 318
  disaster-related disease in, *106*
  environmental justice and, 237
  etiology of diseases in, *292–293*
  from explosion disasters, 83
  fire disasters and, 84
  in flood disasters, 66
  health hazards of, *48, 51*
  industrial disasters from, 89, 90
  from mine disasters, 92
  from structural collapse disasters, 82
hazardous materials (hazmat), 52, 86, 318
hazardous substance, 51–52, 318
health. *See also specific topics*
  defined, 28–32, 318
  legal right to, 5
health determinants. *See* determinants of health
health effects, 27, 318
  disaster-related diseases and, 103, *104–108,* 107–109
  disease prevention for, 16
  in poisoning disaster, 94
  provision of care for, 20
health equality, 318
  heath equity and, 211–212
  outcomes and, 172
  quaternary prevention and, 221
health equity, 169–173, 211–212, 318
  ecosocial model of health for, 169–172, *170–172*
  in health promotion, 18
  health promotion and, 19, 225, 229
  justice and, 173
  quaternary prevention and, 216
  susceptibility and, 172–173
  vulnerability and, 169, 172–173

health hazard, 47–48, 319
disaster hazards and, *48–51*
disaster-related diseases and, 103, *104–107*
in health protection, 20
protection from, 5
health impact assessment, 319
DoH and, 177
health in all policies (HiAP), 208, 225–226, 319
emergency health professionals and, 264
health literacy, 225, 227, 319
health promotion, 223–229
in emergency health, 18–20, *19,* 319
prevention in, 224–225, *225*
health protection, 233–238, *236*
in emergency health, 20
health risk, 319
disaster risk and, 194
in drought disasters, 61
Healthy People 2020, 211
Healthy People 2030, 31, 281
healthy settings, 225, 319
heat index, 67, 319
heat wave disaster, *43,* 67–68, 319
causal pathway of disease in, 129, *129, 136,* 136–137
disaster-related disease in, *105*
etiology of diseases in, *289*
health hazards of, *48, 50*
hierarchy of process control, 132, *132,* 319
high explosives, 83, 84
holistic, 163, 319
homeostasis, 319
health and, 28
hormesis, 53, 319
household goods, 319
public health consequence of, *148*
public health impact of, *142, 146*
humanitarian assistance, 320
in emergency health, 15, 208
mass care for, 248–249
provision of care for, 21
Humanitarian Charter, 249, 320
hurricane disasters, 9, 59, 320. *See also* cyclone disasters
disaster-related disease in, *104*
emergency health for, 21
quaternary prevention in, 220
hydrological disasters, *7, 42,* 320
hydrometeorological disasters, 7, 41, *43,* 320

I

illness, 320
emergency health for, 15
health promotion and, 19
quaternary prevention and, 220
wellness and, 27, *27*
immunization, for disease prevention, 16
impact, 320. *See also* public health impact
disaster risk and, *193,* 193–194
in emergency health, 277–278
environmental impact assessment, 14, 316
of epidemic, 65
hazard-impact matrix, 199, *199,* 318
of hazardous exposure, 46–47
health impact assessment, 319
DoH and, 177
in health protection, 20
of mass gathering disasters, 91
of natural disasters, *158*
on public health, 47, 141–147, *142–144, 146,* 277–278
research for, 278–279
of structural collapse disasters, 82
of technological disasters, *158*
on wellness, 178
impact analysis, 320
for disaster risk assessment, 198
in disaster risk management, *185*
in environmental health, 14
in risk assessment, 193
incidence, 320
disaster risk assessment for, 198
of disasters, 38, 153
exposure and, 54
of natural disasters, *154*
risk management and, 183
of technological disasters, *154*
incident command system (ICS), 40, *244,* 320
in public health, 245
incident continuum, 320
in disaster, 39–41, *40*
incubation period, 320
for epidemics, 64
of infectious diseases, 33–34
index, 320
EHF as, 67
heat, 67, 319
for landslide intensity, 59, 69
PDSI, 61
risk, 196, 327
indicator-based surveillance (IBS), 242, 320
indivisible self, 321
DoW and, 177
wellness and, *165,* 165–166, *166*
industrial disaster, 89–90, 321
infectious disease, 321. *See also* epidemic
causal factors for, 32
disease prevention for, 16, 17
incubation period of, 33–34
infectious dose, 53, 321
information exchange, 280, 321
injury, 321
in convective storm disasters, 70
as disaster-related disease, *108*
as disease category, 34
from earthquake disasters, 63
emergency health for, 15
in flood disasters, 32, 66
health promotion and, 19
from landslide disasters, 69
from mine disasters, 92

provision of care for, 20
from structural collapse disasters, 81
inputs, 321
of resources, 268–269
Institute of Medicine, 7
International Air Transportation, 86
International Monetary Fund, 226
inundation, in tsunami disasters, 71–72
investment in health, 172, 227, 321
ISO 22300, 234
ISO 31000, 183–184, 281, 321

J

justice, 321
environmental, 212, 237–238, 280
health equity and, 173

K

key performance indicator (KPI), 267, *269*, 272, 321
kinetic disasters/hazards, 41, *42*, *43*, 321
in health protection, 20
mass gathering disasters and, 90
mine disasters and, 92
structural collapse disasters and, 81
transportation disasters and, 94
Klinenberg, E., 129, 136–137

L

lahar, 73, 74, 321
land fire, 74, 321
landslide disasters, 7, *43*, 67–69, *68*, 321
in convective storm disasters, 70
from cyclone disasters, 60
disaster-related disease in, *105*
etiology of diseases in, *289*
health hazards of, 47, *48*
from tsunami disasters, 70
landslide intensity index, 59, 69
La Niña, 59
latency period, 321
in disease management, 34
lethal dose (LD_{50}), 53, 54, 321
life expectancy, 6
low explosives, 83, 84

M

major storms, 60
management, 182, 321. *See also specific types*
management by objectives, 268, 322
mass care, 248–249, *249*, 322
provision of care for, 20
tertiary prevention and, 220
mass casualty incident (MCI), 322
in mass gathering disasters, 91
in mine disasters, 92
resources in, 144
in structural collapse disasters, 81
mass gathering disasters, 90–92, 322
disaster-related disease in, *106*
etiology of diseases in, *293*
health hazards of, *48*, *51*
mass movement (mass-wasting), 322
in landslide disasters, 67, *68*
in mine disasters, 92, 93
measures of effectiveness, 210, 322
measures of efficiency, 210, 322
measures of process, 278, 322
measures of success, 210, 237, 258, 322
mechanical explosions, 82–83
medical care, 246–248
meteorological disasters, *7*, *42*, 322
mine disasters, *43*, 92–93, 322
disaster-related disease in, *106*
etiology of diseases in, *294*
health hazards of, *48*, *51*
mortality from, 93, 157
mitigation, 183, 322
primary prevention and, 219
tertiary prevention and, 220
modeling, 218, 322
dose-responsive, 54, *54*, 315
modifiable risk factor, 132, 322
Modified Mercalli Intensity Scale (MMI), 63–64, 72
monitoring and evaluation, 203, 322
morbidity, 322
disaster-related health risk and, 194
disease prevention and, 17
health promotion and, 19
from heat wave disasters, 67
tertiary prevention and, 220
mortality (deaths), 323
from cold weather disaster, 159
from cyclone disasters, 60
disaster-related health risk and, 194
from disasters, 4, 9, *154*, 155–159, *156*
disease prevention and, 17
from drought disasters, 156
from earthquake disasters, 63, 156, 159
from epidemic, 65, 159
from explosion disasters, 84, 159
from fire disasters, 85
from flood disasters, 32–33, 66, 159
good governance and, 226
health promotion and, 19
from heat wave disasters, 67
from industrial disasters, 90
from mass gathering disasters, 91
from mine disasters, 93, 157
from natural disasters, 153, 159
from poisoning disasters, 94
from structural collapse disasters, 81, 157
from technological disasters, 80, *89*, 153, 159
from transportation disasters, 95, 157, 159
from tsunami disasters, 72, 156
from volcanic eruptions, 74
from wildfire disasters, 75

multisectoral, 229, 323
emergency health professionals, 264
mass care, 248

N

National Academies of Sciences, Engineering, and Medicine, 9
National Biodefense Science Board, 8
National Environmental Health Association, 14
National Prevention Strategy, 281
National Research Council, 9
on risk communication, 203
National Response Framework, 248
natural disasters, 41–43, *43*, 57–75. *See also specific types*
health hazards of, *48–51*
impact of, *158*
incidence of, *154*
mortality from, 153, 159
public health and, 47, 141–147, *142–144*
public health impact of, 141–145, *142–143*
technological disasters and, 155, *156*, *157*
wellness and, 178
natural hazards, 42–43, 47, 58–75, 323
increase in, 6, *6*
natural history of disease, *33*, 33–34, 55, 323
of disaster-related disease, 131–137, *133*, *135*, *136*
quality of life and, 131
noncommunicable disease (NCD), 34, 323
as disaster-related disease, *108*
normative safety, 235, 323
nuclear explosions, 83, 84
fire disasters and, 85, 86

O

objective, 323
in emergency health, 21
wellness, 178
operational objective, 269, 323
operations, 202, 323
operations management, 268–269, 323
operations plan, 269, 323
ordinal scale, 53, 323
Ottawa Charter, 224, 225, 323
outbreak, *43*, 323
causal pathways of disease and, *127*
from poisoning disasters, 94
risk assessment and, 192
risk management and, 183
outcome, 323
crisis management and, 188
determinants of health (DoH) in, 27
of disaster-related diseases, 107–108, *108*
DoH and, 175
effectiveness of, 8
efficiency of, 8
in emergency health, 208–210, *209*
environmental justice and, 212
evidence-based decision-making for, 211
health equality and, 172
health equity and, 212
HiAP and, 225
performance management and, *269*
population heath and, 210
for public health, 47, 141–147, *142–144*
risk and, 183, *184*
outcome measures, 209, 323
outputs, 323
performance management and, *269*

P

Palmer Drought Severity Index (PDSI), 61
pandemic, *43*, 64, 323
from hazardous material release disasters, 86
Pandemic and All-Hazards Preparedness Act of 2006, 237
pathological, 26–27, 324
perceived safety, 235, 324
performance, 324
evidence-based decision-making for, 211
HiAP and, 225
planning for, 269–270
performance indicators, 249, 324
KPI, 267, *269*, 272, 321
performance management, 182, 267–272, *268–271*, 324
for emergency health, 271
performance measurement, 272, 324
pillars of emergency health, 15, *15*, 21, 207, 215, 324
plan, 182, 324
in disaster risk management, *185*
operations, 269, 323
risk retention and, 187
strategic, 269, 329
planetary health, 228, 324
health promotion and, 225
planning, 324
for performance, 269–270
poisoning disaster, *43*, 93–94, 324
disaster-related disease in, 107
etiology of diseases in, *294*
health hazards of, *48*, *51*
mine disasters and, 92, 93
population, 324. *See also* vulnerability
at-risk, 4
in disaster pathway, 38
disaster risk assessment for, 198
DoH and, 177
in earthquake disasters, 63
in epidemics, 64
exposure science and, 53
health protection for, 234
incident continuum and, 40
in volcanic eruptions, 74
population health, 210, 324
disease prevention for, 16
population protection measures (PPM)
disease prevention and, 16, 17, 18
health promotion and, 19
primary prevention and, 219

post-traumatic stress disorder, 178
predictability, 324
  disaster risk assessment and, 195
preparedness, 324
  risk transfer and, 187
Presidential Decision Directive 39 (PDD-39), 188, 324
prevalence, 324
  risk management and, 183
prevention, 325. *See also* disease prevention
  ability for, 333
  capability-based planning and, *254*
  of disease, risk reduction and, 187
  emergency health and, 15, *15*, 213–214
  in health promotion, 224–225, *225*
  public health for, 5
  research for, 279
preventive control, 182–183, 325
  in disease prevention, 16
primary health care, 229, 325
  health promotion and, 225
primary prevention, *17*, 17–18, 216, *216*, 218–219, 325
primordial prevention, 17, *17*, 18, 216, *216*, 218–219, 325
  health promotion and, 224
principles, 325
  of emergency health, 15
process, 325
  evidence-based decision-making for, 211
  measures of, 278, 322
process control, 182, 325
  hierarchy of, 132, *132*, 319
process management, 182, 325
process-person-context-time (PPCT), 28, 31, 134, 325
productivity, 227, 325
program, 225, 268, 325
program logic model, 325
  for emergency health, 21
promotion, 325. *See also* health promotion
  emergency health for, 15, *15*
  health effects and, 27
protection, 325. *See also* health protection; population protection measures
  capability-based planning and, *254*
  in emergency health, 208–209, *209*
  emergency health for, *15*
  in environmental health, 14
  from health hazard, 5
  healthy settings and, 226
  research for, 279
protective factors, 325
  for disease, 32
  of hazardous exposure, 47
  in health promotion, 18
provision of care, 20–21, 241–249, *242–244*, *249*, 325
  case in, *243*, 243–245
  components of, 245
  in disaster, 246–248
  in emergency health, 15, *15*
  in event, 244, 245
  research for, 279
proximate cause of disease, 326
  in health promotion, 19, *19*
public health, 326. *See also specific topics*
  art and science of, 4, 5
  consequence on, *148*
  disasters and, *148*
  DoH and, 177
  in drought disasters, 61
  educational opportunities in, 279–280
  emergency health for, 15
  environmental health and, 14
  environmental justice and, 212
  ICS in, 245
  impact on, 47, 141–147, *142–144*, *146*, 277–278
  integration opportunities in, 281
  intervention opportunities in, 280–281
  natural disasters and, 47, 141–147, *142–144*
  outcome for, 47, 141–147, *142–144*
  for prevention, 5
  professionals in, 261–264, *262–263*
  provision of care and, *242*, 242–245, *244*
  research in, 278–279
  response in, 333
  risk assessment and, 192
  risk reduction and, 187
  technological disasters and, 145–147, *146*
  underfunding of, 7
  vulnerability and, 333
public health impact, 326
  of natural disasters, 141–145, *142–143*
  of technological disasters, 145–147, *146*
  of wildfire disasters, 109
pyroclastic flow, *50*, 72, 73, *105*, *291*, 326

Q

quality, 326
  of response, 249
quality of life, 326
  DoW and, 177
  health effects and, 27
  health promotion and, 19
  healthy settings and, 226
  natural history of disease and, 131
quaternary prevention, *17*, 18, 216, *216*, 220–221, 326
  health promotion and, 224

R

radioactive contamination, 42
  industrial disasters from, 89
recovery, 326
  capability-based planning and, *254*
  of functional ability, 253
  mass care and, 248
  risk retention and, 187
  wellness and, 178
relative frequency, of disasters, 153, *153*, 326
reliability, 326
  in disaster risk assessment, 196

residual risk (accepted risk), 326
  risk retention and, 187
resilience, 326
  of at-risk populations, 4
  consequence and, 9
  DoH and, 175
resource, 326
  in disaster pathway, 38
  incident continuum and, 39, 40
  inputs of, 268–269
  mass gathering disasters and, 90
  in MCI, 144
  performance management and, 269, *269*
resource allocation, 196, 326
resource management, 269, 326
response, 327
  in public health, 333
  quality of, 249
  risk retention and, 187
responsible party, 270, 327
results-based protection (RBP), 208–209
Richter scale, 63, 70, 74
Ring of Fire (Circum-Pacific Belt), 62, *62*, 74, 327
risk, 327. *See also specific types and topics*
  in disasters, 38
  DoH and, 175–176, *176*
  in emergency health, *209*
  emergency health and, 213–214
  environmental justice and, 237–238
  in epidemic, 65
  of hazardous exposure, 47
  from heat wave disasters, 67
  incident continuum and, 39
  of landslide disasters, 69
  mine disasters and, 93
  outcome and, 183, *184*
  VEI, 74
risk acceptance, 184, 186, 187, 213, 327
risk assessment, 184, 191–199, 327
  research for, 278
risk avoidance, 186
risk characterization, 327
  for disaster risk assessment, 198
risk communication, 184, *185*, 201–204, 327
  cardinal rules of, 203
  ecosocial model of health for, 203–204
  primary prevention and, 219
  tertiary prevention and, 220
  theories of, 202
risk equation, 194, 327
risk factors, 327
  disease prevention and, 16, 17
  modifiable, 132, 322
  risk reduction and, 187
risk index, 196, 327
risk management, 183–184, *184*, 327
  effectiveness and, *186*
  research for, 279
  standards for, 8
risk messaging, 202
risk perception, 144, 327
risk ratio scale, 196, 327
risk reduction, 187, 327
  of disasters, 9
  vulnerability and, 9
risk retention, 187
risk transfer, 187, 327
risk treatment, 184, 327
  risk retention and, 187
riverine flood, 65
routes of human exposure, 52, 327

S

safety, 327
  in convective storm disasters, 70
  in emergency, 235
  in environment, primary prevention and, 219
  in flood disasters, 66
  in landslide disasters, 69
  mine disasters and, 92
  social, 235, 328
safety standards, 235–237, 328
Saffir-Simpson scale, 60
sanitation, 144, 328
  in convective storm disasters, 70
  disease prevention and, 17
  in earthquake disasters, 63
  in flood disasters, 66
  healthy settings and, 226
satisfaction, 328
  of stakeholders, *269*
scenario, 141, 328
Schultz, J., 131, 166
seasonal floods, 65
secondary prevention, *17*, 18, 219, 328
security, 234–235, *236*, 328
sediment flow, 67, 328
Sendai Framework for Disaster Risk Reduction, 8, 9, 47, 328
Serling, Rod, 195
Shanghai Declaration, 227, 328
shelter in place, 219, 328
Six Sigma, *270*, 270–271, 328
slope failure, 67, *68*, 328
SOARR planning format, 269–271, 328
social determinants of health (SDoH), 31
social safety, 235, 328
socio-politicization of risk, 237, 328
South Asia haze, 75
special cause variation, 26, 28, 38, 328
Sphere Project, 249, *249*, 281
stakeholders, 5, 328
  HiAP and, 208
  incident continuum and, 40
  in performance measurement, 272
  satisfaction of, *269*
standards, 329
  for competency, 280
  incident continuum and, 40
  for risk management, 8
  for safety, 235–237, 328

stochastic, 329
health effects, 27
storm surge, 329
from cyclone disasters, 60
health hazards of, 47
strategic goal, 269–270, 329
strategic plan, 269, 329
strategy, 329
in emergency health, 21
for reduction of disaster-related mortality, 9
structural collapse disasters, *43*, 81–83, 329
disaster-related disease in, 107
etiology of diseases in, *295*
explosion disasters from, 83
fire disasters and, 85
health hazards of, *48, 51*
industrial disasters from, 89
mass gathering disasters and, 91
mine disasters and, 92
mortality from, 81, 157
transportation disasters and, 95
subclinical disease, 26, 329
subduction zone, 71, 329
substantive safety, 235, 329
supportive environment for health, 226, 329
susceptibility, 329
disease prevention and, 16
health equity and, 172–173
sustainable development, 8, 227, 329
health promotion and, 225
sustainable development goal (SDG), 228, 329
syndrome, 329
epidemic of, 64
systems management, 182–183
systems theory, 267, 329

T

Target Capabilities List (TCL), 253
target capability, 175, 253, 329
task analysis, 280, 329
technological disasters, 41–43, *42, 43, 79–95, 80. See also specific types*
health hazards of, *48–51*
impact of, *158*
incidence of, *154*
mortality from, 80, *89*, 153, 159
natural disasters and, 155, *156, 157*
public health and, 145–147, *146*
public health impact of, 145–147, *146*
technological hazards, 47, 329
increase in, 6, *6*
tectonic plate, 62, *62*, 330
volcanic eruptions and, 74
tephra, 72–74, 330
Terrorism Incident Annex, 188–189, 330
tertiary prevention, *17*, 18, 19, 216, *216*, 220, 330
thermal disasters, 41, *42, 43*
thermal hazards, 330
explosion disaster and, 83
fire disasters and, 84
mass gathering disasters and, 90
mine disasters and, 92
transportation disasters and, 94
thunderstorms. *See* convective storm disaster
tornado disasters, 69–70, 330
disaster-related disease in, *105*
health hazards of, *48, 50*
toxic hazards, 330. *See also* hazardous materials; poisoning disaster
in flood disasters, 66
industrial disasters and, 89–90
mass gathering disasters and, 90
mine disasters and, 92
transportation disasters and, 94
toxicological disasters, 41, *42, 43*
transocean tsunamis, 71
transportation disasters, *43*, 94–95, 330
disaster-related disease in, 107
etiology of diseases in, *295*
explosion disasters and, 83
from hazardous material release disasters, 87
health hazards of, *48, 51*
from industrial disasters, 90
mortality from, 95, 157, 159
from structural collapse disasters, 81
tropical cyclone disasters, 40, 59, 330. *See also* hurricane disasters
tsunami disasters, *43*, 70–72, 330
disaster-related disease in, *105*
etiology of diseases in, *290*
health hazards of, *48, 50*
incident continuum in, 40
mortality from, 72, 156
typhoon disasters, 59, 330. *See also* hurricane disasters

U

uncertainty, 330
disaster risk assessment and, 195
in disasters, 38–39
quaternary prevention and, 220
risk management and, 183
unified command, 330
incident continuum and, 40
United Nations, 5
good governance and, 226
Universal Declaration of Human Rights, 5
Universal Task List (UTL), 254
utility, 330
disaster risk assessment and, 195
evidence-based decision-making for, 211

V

validity, 330
of uncertainty, 38
variability, 331
evidence-based decision-making for, 211
incident continuum and, 39

volcanic eruption, *43,* 72–74, 331
disaster-related disease in, *105*
from earthquake disasters, 62–63
etiology of diseases in, *291*
health hazards of, *48, 50*
Volcanic Explosivity Index (VEI), 74
vulnerability, 331
of at-risk populations, 4
disaster risk and, 194
in disaster risk management, *185*
disease prevention and, 16
to hazardous exposure, 46–47
to hazards, 9
health equity and, 169, 172–173
public health and, 333
risk avoidance and, 186
risk reduction and, 9, 187

W

Waeckerle, Joseph, 247
well-being, 331
environmental health and, 14
health equity and, 172
in health promotion, 18
health promotion and, 225, 229
wellness, 163–168, 331. *See also* determinants of health, wellness, and equity; determinants of wellness
in disasters, 167–168
disasters and, 178–179
ecosocial model of health for, *164,* 164–165
in disasters, 167–168
emergency health and, 15, 179, 213–214
in flood disasters, 66
health promotion and, 19
illness and, 27, *27*
indivisible self and, *165,* 165–166, *166*
quaternary prevention and, 216
Whitehead, Margaret, 211
wildfire disasters, *43,* 74–75, 331
in convective storm disasters, 70
disaster-related disease in, *106*
etiology of diseases in, *291*
health hazards of, *48, 50*
in heat wave disasters, 67
public health impact of, 109
wildland, 74, 75, 331
wind chill effect, 58
Winslow, C.-E. A., 4, 5, 14
winter storm disasters, 331
etiology of diseases in, *285*
World Bank, 42, 155, 226
World Health Assembly Resolution 58.33, 5
World Health Organization (WHO), 14
on DoH, 30, *30*
on epidemic, 65
on health, 28
on health hazards, 48
on health promotion, 224
on risk communication, 201
on security, 234
on wellness, 163
World Meteorological Organization, 153